BASIC CONCEPTS IN
EMBRYOLOGY

Notice

Medicine is an ever-changing science. As new research and clinical experience broaden our knowledge, changes in treatment and drug therapy are required. The author and the publisher of this work have checked with sources believed to be reliable in their efforts to provide information that is complete and generally in accord with the standards accepted at the time of publication. However, in view of the possibility of human error or changes in medical sciences, neither the author nor the publisher nor any other party who has been involved in the preparation or publication of this work warrants that the information contained herein is in every respect accurate or complete, and they are not responsible for any errors or omissions or for the results obtained from use of such information. Readers are encouraged to confirm the information contained herein with other sources. For example and in particular, readers are advised to check the product information sheet included in the package of each drug they plan to administer to be certain that the information contained in this book is accurate and that changes have not been made in the recommended dose or in the contraindications for administration. This recommendation is of particular importance in connection with new or infrequently used drugs.

BASIC CONCEPTS IN
EMBRYOLOGY

A STUDENT'S SURVIVAL GUIDE

Written and Illustrated by

LAUREN J. SWEENEY, Ph.D.

Department of Biology
Bryn Mawr College
Bryn Mawr, Pennsylvania

Series Editor
Hiram T. Gilbert, Ph.D.

The McGraw-Hill Companies
Health Professions Divison
New York   St. Louis   San Francisco
Auckland   Bogota   Caracus   Lisbon   London   Madrid
Mexico City   Milan   Montreal   New Delhi   Paris   San Juan
Singapore   Sydney   Tokyo   Toronto

•   •   •   •   •   •   •   •   •   •   •   •

McGraw-Hill

*A Division of The **McGraw·Hill** Companies*

BASIC CONCEPTS IN EMBRYOLOGY:
A STUDENT'S SURVIVAL GUIDE

Copyright © 1998 by the McGraw-Hill Companies, Inc. All rights reserved. Printed in the United States of America. Except as permitted under the United States Copyright Act of 1976, no part of this publication may be reproduced or distributed in any form or by any means, or stored in a data base or retrieval system, without the prior written permission of the publisher.

1 2 3 4 5 6 7 8 9 0 DOC DOC 9 9 8 7

ISBN: 0-07-063308-8

This book was set in Times Roman by Better Graphics, Inc. The editors were James Morgan and Pamela Touboul; the series editor was Hiram F. Gilbert, Ph.D.; the production supervisor was Richard Ruzycka; the project manager was Hockett Editoral Service; the cover designer was Marsha Cohen.

R. R. Donnelley & Sons Company was printer and binder.

This book is printed on acid-free paper.

Library of Congress Cataloging-in-Publication Data

Sweeney, Lauren J.
    Basic concepts in embryology : a student's survival guide / Lauren J. Sweeney.
        p. cm.
    ISBN: 0-07-063308-8
    1. Embryology, Human. 2. Embryology.   I. Title.
    [DNLM: 1. Embryo—embryology.   2. Fetal Development—physiology.
3. Cell Differentiation—physiology.   QS 604 S974b 1998]
QM601.S94   1998
612.6′4—dc21
DNLM/DLC
for Library of Congress   97-26599

• C O N T E N T S •

· P R O L O G U E ·

Basic Concepts in Embryology: A Student's Survival Guide is designed to serve several purposes missing in available embryology books. It can be used as a primary text, a review book, or as a reference for those who occasionally find themselves in need of a quick understanding about a specific point of embryonic development without delving into the whole field.

Embryology has traditionally been a difficult subject for most students to grasp. That difficulty turns off many students to the intriguing story that it tells. After all, we're talking about how a single cell can contain (and correctly express) all the instructions to cause daughter cells to "germinate" into the correct tissues in the correct locations, and how these tissues then interact to form all the specific organs which compose an entire human being.

As the number of embryology lectures in medical curricula decrease, the burden placed on students actually increases, as they are forced to absorb *greater* numbers of new terms and unfamiliar visual pictures per class "contact hour", leaving less time for explanations which tie the facts together. This also means that students learn embryology less thoroughly the first time around, placing more demands on their time as residents and fellows when some of this material becomes clinically relevant.

All of this puts a greater premium than ever on having a short source book which contains just enough of a description of events so that the facts are tied together into a conceptual framework which tells the story of embryonic development. This book is designed to fill that need.

BASIC CONCEPTS IN
EMBRYOLOGY

· C H A P T E R · 1 ·

INTRODUCTORY
FRAMEWORK

·

HOW TO MAKE MAXIMAL USE OF THIS BOOK
Where to start

Constantly remind yourself *why* you have opened this book, and zero in on just the material relevant to that purpose. Are you trying to clarify a particular point of basic embryonic development? Are you trying to understand the embryonic basis for a specific congenital defect? Or are you trying to learn the full story of embryology for a current course? Your plan of attack will depend on your goal.

Use the chapter subheadings as a preview

Each chapter begins with a detailed outline of its contents, and each section of the chapter contains many headings and subheadings. Most of the subheadings summarize the embryonic story in the text that follows. If you already know the story summarized in the heading, or it's not relevant to your specific quest, you can proceed on to the next heading. The chapter outline and its headings can be used as a preview or overview of the entire chapter. In many cases, that may be all the detail you need on that area.

Key in on the information in boxes

> Boxes surround key pieces of material within each section. In particular, descriptions of congenital defects and their causation are "boxed up" for ready identification.

Text and illustrations are always on facing pages

The format of this book eliminates the need to constantly flip back and forth between figures and the text that explains them.

TRIVIA SORTER

Focus on the story that ties together the facts

This book contains just the bare bones facts of embryology to which everyone should have ready access. The text concentrates on outlining the story which connects these facts. However, to the uninitiated, the facts can still overwhelm the story. For example, if you have never studied embryology before, you are unlikely to know what the *primitive streak* or *buccopharyngeal membrane* are, or what role they play in development. Here are some suggestions to take such detail out of the level of apparent trivia and connect it into a story.

Break down development into categories, and then ask what you need to know about each

Chapter 2 provides you with the overview you will need to divide development into the following categories. Concentrate on answering the following questions in each category, and you will spend a lot less time memorizing facts:

Developmental events

Embryonic versus *fetal* stages of development:

- What are the major developmental events that occur in each of these stages?
- Which period is more susceptible to formation of congenital defects?

Development of *extraembryonic* "support" structures: yolk sac, amnion, chorion, placenta, and umbilical cord:

- Which extraembryonic structures are formed by embryonic contributions and which by maternal uterine tissues?
- What role does each extraembryonic structure play in embryonic development?

Formation of the germ layers: ectoderm, mesoderm, and endoderm:

- What is the origin of each germ layer?
- How does body folding change the relationship of these layers?
- What are the derivatives of each germ layer?
    Specifically, what are the *tissue* derivatives of each germ layer?
    For this, you have to know only the basics of the *four* tissue categories in the body: this is introduced in Chap. 5.

Organogenesis: the formation of organs from tissues:

• What tissue types are part of each organ system?
• What germ layers are involved in forming each organ system? To answer this, start by asking:
• Which germ layers give rise to each of the tissue types in the organ?

Germ layer derivatives provide a *conceptual framework* for learning embryology. If you can learn the tissue derivatives of each germ layer, you can use them to build organs from their respective tissues.

Congenital defects

• What do the descriptions of the features, causes, and development of congenital defects tell you about *normal* development? The descriptions of defects in this book are intended as a wake-up call that alerts you to the importance of that particular aspect of normal development. Do not try to memorize each defect, unless you are receiving such feedback from a professor. You will have plenty of time in your clinical years to relearn the names and details of congenital defects.

Transient structures created during embryonic development. Short-lived structures are one of the biggest headaches that students of embryology encounter. They have strange names, they often don't appear to bear any direct relation to the mature structures of the body, and yet they pop up constantly throughout the story of embryonic development. Ask yourself the following questions to determine the level of importance you should attach to learning about these structures:

• Does the transient structure get incorporated into a major permanent structure?
• Does the transient structure serve only as a landmark in development and then disappear? Is learning the name of the transient structure less cumbersome than its description? For example, *stomodeum* is shorter than *spot marking future mouth opening.*
• Does the transient structure play a role in the development of any congenital defects?

Timing of development

Specific timing is often mentioned within the text, but mostly as a frame of reference. This lets you know which events are contemporaneous and whether a series of events take days, weeks, or months to complete. It's not very informative to say "a little later" or "much later."

Chapter 2 breaks down the timing of developmental events into the following major divisions which should be sufficient for you to learn the broad picture:

- The embryonic period: from fertilization through 2 months:
  Know developments in the first month on a week by week basis.
  Know that month 2 is the time of all organ *formation*.
- The fetal period: month 3 through birth:
  Know that this is the period of organ growth.

Reinforce what you're learning by color coding the diagrams

Turn this book into a coloring book by color coding the derivatives of each of the germ layers. This should reinforce your knowledge of the germ layers and their derivatives, just as diagramming material does in other, less visual, subject areas. (This should also help to keep you from using your highlighters on the text itself, a habit that is notoriously hard for students to break.) I suggest the following scheme, although you can certainly come up with your own personalized scheme:

Embryonic tissues
   Ectoderm: blue
      Surface ectoderm: blue
      Neural ectoderm: green
   Mesoderm: reds
      There aren't enough colors for all the separate mesoderm subregions. I suggest bright red for somites, maroon or purple for intermediate mesoderm, and pink for lateral plate.
   Endoderm: yellow
Extraembryonic tissues: Orange and brown
   Trophoblast derivatives: orange
   Amnion: brown
   Yolk sac: yellow orange

· C H A P T E R · 2 ·

DEVELOPMENTAL PERIODS AND CONGENITAL MALFORMATIONS

·

·   ·   ·   ·   ·   ·   ·   ·   ·   ·   ·   ·

DEVELOPMENTAL PERIODS

Humans are complex organisms, whose development begins at fertilization, and continues on some levels throughout life. The study of *embryology* focuses on the development that occurs in the *prenatal* period, that is, before birth. This can also be referred to as the *gestational* period. Prenatal development can be divided into the embryonic and fetal periods. The embryonic period extends from fertilization through 8 weeks, while the fetal period extends from week 9 until birth.

Embryonic period: Fertilization through 8 weeks

Each of the first 3 weeks is characterized by specific developments. Week 1 starts with *fertilization* and extends through the first cell divisions that produce an embryo with one germ layer. Week 2 produces two germ layers. Week 3 produces three germ layers and folds those layers into a recognizable three dimensional body form.

• **Weeks 4 through 8 (month 2) are the period of organogenesis.**

> All the major events of organ formation and formation of body regions occur during the period of *organogenesis*, which is completed in the *embryonic* period.

Week 4 is particularly important, as the initial set-up of all organ systems is completed in this week. In most cases, it will be sufficient to know that establishment of other structures occurs in the remaining weeks of month 2.

Fetal period: Month 3 to birth

The major events that occur during the fetal period involve growth in size (*hypertrophy*) of organs by rapid increase in cell number (*hyperplasia*), as well as biochemical and functional maturation. Most organ systems begin a rudimentary form of functioning during the fetal period, but this usually is important only for the development of the organ itself. The most important exception is the cardiovascular system. The heart begins pumping blood to all organs as they are first forming. Without this circulation, organs would not be able to develop. Mature functional status is not achieved in most organ systems until after birth. This explains why you will find so little discussion of physiologic maturation in any embryology book, and so much discussion of physiology in pediatrics and neonatology books.

EMBRYONIC BODY AXIS TERMINOLOGY

As the embryo forms, it rapidly develops several axes (see Fig. 2-1). It is impossible to get very far into the description of any aspect of embryonic development without referring to these axes, so it will make life easier to spend a few minutes now familiarizing yourself with axis terminology.

• **The first axis formed is the cranial-caudal axis.** The cranial-caudal axis is established while the embryo is still a flat disk or sheet of cells, long before it folds into the three-dimensional structure we recognize as the embryonic body. This axis runs from the future head (cranium) to the future "tail" end (caudum).

• **The dorsal-ventral axis is established very shortly thereafter.** The second major axis, the dorsal-ventral, is formed as the body folds. This axis defines, respectively, the future "back" and "front" (or "stomach") sides of both the

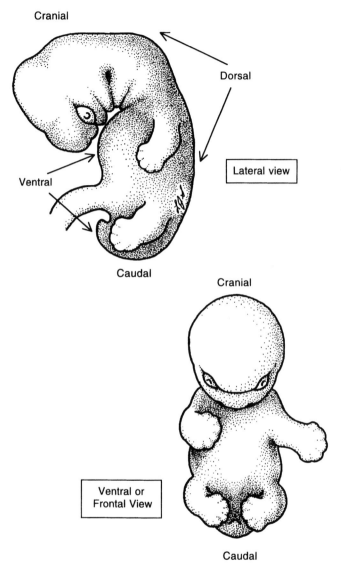

Figure 2-1
Embryonic body axes.

embryonic and adult bodies. This axis is also called the *posterior-anterior* axis in the adult, but since that term actually applies to the cranial-caudal axis in the embryo (!), it is not used in this book.

• **Terminology used in sectional views of the embryo.**   The terminology used for viewing the embryo from different angles is the same as that for viewing the adult (see Fig. 2-2). A *sagittal* plane of section runs the length of the embryo, splitting the embryo into left and right portions. If the section runs right along the middle of the body, then it is a *medial* or *midline sagittal* section. Sagittal sections are often also referred to as longitudinal sections. However, *longitudinal* properly refers to any section that runs along the long axis of an organ or region of the body, without regard to the body's overall axes.

A *transverse* or *cross* section runs across the embryo, transecting it into cranial and caudal portions. (*Transverse* or *cross section* can also refer to the plane of section across the short axis of an organ or region of the body.)

A *frontal* section runs the length of the embryo, as does a sagittal section, but at right angles to it, so that it cuts the embryo into dorsal and ventral portions. This view is used infrequently in this book.

In addition to these terms, there are several sets of directional terms which are used frequently when describing the location of embryonic structures in relation to some point of reference. First, the terms *medial* and *lateral* refer to structures which are, respectively, closer to or farther from the midline sagittal axis of the body. For example, the two ears are lateral to the eyes (and the eyes are medial to the ears). A second set of terms, *proximal* and *distal,* refer to structures which are, respectively, closer to or farther from a fixed point, such as the point of attachment of a limb. For example, the elbow joint of the arm would be described as proximal to the wrist joint, because it is closer to the point of attachment of the arm to the body, while the wrist would be described as distal to the elbow.

All of these definitions may not make a permanent impression on you now from just one read-through. Just remember that they are here in case you run into some confusion later on in the book.

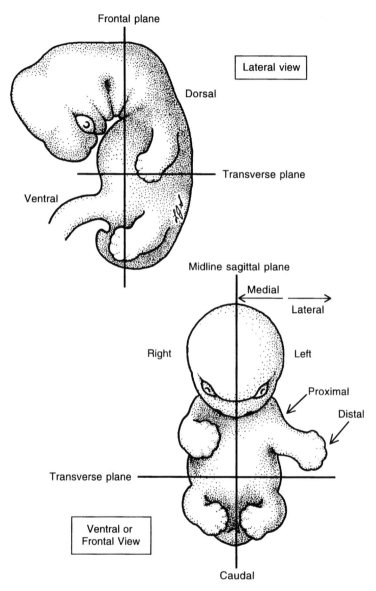

Figure 2-2
Terminology used in planes of section.

CONGENITAL ABNORMALITIES

• **Congenital abnormalities develop during gestation.** *Gestation* refers to the period of development prior to birth, which occurs within the mother's uterus. One of the most important reasons for learning about embryonic development is the basis it gives the clinician (and the clinician-in-training) for understanding both the causes and anatomy of congenital abnormalities.

Clinically, congenital abnormalities are abnormalities or malformations detected either at birth, or shortly thereafter. Sometimes this period is extended to include abnormalities detected in the first year or two after birth. The thinking is that abnormalities that develop during gestation should not be excluded simply because they may not be detected right away. Congenital abnormalities include not only gross structural defects, but also defects in cellular metabolism or functioning. These metabolic defects are the province of biochemistry and genetics texts. Most occur without associated structural defects.

• **Congenital abnormalities can be serious malformations, or they can be "variations" with little or no clinical significance.** These variations are often worth noting, however, since they can provide a major surprise to the physician who is not aware of the potential for their existence. For example, many variations on blood vessel patterning occur and, while they are perfectly functional, their existence should be known to any surgeon planning an operation in that field of blood supply.

• **Syndromes are "packages" of congenital abnormalities that occur in several organ systems as the result of a single factor.** Little is currently known about how the separate defects that compose most syndromes are caused to develop together. Most syndromes have been described on the basis of the frequency with which their individual defects occur together, which statistically suggests that they are all due to a common causative factor. Only the most common and serious syndromes are mentioned in this book, since this is more properly the province of clinical training than basic embryology. Without an immediate clinical application or explanation that ties their causation together, learning the list of defects in a syndrome is just memorization.

• **Causation or etiology of congenital abnormalities.** Congenital abnormalities are detected in approximately 2 to 3 percent of newborns, and another 2 to 3 percent of infants in the first years of life. These numbers may seem low, but congenital abnormalities are the cause of as much as one-fifth of all infant mortality and one-third of all neonatal hospitalization.

The etiology, or cause, of fully half of all congenital abnormalities remains unknown. We do know that environmental agents alone induce as many as 10 percent of all congenital anomalies, and genetic abnormalities induce another 15 to 25 percent. Interaction of the two factors induces an additional 15 to 25 percent of defects. This interaction is referred to as *multifactorial causation.* This means environmental factors interact with a genetic "predisposition." We still have a long way to go in sorting out just what the nature is of the genetic changes that predispose an individual to developmental abnormalities in response to environmental factors. At present, the existence of these interactions can often only be deduced from analysis of statistical data which demonstrates higher incidence in affected families than observed in the general population. Finally, it is likely that most of the congenital abnormalities of "unknown" causation have a genetic basis which has yet to be discovered.

Genetic causes of congenital abnormalities

Genetic abnormalities can arise in several ways. They can be inherited, or they can be created anew with the generation of gametes. The distinction should be made between *defects in chromosomes*, and defects in single *genes.*

Studies have shown that the majority of fertilized eggs with chromosomal abnormalities either don't successfully implant at all, or spontaneously abort shortly after implantation. Many spontaneous abortions (or miscarriages) occur in the first three weeks, and so may not be recognized as anything other than a late menstrual cycle.

In *chromosomal defects,* whole chromosomes can be missing or duplicated, or parts of chromosomes can be missing or duplicated.

• **Abnormal chromosome numbers are called** *aneuploidy.* Abnormal numbers are usually caused by an error in separation of chromosomes into appropriate daughter cells during meiotic division, a defective process called *nondisjunc-
tion.* This will be clearer when you read about the steps in meiosis in the next
chapter. Aneuploidy can occur in either sex chromosomes, or in autosomes (non-
sex chromosomes). The most common abnormalities are *monosomy,* in which
only one copy of a chromosome pair is present, and *trisomy,* in which three members of a chromosome pair are present. Most monosomies are not viable. The one
major exception is that of XO individuals, who have one X chromosome and no
second sex chromosome. This is referred to as *Turner's syndrome,* in which individuals have a female phenotype but are sterile.

Several types of trisomy do survive. Three major trisomies of the sex chromosomes occur. Individuals with XXY trisomy (*Klinefelter's syndrome*) have a
male phenotype, but are infertile. Individuals with XYY trisomy also have a male
phenotype and frequently demonstrate impulsively aggressive behavior. XXX
individuals have a female phenotype and are often retarded. There are three major
autosomal trisomies. The most common is trisomy 21 (*Down syndrome,* with
three copies of chromosome 21). It is characterized by varying degrees of mental
retardation, abnormal facial features, and, in as many as one-third of cases, serious congenital heart defects. Trisomies 13 and 18 result in severe retardation and
structural central nervous system defects, as well as serious cleft lip and palate
defects. Most of these individuals die within the first few months after birth.

• **Abnormal chromosome structure can also occur.** Abnormalities can
include deletion or duplication of portions of chromosomes, translocations of
portions between chromosomes, or inversion of sequences (reversal of normal
orientation within the chromosome). These changes are due to chromosome
breaks, followed by abnormal reattachments. Breaks are usually generated by
environmental insults such as radiation, drugs or chemicals during meiosis, or
they can occur spontaneously.

Translocations, inversions, and duplications are most compatible with survival, since a full complement of the genome is still present. Some affected individuals have no abnormalities. However, they have a higher tendency to produce gametes with an abnormal chromosome number or structure. Conversely, individuals with only a few deletion abnormalities have been shown to survive. New methods have allowed detection of microdeletions, which span only several contiguous genes. Several syndromes have now been determined to be the product of such microdeletions. Microdeletions bridge the clear distinctions that have traditionally existed between chromosomal defects and single gene defects.

• **A number of mutations in single genes have been documented to cause abnormal development.**   The mechanism by which any single abnormal gene produces defects is largely unknown, even in those cases in which the abnormal gene has been identified and cloned and its product identified. Autosomal and sex chromosome–linked mutations have been identified. Mutations of single genes cause several defects, including achondroplasia and polydactyly (defects in limb development, covered in Chap. 7), and polycystic kidney disease (covered in Chap. 14). They are also one cause of microcephaly (covered in Chap. 10).

For a full description of the genetic causes of congenital defects, see a clinical textbook on congenital defects or a genetics textbook.

A number of environmental agents cause congenital abnormalities

Environmental agents that cause congenital abnormalities are called *teratogens*. This unfortunate term is derived from the Greek word for monster (*teratos*). While modern society has a more compassionate view of the individuals who are born with congenital abnormalities, the term for their causative agents remains in use.

> The embryonic period (through 8 weeks) is the critical period of susceptibility to teratogens.

Exposure to teratogens during weeks 1 and 2 interferes with implantation or kills the embryo directly, but does not interfere with organ system development, since that hasn't begun yet. Exposure during weeks 3 through 8 results in organ system–specific malformations, since this is the period of organ formation. Exposure during the fetal period can interfere with growth and maturation of organs but doesn't cause primary structural malformations. However, changes in growth may result in serious underdevelopment, and that, by itself, may cause some lesser structural defects. Alternatively, retardation of fetal growth can result in serious functional underdevelopment. For example, underdevelopment of the nervous system during the fetal period can result in mental retardation.

Each teratogen has its own peak period of effectiveness on the embryo as a whole and on particular organ systems. Each organ has a slightly different period of peak susceptibility to teratogenic insults. The heart, for example, develops earlier and more rapidly than other organs and so defects will be caused by exposure at earlier times than other organs. The brain, alternatively, undergoes such a prolonged period of development through the embryonic and fetal periods that defects can be caused over a very long time.

We know from studies that each teratogen has preferred organ systems it affects and different peak periods of effectiveness. Very little is known about how most of these factors work, however. In this book, particular attention is paid to the few teratogens for which mechanisms of action are becoming clear.

• **Known teratogens include chemicals (many of them drugs), infectious agents, radiation, and mechanical factors.** Drugs that are teratogenic include many antibiotics (tetracycline and streptomycin), anticoagulants, anticonvulsants, antitumor agents, some sedatives and tranquilizers, some hormones (androgens used to prevent spontaneous abortion or birth control pills taken before pregnancy is detected), folic acid, alcohol, and vitamin A in excess.

Particular attention is currently being paid to the dangers of alcohol, as it has been recognized that it can produce a number of defects that comprise *fetal alcohol syndrome*. The defects include mental retardation, slow growth, heart defects, underdevelopment of facial structures, and lifelong behavioral and learning problems.

> Maternal alcohol abuse is now thought to be the most common cause of mental retardation.

Attention is also being paid to retinoic acid (vitamin A), which can produce neural tube defects, cleft palate, underdevelopment of facial structures, defects of the heart and thymus, and limb defects. The mechanism of action of vitamin A is actually becoming understood and is described in chapters on development of both the limbs (Chap. 6) and central nervous system (Chap. 9).

> Evidence indicates that even very low doses of vitamin A, equivalent to only 2 to 3 times the recommmended daily allowance in a vitamin tablet, can produce defects.

This quantity of vitamin A can easily be ingested if a woman continues to take antiacne medications that contain vitamin A during the early stages of pregnancy when she may not yet be aware that she is pregnant.

• **Infectious agents that can induce defects are mostly viruses.** They include the rubella virus (which causes German measles), the cytomegalovirus, the herpes simplex virus, the varicella virus (which causes chickenpox), and HIV (human immunodeficiency virus) which causes AIDS (acquired immune deficiency disease). Two notable exceptions are the spirochete, which causes syphilis, and the protozoa, which causes toxoplasmosis. These agents actually do their damage by crossing the placenta during the fetal period and destroying existing structures.

• **There are several other important teratogenic factors.** Radiation (above diagnostic levels) can produce congenital defects in many systems, particularly the central nervous system (producing defects in the neural tube that forms the brain and spinal cord). Ionizing radiation acts by causing breaks in chromosomes and mutations in single genes. Mechanical factors in utero can produce excessive pressures that can reduce fetal mobility. This can lead to defects such as congenital dislocation of the hip or club foot. Pressure can come from several sources, including bands of the amniotic sac twisting around the foot or arm and reduced quantities of amniotic fluid (oligohydramnios), which can occur as the result of several types of fetal defects. This produces pressure by giving the fetus less of a flotation sac to move around in.

Other important factors include high temperatures, as may occur when a maternal infection produces a maternal fever. Another factor may be poorly controlled maternal diabetes (mellitus), which can lead to stillbirth, high birth weight, and some structural defects. In addition, many factors cause fetal growth retardation and low birth weight, including maternal cigarette smoking, malnutrition, and alcoholism.

> Low birth weight and growth retardation are not trivial; they are associated with a high incidence of neonatal death and susceptibility to disease.

• **The basis for coverage of congenital defects in this book.**   Defects are covered in this book for any one of several reasons. Emphasis is placed on common defects, as well as on abnormalities that are compatible with a normal life span, since these individuals will be encountered as patients by physicians. Alternatively, a few uncommon or fatal defects are described, because they reveal something about the underlying mechanisms of development.

PRENATAL DIAGNOSTIC TECHNIQUES

Fetal abnormalities in chromosome number, size, and shape can be detected by *karyotyping,* or the analysis of chromosomes taken from fetal cells. These cells are acquired by one of two methods: *amniocentesis* or *chorionic villus sampling.* In amniocentesis, samples of fetal cells are obtained by withdrawal of amniotic fluid surrounding the fetus. This fluid contains some fetal cells, which are then cultured to multiply their numbers. Amniocentesis also permits biochemical analysis of the fluid contents, permitting diagnosis of several inborn (genetic) errors of metabolism and some structural defects such as neural tube defects. The latter defect is picked up by abnormal levels of alphafetoprotein, which leaks from the open spinal canal. Amniocentesis is ideally timed for weeks 12 through 14 of gestation, to maximize chances of getting adequate amniotic fluid volume and fetal cell number, while minimizing chances of injuring the fetus. Chorionic villus sampling provides direct samples of fetal tissues from the *chorionic villi* of the placenta for analysis. (The structure of the placenta is described in Chaps. 4 and 18.) The advantage of this technique is that results are available quickly, since cells don't have to be cultured. The major concern with this technique is that there is some risk of causing fetal loss, although it is less than 1 percent. In both cases, considerable experience in these procedures on the part of the physician is critical.

Noninvasive visualization of the fetus is also an invaluable tool. It can be accomplished by modern imaging techniques, such as ultrasound, magnetic resonance imaging (MRI), and computed tomography.

· C H A P T E R · 3 ·

FERTILIZATION

·

· · · · · · · · · · · ·

The study of embryonic development begins at fertilization. However, the process of fertilization is best understood by starting with the development of the gametes, and following that development through until the point at which egg and sperm meet. Thus, this chapter begins with a prologue to fertilization, in which the processes of gamete development are covered. These processes include both *meiosis*, in which the proper genetic content for each gamete is created, and cellular maturation, in which the cytoplasmic contents are specialized for the different roles of egg and sperm. Then the events of fertilization are covered, from the point of contact between egg and sperm, through the formation of a single celled *zygote*.

PROLOGUE TO FERTILIZATION

Gamete development: meiosis and cellular maturation

Gamete is the "sex-neutral" term for both the egg (ovum) and sperm. Gametes must undergo both meiosis and cellular maturation to complete development. Meiosis halves the number of chromosomes found in typical body (somatic) cells, while cellular maturation modifies the "generic" cell structure of the gamete for the unique functions of egg or sperm.

Meiosis

> The objective of *meiosis* is to put just one copy of each of 23 chromosomes in each gamete. Meiosis does this by a single duplication of DNA, followed by two rounds of nuclear and cell division. This produces (a maximum of) 4 gametes, each with half the number of chromosomes in mature body cells. *Fertilization* will restore the full complement of DNA by uniting sperm and egg nuclei.

• **STAGES OF MEIOSIS**   Duplication of DNA is the first step in both meiosis and mitosis (see Fig. 3-1). Primitive sex cells ready to begin meiosis are called *oogonia* in the female, and *spermatogonia* in the male. When these gametes begin to duplicate DNA, they enter the primary oocyte and primary spermatocyte stages in the female and male, respectively.

Chromosome division follows duplication in both meiosis and mitosis. Both processes go through the same phases of division: prophase, metaphase, anaphase, and telophase. There's one big difference: meiosis goes through this cycle twice. The gametes have different names in each cycle. They remain primary oocytes and primary spermatocytes from the time they enter meiosis until they complete the first meiotic division. They become secondary oocytes and secondary spermatocytes from the time they enter the second meiotic division until they complete meiosis.

Another important difference is that four sperm are formed from each spermatogonium that enters meiosis, while only one egg or oocyte is formed from each oogonium. The "excess" DNA in the oocyte is cast off into polar bodies, which rapidly disintegrate.

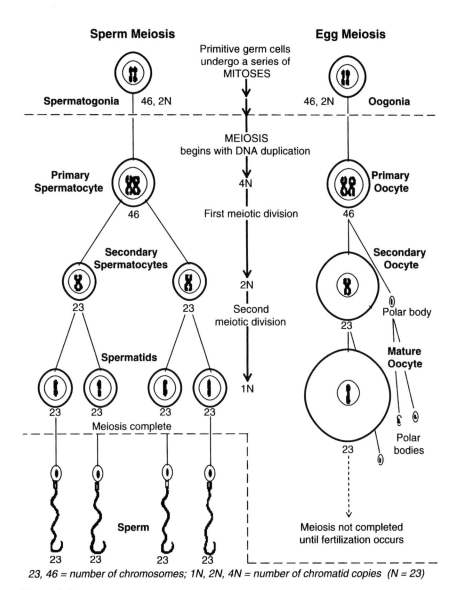

23, 46 = number of chromosomes; 1N, 2N, 4N = number of chromatid copies (N = 23)

Figure 3-1
Stages of meiosis in sperm and egg.

• DNA TERMINOLOGY DURING MEIOSIS (SEE FIG. 3-2)   This terminology is always a source of confusion, so it is reviewed in detail here. A nondi-
viding (interphase) human body cell contains 23 *pairs* of chromosomes. The 2
chromosomes of each pair are called *homologous* chromosomes. Each chromosome consists of a single DNA double-helix strand called a *chromatid.*

> Interphase cells contain a *diploid* number of chromosomes and $2N$ chro-
> matid strands. *Ploid* designates the number of homologous chromosomes
> present: diploid (double), haploid (single). $1N$, $2N$, $4N$ refer to the number
> of copies of chromatids present, where $1N = 23$. These two measures are
> *not* always the same during meiosis.

     When chromosome duplication occurs, an identical daughter chromatid is
formed. In meiosis, the two chromatids initially remain attached at one point,
called the *centromere.* This transient attachment creates a cell which is $4N$ but
still diploid. How is this possible? Twice the normal number of chromatid strands
are present ($2 \times 2N = 4N$). But because the daughter chromatids remain
attached, there are still only *pairs* of homologous chromosomes, or a diploid
number of chromosomes. When the two separation divisions of meiosis are completed, each gamete has only one chromosome of each pair, composed of one
chromatid each. Gametes are thus haploid and $1N$.

**• MEIOSIS RESULTS IN GENETIC VARIABILITY BY TWO METH-
ODS: CROSSING OVER AND INDEPENDENT ASSORTMENT.**   Each
gamete will contain a unique combination of paternally and maternally derived
genetic material as a result of two features unique to meiosis. First, *crossing over*,
or exchange can occur between homologous chromosomes. When the homologous chromosomes line up together at the start of the first meiotic division, their
chromatid arms can "cross over" on top of each other. The terminal portions of
these chromatid arms then break off and become exchanged between the homologous chromosomes.
     Variability is also produced by the random or *independent assortment* of the
maternally and paternally derived homologous members of each chromosome
pair to each gamete.

> Errors in chromosome *duplication* can occur in meiosis during crossing
> over, forming incomplete chromosome arms or arms carrying extra bits.

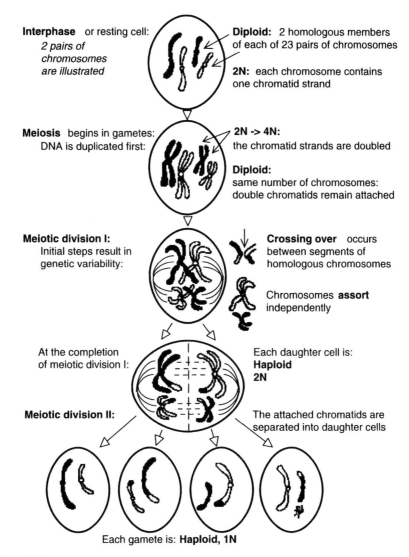

Interphase or resting cell:
    2 pairs of
    chromosomes
    are illustrated

Diploid: 2 homologous members
of each of 23 pairs of chromosomes

2N: each chromosome contains
one chromatid strand

Meiosis begins in gametes:
    DNA is duplicated first:

2N -> 4N:
the chromatid strands are doubled

Diploid:
same number of chromosomes:
double chromatids remain attached

Meiotic division I:
    Initial steps result in
    genetic variability:

Crossing over occurs
between segments of
homologous chromosomes

Chromosomes **assort**
independently

At the completion
of meiotic division I:

Each daughter cell is:
Haploid
2N

Meiotic division II:

The attached chromatids are
separated into daughter cells

Each gamete is: **Haploid, 1N**

Figure 3-2
Chromatid and chromosome structure during meiosis.

Errors in chromosome *assortment* can also occur, putting an extra copy of
a particular chromosome in one gamete and no copies in another. This can
lead to failure of the fertilized egg to develop or to congenital malformations.

Cellular maturation of gametes

- ### DIFFERENCES IN SPERM AND EGG DEVELOPMENT
- **Differences in the timing of meiosis and cellular maturation.** In the male, meiosis (spermatogenesis) and cellular maturation (spermiogenesis) occur in two separate but continuous stages. In the female, oogenesis is a single process in which meiosis and cell maturation overlap.

- **Differences in the supply of gamete precursors.** In the male, a stem cell population continually renews itself as well as generates sperm once puberty begins. Thus, there is theoretically an unlimited supply of sperm "donors." Each primary spermatocyte produces four sperm, maximizing numbers for successful fertilization. By contrast, in the female, a non-renewable population of oocytes is established before birth, from which all mature oocytes are generated. Further, one primary oocyte produces only one mature oocyte.

- ### SPERM DEVELOPMENT
- **Spermatogenesis (meiosis) occurs first.** Sperm development begins at puberty. Primordial stem cells (or germ cells) in the seminiferous tubules of the testes begin to undergo *mitotic* divisions (see Fig. 3-3). Some of the resulting *spermatogonia* replenish the stem cell population, while others enter the meiotic path. Meiosis begins when spermatogonia replicate their DNA to form primary spermatocytes. Completion of the first meiotic division produces *secondary spermatocytes*. The second meiotic division produces *spermatids*. This part of the process takes about two weeks. As spermatocytes mature, they move towards the central lumen of the tubule, enveloped along the way by supporting Sertoli cells.

- **Spermiogenesis is maturation of spermatids to sperm.** Maturation produces a cell specialized as a compact propulsion system designed to deliver paternal DNA to the egg. Development is finished about two months after the start of meiosis. Maturation (1) eliminates all excess cytoplasm and organelles and (2) produces specialized structures organized into head, midpiece, and tail. The tail, or flagellum, propels the sperm through the female reproductive tract to the egg. The midpiece is filled with mitochondria and glycogen to provide energy for this motility. The compact head of the sperm contains an *acrosomal vesicle* cupped around the haploid nucleus.

> The *acrosomal vesicle* is a giant lysosome. Its contents will be released extracellularly to digest materials surrounding the egg.

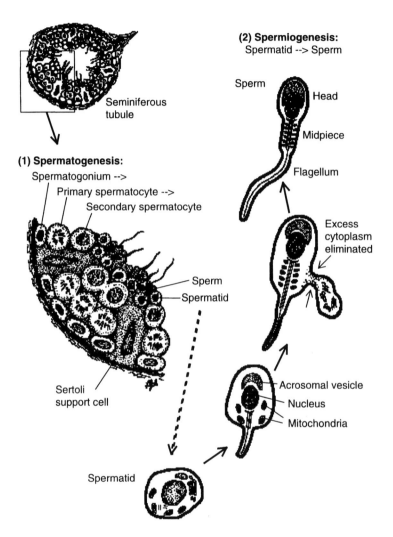

Figure 3-3
Sperm development in the seminiferous tubules.

• **Capacitance prepares sperm for binding to the egg.**   While sperm become fully mature in the male reproductive tract, they must undergo *capacitance* in the female reproductive tract to have the capacity to fertilize the egg. Capacitance involves the removal of cell surface glycoproteins by secretions from the uterus and uterine tubes.

• EGG DEVELOPMENT

• Oogenesis refers to both meiosis and cellular maturation.
Development of the oocyte (or egg) is a prolonged and *discontinuous* process, in which meiosis overlaps with cellular maturation. Thus, the single term *oogenesis* refers to both processes (see Fig. 3-4).

> *Oogenesis* begins during fetal life and is not completed until (and unless) the egg is fertilized.

• Oogenesis starts and stops during fetal development.
During fetal life, each primitive germ cell, or *oogonium,* begins meiosis, but then arrests in the *primary oocyte* stage (specifically, in metaphase of the first meiotic division). Atresia then gradually reduces the number of primary oocytes from a high of 1 to 2 million to only (!) about 40,000 by birth.

• Oogenesis resumes at puberty.
Several *primary oocytes* mature each month under the influence of circulating hormones (estrogen and progesterone). Normally only one oocyte completes the process to be released or ovulated from the ovary. One primary oocyte produces only one egg. The excess DNA generated in each meiotic division is cast off as functionless *polar bodies.* Ovulation continues monthly for 35 to 40 years. Its ceases at menopause.

• Oocytes complete their cellular maturation before they awaken from their meiotic slumber.
Maturation creates a large cell which serves as a storehouse for materials needed during and after fertilization. Cortical granules contain enzymes essential for fertilization. Excess organelles, proteins, ribosomes, and RNAs (ribonucleic acids) are all stored for a burst of protein synthesis after fertilization. Some of these RNAs and proteins activate the first embryonic genes.

• Oocyte maturation is accompanied by formation of an ovarian follicle and protective coatings around the egg.
Ovarian follicular cells that surround each oocyte proliferate to create primary and secondary follicles. (Be alert to the distinction between primary and secondary *follicles* and *oocytes.*) A sticky glycoprotein coat, called the *zona pellucida* or "clear" zone, is formed around the oocyte by these cells. The zona, together with a *corona radiata* (or "radiating crown") of follicular cells surrounding the egg, form a protective coating which stays with the egg when it is ovulated.

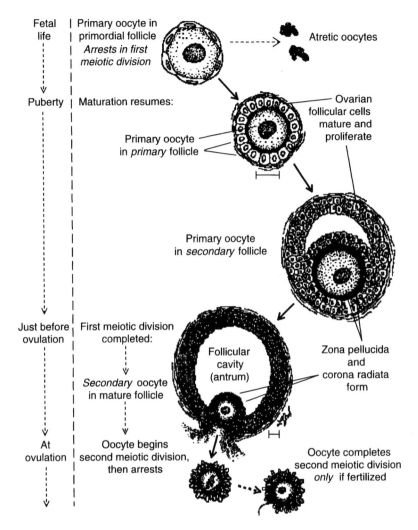

Figure 3-4
Maturation of the oocyte and its ovarian follicle.

• **Meiosis finally resumes just before ovulation.**   The first meiotic division is now completed, producing a *secondary oocyte*. It then immediately enters the second meiotic division and is ovulated at the same time. *Meiosis arrests again until fertilization.*

FERTILIZATION

Fertilization must occur within 24 hours of ovulation. Sperm can remain viable for as long as 6 days in the female reproductive tract, while the egg begins to degenerate within a day.

Gamete contact

• **Sperm meets egg in the uterine tube.**   The egg is ovulated into the pelvic cavity. It is scooped up by the open end of the uterine (or Fallopian) tube, which partially surrounds the ovary like a cupped hand (see Fig. 3-5). Fertilization normally occurs in this open end of the uterine tube. Sperm first contact the corona radiata cells surrounding the egg. Only capacitated sperm can break through the glycoprotein meshwork holding these cells together. The sperm membrane then binds to specific glycoproteins in the zona pellucida surrounding the egg.

• **Sperm-zona binding causes sperm to undergo the acrosome reaction.** The *acrosomal vesicle* in the head of the sperm fuses with the sperm membrane and releases its contents extracellularly. Its enzymes dissolve a path through the zona pellucida. The acrosome reaction occurs in multiple sperm, which together help digest a path through the zona pellucida for the one sperm which will ultimately fertilize the egg.

Sperm and egg membranes fuse

When the first sperm contacts the oocyte's membrane, their two membranes fuse. Fusion triggers extracellular release of the enzymatic contents of the oocyte's cortical granules. These granules cause the zona reaction: biochemical and electrical changes in the zona pellucida and egg membrane which prevent fertilization by more than one sperm (or *polyspermy*).

> While multiple sperm may make contact with the egg, only one fertilizes it.

Sperm contact triggers the oocyte to finally complete its second meiotic division

This creates a single haploid female nucleus. All oocyte chromatin discarded in polar bodies soon disintegrates.

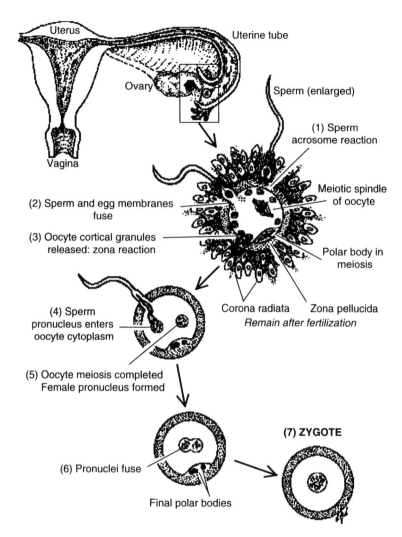

Figure 3-5
Events of fertilization.

Fusion of maternal and paternal genetic material forms the zygote

The contents of the sperm enter the egg's cytoplasm, where everything degenerates except for the sperm's nucleus. Male and female nuclei form condensed *pronuclei*, which swell, migrate toward each other, and fuse. This creates a single nucleus with a full complement of chromosomes (diploid or 2*N*) about 12 h after fertilization. The fertilized egg is now referred to as a *zygote*.

EARLY EMBRYOGENESIS AND IMPLANTATION

•

•   •   •   •   •   •   •   •   •   •   •   •

TIMETABLE OF DEVELOPMENTS

This chapter covers events of embryonic development in the first three weeks, from fertilization through germ layer formation. Germ layers will later "germinate" into specific tissues that interact to form organs during the period of organogenesis.

> The timing of early development is easy to learn: *the embryo forms one germ layer during each of the first three weeks.*

This chapter also briefly covers the events of extraembryonic development, which occur at the same time: the implantation of the embryo in the uterus and initial formation of the placenta that nourishes it. Details of their development are left for Chap. 18.

EVENTS OF EMBRYONIC DEVELOPMENT IN WEEK 1 (SEE FIG. 4-1)

First divisions of the embryo

• CLEAVAGE DIVISIONS PRODUCE A ONE-LAYERED EMBRYO
The first few mitotic divisions of the zygote are called *cleavage* divisions, to indicate that the daughter cells (called *blastomeres*) are created by *cleaving* the parent cell in half. Division thus occurs without any increase in total cytoplasmic mass. This can occur because the daughter cells can initially use mRNAs, proteins, and excess organelles stored for this purpose in the oocyte during its formation. Since storage of all these materials also transformed the oocyte into a really big cell during its development, the series of cleavage divisions progressively reduces blastomeres to a typical body cell size.

• Cleavage divisions produce a solid ball of cells called a morula. The embryo remains a solid ball of cells, or *morula,* through 3 to 4 cleavage divisions (3 days past fertilization). The embryo enters the uterine cavity during this stage.

• A cavity forms within the morula, transforming it into a blastula or blastocyst. The *blastula cavity* begins to form in the interior at 4.5 to 5 days. It rapidly enlarges toward one side and becomes filled with fluid which keeps it expanded. The blastula is still the same size as the single-celled zygote, because the cleavage divisions have continued to reduce the size of the blastomeres. The zona pellucida, which still surrounds the outside of the embryo at the beginning of the blastula stage, now begins to disintegrate. At the end of the blastula stage, the cell divisions become typical mitotic divisions in which daughter cells are built up to the parent's size with new organelles. Only at this point does the embryo begin to grow in size.

• The blastula stage embryo forms into two cell masses. The cells on the interior form the *inner cell mass,* or *embryoblast,* which will form all the components of the embryo.

This inner cell mass constitutes the one-layered embryo stage.

The cells that form the outer wall of the blastula become the *outer cell mass,* or *trophoblast.* The trophoblast will form the extraembryonic tissues, primarily the *placenta,* required to support embryonic development.

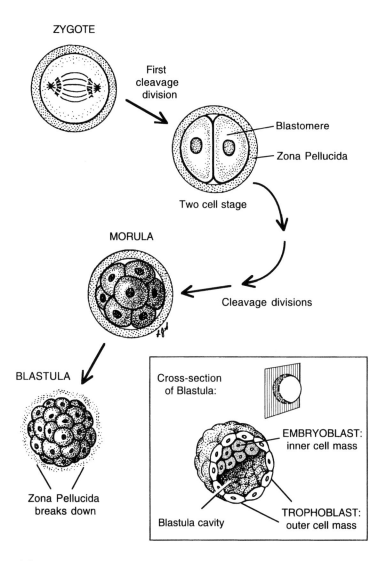

Figure 4-1
Cleavage stages: morula and blastula.

Embryo travels through the female reproductive tract (see Fig. 4-2)

While the embryo is cleaving its way from a single-celled zygote into the morula stage, it is also busy traveling along the uterine (Fallopian) tube to the uterine cavity. The first cleavage division occurs about 30 hours after fertilization. Subsequent cleavage divisions then occur at 12 to 24 hour intervals while the embryo is traveling down the uterine tube towards the uterus. The embryo is still a morula, or solid ball of cells, when it arrives in the uterine cavity about 4 days after fertilization.

Implantation begins in uterus

In the uterine cavity the morula rapidly develops into a blastula (4.5 to 5 days). The blastula stage embryo "hatches" from its zona pellucida coating in the uterus. This is necessary to expose the "bare" surface of its outer (trophoblast) layer to direct contact with the endometrial lining of the uterus. The endometrial layer increases in thickness in preparation for implantation each month under hormonal control. If there is no implantation, this layer is partially shed during menstruation.

As the trophoblast layer of the embryo makes contact with the endometrium, it is busy forming into two separate components. The outermost portion, called the *syncytiotrophoblast*, begins to invade the endometrium during week 1 (5.5 to 6 days).

> The process of the embryo *completely* embedding itself within the endometrium is called *implantation*. The embryo begins implantation during the blastula stage.

• **Normal and abnormal (ectopic) sites of implantation.**   The embryo normally implants in the endometrium of the uterus. Rarely, implantation may occur in one of several abnormal (or ectopic) sites. The most common site is the uterine tube, particularly at the open end where fertilization occurs. If the embryo travels too far, it may implant at the junction of the uterus with the vagina (the *cervix*). If the egg is fertilized before it reaches the uterine tube, the embryo may implant in the peritoneal lining of the abdominal cavity, or even in the ovary. Ectopic pregnancies can result in spontaneous abortion, or produce internal bleeding, which can be fatal to the mother if not treated.

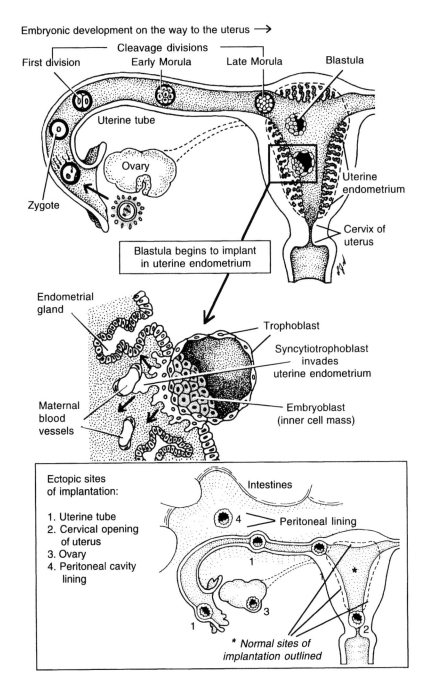

Figure 4-2
Development of the embryo and its travels during week 1.

EVENTS OF DEVELOPMENT IN WEEK 2 (SEE FIG. 4-3)

Formation of the two-layered embryo and completion of implantation

- **EMBRYONIC DEVELOPMENT**
- **The embryo forms into two layers, which are the forerunners of two embryonic "germ" layers.** The inner cell mass, or *embryoblast,* organizes into two flat, oval cell layers, creating the "bilaminar germ disc" stage. The longer axis of this oval will become the cranial-caudal axis of the embryonic body.

> The embryonic layers are called *germ layers* because they will eventually germinate, or give rise to, all the structures of the embryo.

The *hypoblast* (or *primitive endoderm*) layer is formed first by the embryoblast cells facing the blastocyst cavity. The *epiblast* (or *primitive ectoderm*) is formed by the remaining embryoblast cells above the hypoblast. Their formation establishes the future dorsal-ventral axis, with the hypoblast as the ventral layer and the epiblast as the dorsal layer.

- **EXTRAEMBRYONIC DEVELOPMENT**
- **Implantation is completed during week 2.** By 12 days, the embryo burrows completely into the uterine endometrium, which then closes over it to complete implantation. An important area of current research is the examination of how the embryo sets up shop in the immunologically foreign environment of the uterus.

- **Extraembryonic support structures begin to form from the embryonic trophoblast during week 2.** Structures that are essential for the subsequent development of the embryo are collectively described as extraembryonic support structures. They begin to develop in week 2 and are largely established by week 4. However, they continue to develop along with the embryo itself throughout the pregnancy. Therefore, implantation and the initial formation of these structures are described briefly at the end of this chapter, but the details are left for Chap. 18.

> It is important to keep in mind that the trophoblast is embryonic tissue: it has the embryo's genome and not the mother's.

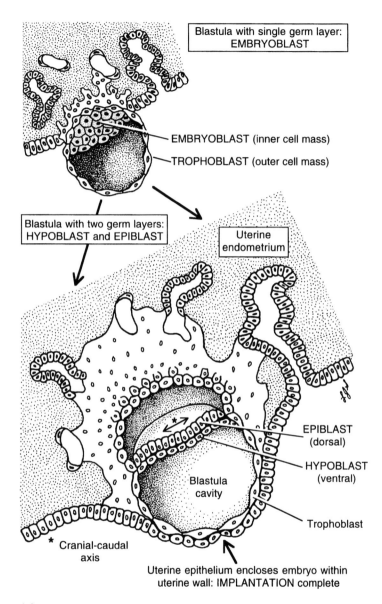

Blastula with single germ layer:
EMBRYOBLAST

EMBRYOBLAST (inner cell mass)

TROPHOBLAST (outer cell mass)

Blastula with two germ layers:
HYPOBLAST and EPIBLAST

Uterine
endometrium

EPIBLAST
(dorsal)

HYPOBLAST
(ventral)

Blastula
cavity

Trophoblast

* Cranial-caudal
axis

Uterine epithelium encloses embryo within
uterine wall: IMPLANTATION complete

Figure 4-3
Week 2: formation of two embryonic germ layers and completion of implantation.

EVENTS OF EMBRYONIC DEVELOPMENT IN WEEK 3 (SEE FIG. 4-4)

Formation of the three-layered embryo by gastrulation

The flat two-layered embryo becomes a flat three-layered embryo (or "trilaminar germ disk") by a process of cell migration called *gastrulation.* The first sign that this is about to happen is the formation of the *primitive streak,* a thickening of the epiblast along the future cranial-caudal axis. Its prominent cranial end forms the *primitive node.*

• **The primitive streak is the target for gastrulating cells.** Gastrulation begins when epiblast cells migrate toward, and then move through, the primitive streak. This process is called *ingression.* (The term *invagination* is often inaccurately used for this process.) Gastrulating cells leave the epiblast to form the definitive germ layers.

• **GASTRULATION RESULTS IN THE FORMATION OF THE THREE DEFINITIVE GERM LAYERS: ENDODERM, MESODERM, AND ECTODERM.**

> The definitive endoderm is formed by gastrulating cells that invade and replace the entire hypoblast layer.

The new endoderm cells enter the hypoblast layer in the midline, displacing the hypoblast cells laterally. The hypoblast cells now enter their second career: they migrate out to line the blastocyst cavity, transforming it into the *primary yolk sac.*

> The mesoderm layer is formed by gastrulating cells that migrate between the two existing layers.

The mesoderm forms a *mesenchymal* layer: loose cells separated by an extensive extracellular matrix. A number of different regions will coalesce within this layer. One mesoderm region is important to take note of as gastrulation occurs: the *notochord.* The notochord forms a long cord along the cranial-caudal axis of the embryo. It serves an important function while the germ layers are still forming: it signals the ectoderm directly overlying it to become *neural tissue* (see Chap. 5).

> The definitive ectoderm layer is formed by the cells that remain in the epiblast after gastrulation is complete.

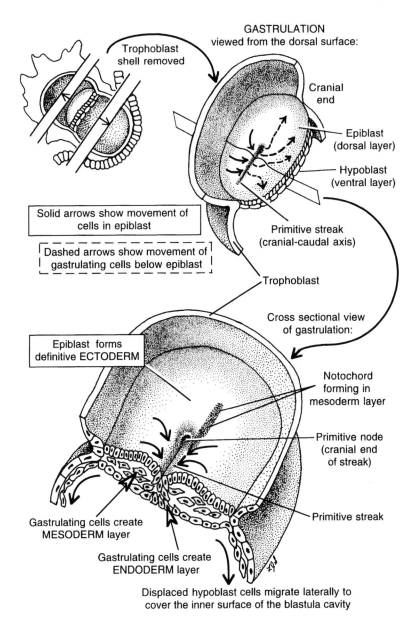

GASTRULATION
viewed from the dorsal surface:

Trophoblast
shell removed

Cranial
end

Epiblast
(dorsal layer)

Hypoblast
(ventral layer)

Solid arrows show movement of
cells in epiblast

Dashed arrows show movement of
gastrulating cells below epiblast

Primitive streak
(cranial-caudal axis)

Trophoblast

Cross sectional view
of gastrulation:

Epiblast forms
definitive ECTODERM

Notochord
forming in
mesoderm layer

Primitive node
(cranial end
of streak)

Gastrulating cells create
MESODERM layer

Primitive streak

Gastrulating cells create
ENDODERM layer

Displaced hypoblast cells migrate laterally to
cover the inner surface of the blastula cavity

Figure 4-4
Week 3: formation of three germ layers by gastrulation.

The three germ layers form (or "germinate" into) all tissues of the body.
Each germ layer gives rise to specific tissues.

Events initiated at the end of week 3

- **BODY AXES ARE ESTABLISHED EARLY (SEE FIG. 4-5)**
- **The cranial-caudal axis is established as the embryoblast organizes.**   As the embryoblast forms, it has a long axis, called the *cranial-caudal axis.* The primitive streak forms along this axis at the beginning of gastrulation, with its cranial end defined by the primitive node.

- **The dorsal-ventral axis is established by the formation of two germ layers in week 2.**   As the embryoblast cells organize into two layers, the hypoblast layer facing the blastocyst cavity becomes the ventral layer, and the epiblast becomes the dorsal layer.

- **INITIAL BODY SHAPE IS FORMED BY FOLDING**   A recognizable body shape is created by folding, which rearranges the three flat germ layers into tubes within tubes. Body folding is largely the result of rapid, differential growth of some germ layer regions more than others. You will need to be able to visualize this folding process in order to understand the major events of early embryogenesis, since folding starts during gastrulation at the end of week 3 and continues while the first structures of most organs are being established in week 4.

- **Lateral body folds cause the three germ layers to encircle each other.** Lateral folds are best illustrated in cross sectional views. The lateral edges of all three germ layers grow rapidly, curling around each other to the ventral embryonic surface. This changes their relationships:

1.   The *endoderm* becomes folded into a long, narrow tube, which is incorporated into the interior of the body.
2.   The middle *mesoderm* layer continues to separate endoderm from ectoderm. It remains thickest along the dorsal midline.
3.   The *ectoderm* completely encircles the other two layers, forming the outer covering of the embryo.

- **Cranial and caudal folds create identifiable head and tail regions.**   These folds are best illustrated in longitudinal (or midline sagittal) views. Rapid growth causes the head and tail ends of the flat embryonic disk to curl toward the ventral surface, creating a C-shaped body.

> Folding creates a single point at which the three germ layers are connected to extraembryonic tissues: the ventral yolk stalk.

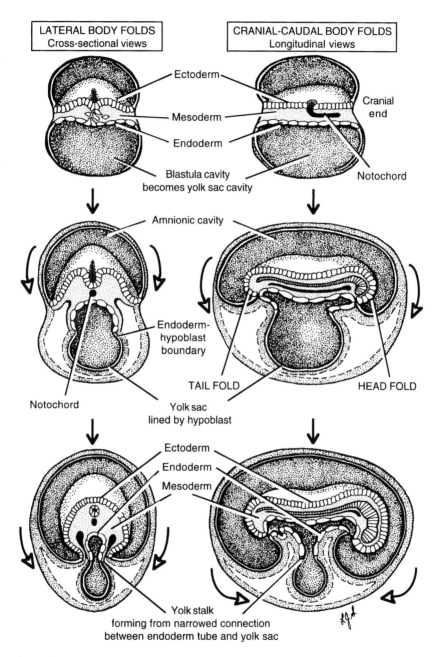

LATERAL BODY FOLDS
Cross-sectional views

CRANIAL-CAUDAL BODY FOLDS
Longitudinal views

Ectoderm

Mesoderm

Endoderm

Cranial
end

Blastula cavity
becomes yolk sac cavity

Notochord

Amnionic cavity

Endoderm-
hypoblast
boundary

TAIL FOLD

HEAD FOLD

Notochord

Yolk sac
lined by hypoblast

Ectoderm
Endoderm
Mesoderm

Yolk stalk
forming from narrowed connection
between endoderm tube and yolk sac

Figure 4-5
Process of body folding at the end of week 3.

EXTRAEMBRYONIC DEVELOPMENTS IN WEEKS 1–3
Implantation (see Fig. 4-6)

Implantation of the embryo in the uterine wall is achieved by cells of the outer cell mass or trophoblast. The trophoblast forms into two layers as the blastula-stage embryo moves toward the uterine wall. Implantation begins in week 1 and is completed in week 2.

• **An outer trophoblast layer called the syncytiotrophoblast is formed.**   This is the trophoblast component which comes into direct contact with the uterine tissues and is the component that does the actual work of burrowing into the uterine wall. "Syncytio" tells you that it is a multinucleated mass, or *syncytium*. It is formed by cells leaving the cellular trophoblast layer and fusing together into a syncytium.

• **Cytotrophoblast is the new name for the original trophoblast layer.**   This layer continues to be a cellular layer that divides to increase its own cell number, as well as contributing to the new syncytium. This layer is closest to the embryo.

Implantation occurs when the syncytiotrophoblast produces proteases that erode the uterine endometrium, causing the embryo to become completely embedded (or implanted) within the endometrium, which then closes over it.

The beginnings of *uteroplacental circulation* are established when the syncytiotrophoblast erodes the walls of maternal blood vessels and nutrient glands in the endometrium, forming lacunae (spaces) into which maternal blood and glandular secretions empty. Maternal fluids are then in direct contact with the membrane of the embryonic syncytiotrophoblast. Transport of nutrients and oxygen across this membrane is the beginning of uteroplacental circulation. These materials are transported through the syncytiotrophoblast to the cytotrophoblast. From there, they diffuse into the embryonic germ layers as they form.

Figure 4-6 reexamines the same drawings seen in Fig. 4-3, concentrating this time on the extraembryonic structures.

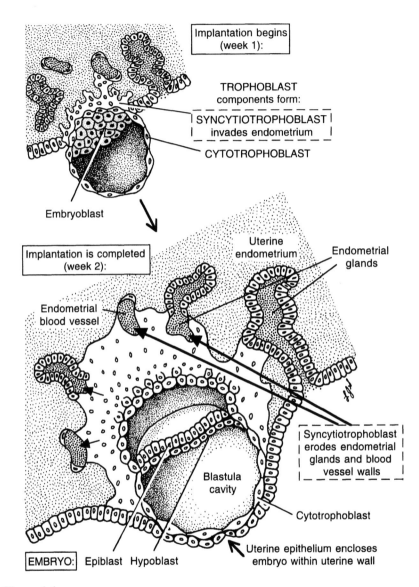

Figure 4-6
Implantation and establishment of trophoblast layers.

Establishment of extraembryonic support tissues (see Fig. 4-7)

The extraembryonic support tissues develop right along with the embryo proper. Their development begins in week 2 and is largely established by week 4. These structures consist of the *chorion* (future *placenta*), future *umbilical cord,* and *amnion.* It is essential that the support tissues develop early, because the embryo can't get beyond the formation of its three germ layers relying simply on diffusion of nutrients and oxygen. The placenta must be set up to provide circulatory input from the maternal vasculature. The structures of the umbilical cord must be set up to connect the placenta to the embryo. Finally, the embryo must develop a flotation sac (amnion).

The extraembryonic support tissues are formed largely by the embryonic trophoblast and its derivatives, with some contributions from the embryonic germ layers and maternal endometrium.

All of these structures initially appear while the embryo is still a two-layered embryonic disk (i.e., in the second week of development).

• **The embryonic connection to the yolk sac becomes a narrow stalk.**   The blastula cavity is transformed into the yolk sac cavity when the cells of the original hypoblast layer migrate out to line the inside of the blastula cavity. The yolk sac lining remains continuous with the endoderm that replaces it. The connection between the endoderm and yolk sac gradually becomes narrowed as the result of body folding into a long, thin yolk sac stalk (see also Fig. 4-5).

• **THE EMBRYO FORMS A PERSONAL FLOTATION SAC CALLED THE AMNION.**   The embryo will eventually float in a fluid-filled sac called the *amnionic sac.* During the blastula stage, the amniotic cavity begins to form between the epiblast and the trophoblast. The cavity becomes lined by the amnionic membrane, which is (probably) formed by cells moving out from the epiblast in a mirror image of the way in which the yolk sac becomes lined by the hypoblast. The amnionic sac expands enormously as the embryo develops. The embryo will become suspended in the amnionic sac, and then the amnionic sac will become suspended within the chorionic cavity.

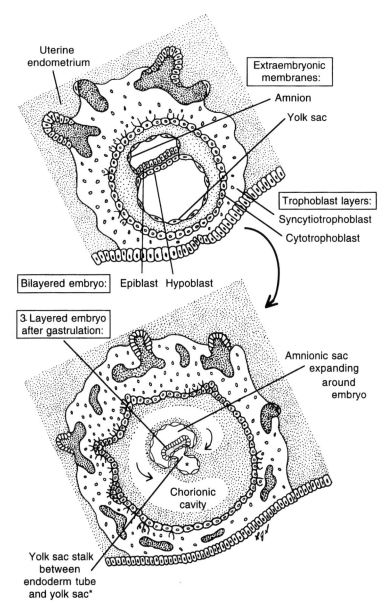

Figure 4-7
Initial development of extraembryonic support structures.

**• THE PLACENTA IS A JOINT VENTURE BETWEEN THE EMBRYO
AND ITS MOTHER (SEE FIG. 4-8).** The maternal contribution to the placenta is formed by the endometrial lining of the uterus. This part of the
endometrium is renamed the *decidua* with the onset of pregnancy.

> The fetal contribution to the placenta is called the *chorion.* It is formed
> from *both* trophoblast layers, and a portion of another embryonic deriva-
> tive called the *extraembryonic mesoderm.*

**• Extraembryonic mesoderm forms between the embryo and the cytotro-
phoblast.** While it is clear that this is an *embryonic* derivative, its specific origins are currently a matter of dispute. It is formed by cells derived either from the
cytotrophoblast, the epiblast, or the hypoblast.

• A chorionic cavity forms within the extraembryonic mesoderm. This
cavity separates the embryo from the developing placental tissues. It also separates the extraembryonic mesoderm into two arms. One wraps around the outer
surface of the embryo, its amnion, and yolk sac. The other hugs the inner surface
of the trophoblast layers. It is this latter bit that becomes part of the chorion.

**• The embryo establishes a connection with the developing placenta via the
umbilical cord during weeks 3 and 4 (Fig. 4-8).** First, a connecting stalk is
formed by extraembryonic mesoderm, which remains continuous across the
developing chorionic cavity. The connecting stalk eventually becomes the connective tissue core of the umbilical cord. This core forms around the embryonic
yolk sac. Umbilical blood vessels grow into this connective tissue core from the
embryo to form the fetal arm of the placental circulation. As the amnion expands
around to the ventral surface of the embryo, it eventually becomes plastered
against the outer surface of the umbilical cord.

**• The edges of each of the germ layers are connected to extraembryonic
structures at the umbilical cord.** The preceding descriptions demonstrate that
the edges of the embryonic germ layers don't simply end in free space. It makes
it easier to visualize the events of early embryonic development if you understand

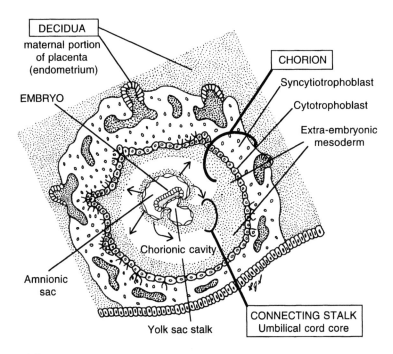

Figure 4-8
Development of placenta and umbilical cord.

the extraembryonic structures to which the lateral "edges" of each germ layer are attached:

1. The ectoderm is continuous at its edges with the amnionic membrane, which forms the covering of the umbilical cord.
2. The endoderm is continuous with the yolk sac lining, which extends into the core of the umbilical cord.
3. The embryonic mesoderm is continuous with the extraembryonic mesoderm, which forms the core of the umbilical cord.

This is the state of development of the extraembryonic structures at the time that the embryonic germ layers begin to differentiate into tissues. To finish this story, proceed directly to Chap. 18; to continue the story of embryonic development, proceed to Chap. 5.

· C H A P T E R · 5 ·

GERM LAYER DERIVATIVES

·

· · · · · · · · · · · · ·

GERM LAYERS: THE BUILDING BLOCKS OF ORGANS

Learning the embryonic origins of each organ system is easier if you start by thinking in terms of the tissues that build them. This is because there are only four basic tissue types, and each of them originates from specific germ layers.

> The three germ layers give rise to four basic tissue types. These organize in specific combinations and interact to build all organs during the period of *organogenesis* (4 to 8 weeks).

Each of the points covered in this chapter will come up again as you go through the specific development of each organ system. This chapter gives you an *overview* of these points, as well as a *review* to which you can come back as you are studying the development of each organ system.

BODY FOLDS REARRANGE GERM LAYERS

• **Folding creates the final three-dimensional body form from which tissues and organs originate.** The folding process, which the embryo undergoes beginning in week 3, rearranges its three flat germ layers into a three-dimensional C-shaped body (think of this as a trio of threes). As described in the last chapter, this results in the *ectoderm* covering the entire outer surface of the embryo, the *mesoderm* forming a wide middle layer, and the *endoderm* fusing into a narrow tube which runs the length of the embryo on its interior. This folding is still underway while the germ layers form the first tissue components in week 4, so it is worth spending a little time reviewing this folding in order to understand the major events of early embryogenesis.

ORIGINS OF FOUR BASIC TISSUE TYPES

The great complexity of the body can be broken down into four basic categories called *tissues* (see Fig. 5-1). A tissue is a group of cells that have common structural features and perform common functions. The key word here is "group": cells of most tissues must live and work together in groups for them to perform their functions.

> The four basic tissue types are *nerve, muscle, connective tissue,* and *epithelium.*

Each germ layer gives rise to specific tissue types:

Ectoderm forms all *nerve* and some *epithelia.*
Mesoderm forms all *connective tissues,** *muscle,* and some *epithelia.*
Endoderm forms some *epithelia.*

Each tissue type therefore originates from specific germ layers:

> Three tissues each originate from a single germ layer. *Nerve* is derived from ectoderm. *Muscle* and *connective tissues** are derived from mesoderm. By contrast, *epithelia* are derived from all 3 germ layers.

---

*You knew there had to be at least one exception: the head, as befits its special status, forms some of its connective tissue from a specific ectoderm derivative called *neural crest.* More about this later in this chapter and in Chap. 10.

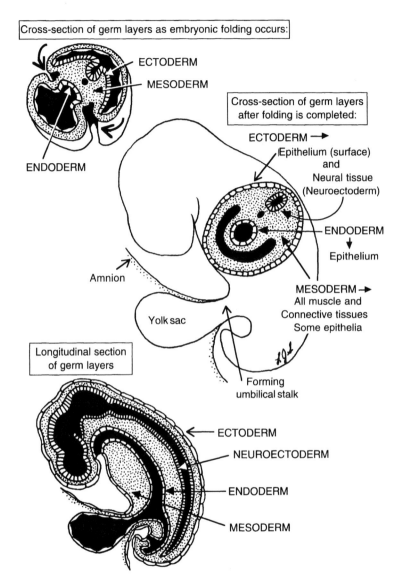

Figure 5-1
Overview of germ layer origins of the four basic tissue types.

DISTINGUISHING BETWEEN TISSUE TYPES

• **The four basic tissue types can be distinguished without completing an entire histology course.**   Remember that the objective here is to know enough about each tissue type to be able to sort out which tissue components are likely to be present in each organ. While each tissue type has subtypes, and many of those subtypes are composed of multiple cell types, you can nevertheless readily learn the essential features that distinguish each tissue category.

• **Use this section as a review or as an introduction if you need it.**   If you are confident of your knowledge of the existence of all the different tissue types and their main histologic characteristics, then by all means proceed to the next section of this chapter, which describes how each germ layer gives rise to specific tissues.

• **The development of tissues is referred to as *histogenesis*.**   The histogenesis of each tissue is covered in more detail in the first relevant chapter for that tissue, as indicated on the following pages.

Muscle: cardiac, skeletal, and smooth

Muscle is a tissue composed of elongated cells that are specialized to contract or shorten. There are three major types of muscle, each performing a different job when it contracts (see Fig. 5-2). *Skeletal* muscle tissue is the major tissue that forms individual skeletal muscles (such as the biceps or deltoid). Skeletal muscle contraction moves the body by its attachment to the skeleton. *Cardiac* muscle forms the bulk of the heart wall. Its contraction propels blood into blood vessels. *Smooth* muscle forms part of the walls of many organs, from the gastrointestinal tract to blood vessels. Its contraction performs many functions, primarily by changing the diameter of the cavity (or lumen) within that organ. Muscle development is covered in Chap. 8 (skeletal muscle) and Chap. 11 (cardiac and smooth muscle).

> While all muscle types are derived from mesoderm, each type is derived from a different region of the mesoderm. Smooth muscle originates from several subregions of mesoderm because it is usually derived from the "local" mesoderm of each organ.

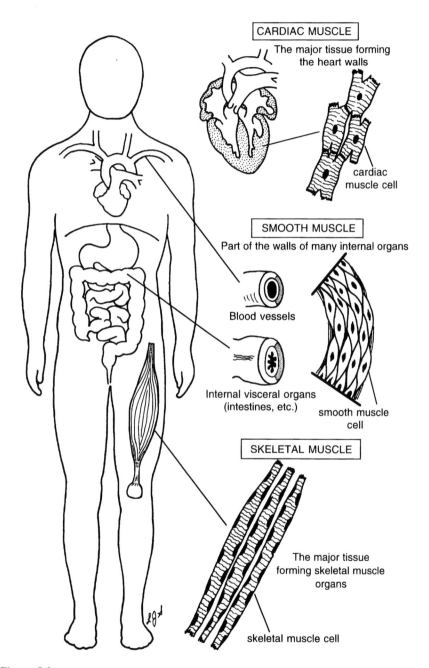

Figure 5-2
Muscle subtypes: skeletal, cardiac, and smooth.

Nerve

Nerve is a tissue composed of large irregularly shaped cells with very long cellular processes (see Fig. 5-3). Nerve cells (or neurons) function to receive, generate, and transmit signals to target tissues. The targets that they innervate include other nerve cells and all types of muscle. Nerve cells innervate muscle in distant organs by extending processes out from their cell bodies, which stay in the nervous system. The development of nerve tissue and the nervous system is introduced in this chapter and covered in detail in Chap. 9.

> While the development of the nervous system is complex, its origins are simple: all nerve tissue is formed from a specialized part of the ectoderm called the *neuroectoderm.*

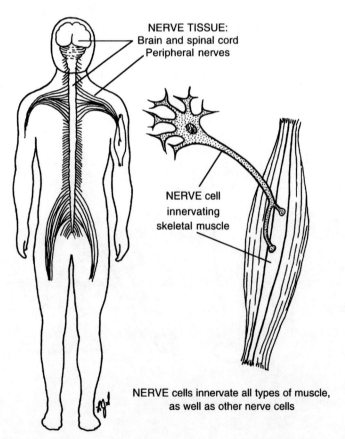

NERVE TISSUE:
Brain and spinal cord
Peripheral nerves

NERVE cell
innervating
skeletal muscle

NERVE cells innervate all types of muscle,
as well as other nerve cells

Figure 5-3
Nerve tissue.

Connective tissue

Connective tissue does just what the name implies: it connects other tissues together. To do this, connective tissue makes use of a major cell type, the *fibroblast*, and a significant amount of extracellular matrix material created by those fibroblasts (see Fig. 5-4). Variations in the matrix components are important factors in the type of connective tissue formed. Connective tissue contains a number of different subtypes.

All connective tissue types are formed by mesoderm, except for some neural-crest-derived components in the head (which are covered in Chap. 9). Connective tissue is usually derived from the "local" mesoderm of that organ. Thus, it originates from many mesoderm subregions.

"General" connective tissue elements are distributed throughout the walls of many organs, where they are essential in binding the other tissues together. General connective tissue is also organized into *fascia, tendons, ligaments,* and *joint capsules.* The histogenesis of general connective tissue is covered for the first time in Chap. 6 and in more detail in Chap. 7.

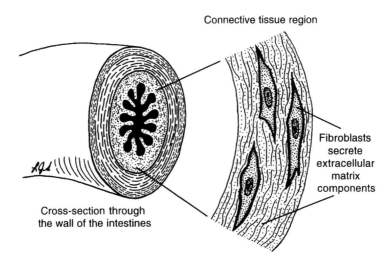

Connective tissue region

Fibroblasts secrete extracellular matrix components

Cross-section through the wall of the intestines

Figure 5-4
General connective tissue.

• SPECIALIZED CONNECTIVE TISSUES

• **Cartilage and bone.**   There are also several specialized types of connective tissues (see Fig. 5-5). Cartilage and bone are rigid connective tissues that form the internal skeletal framework of the body. Specialized cartilage and bone cell types generate a dense matrix which gives each of these connective tissues its unique properties. With regard to embryology, it is important to realize that much bone formation occurs by the initial formation of cartilage "templates" which are then replaced by bone during subsequent embryonic and fetal development.

> Cartilage and bone form during embryonic life from condensations of mesoderm. Distinct, separate subregions of mesoderm give rise to specific cartilages and bones of the body (trunk), limbs, and head.

Again, the disclaimer must be inserted here that some cartilage and bone in the head are derived from the neural crest. Their formation occurs in a similar manner to mesoderm-derived cartilage and bone. The development of both cartilage and bone is described in Chap. 7.

• **Blood cells.**   The circulatory system contains a number of cells, collectively referred to as *blood cells* or *blood-borne elements.* These cells are classified as connective tissue components, in part because they develop throughout life within (largely) mesodermally derived organs. They include red blood cells (*erythrocytes*), *platelets,* and white blood cells, or *leukocytes.* The latter are subdivided into several different types of granular and agranular leukocytes (or lymphocytes). These cells perform a number of functions, either while in the blood stream, or after entering the surrounding connective tissues. Blood cells continue to be produced throughout life from self-renewing hematopoietic stem cells (or precursor cells), which reside within host organs. The principal host organ for most blood cells is the bone marrow, while lymphocytes are also hosted by lymphoid organs such as the thymus and lymph nodes. During embryonic development, blood cell precursors home in on a series of host organs in the embryo before settling into the developing bone marrow or (later) the lymphoid organs. The histogenesis of these cells within their host organs is covered in Chap. 17.

> The origins of blood cells themselves are still a matter of dispute, but the evidence suggests they originate in the mesoderm.

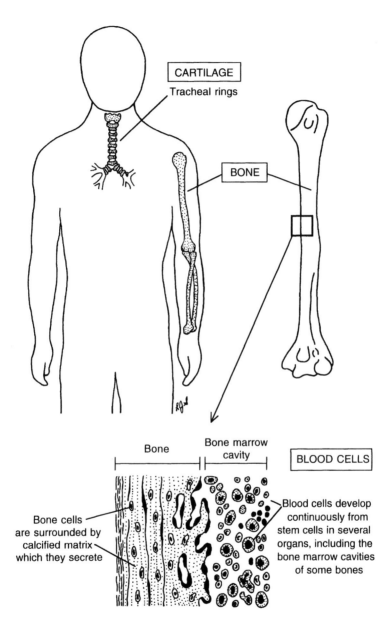

Figure 5-5
Specialized connective tissues: cartilage, bone, and blood cells.

Epithelia

Epithelium is a tissue type that is composed of sheets of attached cells. The operative word here is *sheet*: epithelial cells must function in tight association with other epithelial cells. These sheets line or cover the boundaries between the "outside" environment and other tissues (see Fig. 5-6). *Outside* refers not only to the world outside the body, but also to the cavity (lumen) of any tube or space within the body, such as blood vessels, the GI tract, or body cavities. Epithelia isolate these spaces in an important functional sense by controlling transport across their sheets. Epithelia thus protect the underlying tissues. Connective tissue usually anchors epithelia to the underlying structures. In addition, many epithelia secrete important products, ranging from digestive enzymes to hormones. Some secretory epithelia form collections of epithelial tubes called *glands*. The many specializations of epithelia are covered in their respective organ systems.

> The derivation of epithelia is the most complex: all three germ layers give rise to epithelia. Specific epithelia originate from each germ layer.

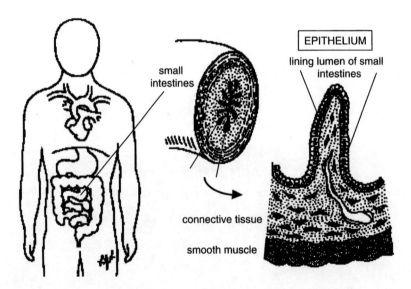

Figure 5-6
Epithelium lines structures such as the lumen of the gastrointestinal tract.

• **All embryonic germ layers are initially organized as either** *epithelia* **or** *mesenchyme,* **a primitive form of connective tissue.**   Ectoderm and endoderm are formed as epithelial sheets. Most (but not all) of their derivatives differentiate directly into epithelia. Mesoderm, however, is formed as a *mesenchyme,* which means separate cells are surrounded by a hydrated (watery) matrix. This state is really a primitive form of connective tissue; the extensive matrix facilitates migration of cells through it to their target destinations.

Transformations back and forth between mesenchymal and epithelial states are common during early embryonic development, particularly in cells of mesodermal origin. The first of these transformations occurs in the creation of the mesoderm germ layer during gastrulation (see Fig. 5-7).

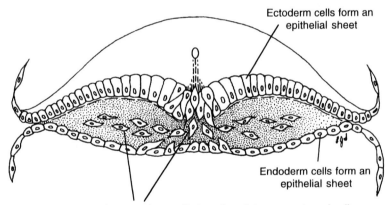

Ectoderm cells form an epithelial sheet

Endoderm cells form an epithelial sheet

During gastrulation, ectoderm cells transform into mesenchymal cells.
Then they migrate between the two existing germ layers to form the mesoderm.

Figure 5-7
Epithelial-mesenchymal transformations during gastrulation: cross-section of embryo.

> *Putting it all together:* tissues are formed from specific germ layers, and organs are formed from specific combinations of those tissues.

BUILDING ORGANS FROM TISSUES

If you study this chapter before you study the chapters on individual organ system development, you should be able to limit the amount of memorization required because you will learn to ask questions such as, "What tissues form this organ or system?" and "What germ layers must have contributed to their formation?"

• **The following are the general principles in building organs from tissues:**

1. Virtually all organs and structures in the body will require a mesoderm contribution, since all muscle and almost all connective tissues are derived from mesoderm. The only exception to this is the central nervous system, which is formed almost entirely by ectoderm (see Chap. 9).
2. Epithelia will be present in any organ or structure that has a lumen or that is covered by a membrane. The trick to learning the origins of any organ is to learn the germ layer origins of its epithelia. As you will see in the rest of this chapter, the best plan of attack is to learn the organ systems whose epithelia are derived from endoderm or ectoderm. The other systems will have epithelia derived from mesoderm.
3. While nerve innervates all organs, it arrives only after other tissue components are on their way to forming the organ's mature structure. It doesn't really contribute to the "architecture" of organs. Nerve innervates target organs by extending cell processes into the organ, either from outside or from small groups of nerve cells which take up residence in the organ. In either case, the presence of nerve cells or processes is not integral to the architecture of the organ as is the presence of smooth muscle or connective tissue elements. This is why you will not find a lot of discussion in this book about innervation of organs. You should, nevertheless, understand that arrival of nerve is essential to the final development of organs, as well as to the onset of full function.

• **A word about the formation of blood vessels.**   Blood vessels, like nerves, grow into organs as they form. However, blood vessels (like the rest of the cardiovascular system) are composite structures, or organs, made of several tissue types (epithelial linings, connective tissue, and smooth muscle walls). Their formation is described in Chap. 11. Conveniently, however, all blood vessel components are formed from a single germ layer: mesoderm.

Subdivision of germ layers into different regions marks commitment to specific tissues.

The formation of grossly visible subdivisions in each germ layer reflects major events going on at the biochemical and genetic level. The cells within these regions are "induced" to "commit" to specific fates during this period. Committed cells have received instructions that "tell" them to differentiate into specific cell types. Usually the cells also must receive a separate stimulus to actually begin differentiation.

The field of developmental biology today is focused on determining the identity of the inducing signals that cause commitment, their mechanisms of action on the genome, and the specific alterations that are triggered in gene expression. The focus in this book is on the *events* of development, not on the *mechanisms* behind those events. Hence, the attention given to induction in this book is largely limited to pointing out which specific germ layer components induce commitment of other components and when this occurs. The first major inducing component has already been introduced: the notochord. In case you've forgotten it, it makes a return engagement on the very next page.

Do not try to memorize everything in this chapter. It is intended as a preview to help you focus as you proceed, as well as a review you can come back to for clarification throughout your studies.

ECTODERM DERIVATIVES

The ectoderm gives rise to two subdivisions: neuroectoderm, which forms all neural tissue, and one specific epithelium, the epidermal covering of the body.

Neuroectoderm forms all neural tissue

• **Neuroectoderm, the neural tissue precursor, is formed from midline ectoderm (see Fig. 5-8).**   Neural tissue is the first tissue type to be committed to its fate. It is important to learn the basics of the formation of the neuroectoderm now, because it forms while the other germ layers are still forming. It begins to form at the end of week 3, while the embryo is still a flat disk, and continues throughout gastrulation and the body folding process (week 4 and early week 5). (The complete development of the nervous system is covered in Chap. 9.)

   The first sign that a part of the ectoderm has been induced to start forming neural tissue comes when the ectoderm cranial to the primitive streak thickens along its midline (cranial-caudal) axis. This thickened region is the neural plate, or neuroectoderm.

The notochord induces the ectoderm overlying it to form the neural plate and commits it to neural tissue fate.

   Do you remember the notochord from the last chapter? It's that dense cord of mesoderm that forms under the ectoderm in the midline along the cranial-caudal axis. During gastrulation, it extends cranially from the primitive node (the cranial end of the primitive streak). Both the notochord and overlying neural plate ectoderm continue to grow cranially, whereas the more caudal portions of the embryo in the area of the primitive streak "appear" to shrink. (In fact, this caudal region just grows much more slowly.) The net result is that the primitive streak winds up as a small point at the most caudal end of the embryo, while the neural plate extends along most of the length of the embryo, with the notochord lying under it in the mesoderm layer. The rapid growth of the neuroectoderm is largely responsible for the formation of the cranial or head fold and for the overall enlargement of the cranial end of the embryonic disk.

• **Neuroectoderm forms the neural tube and neural crest.**   The neural plate rapidly begins to rise up into two neural folds along its length, creating a neural groove or depression between them. The cells at the crest of each neural fold sep-

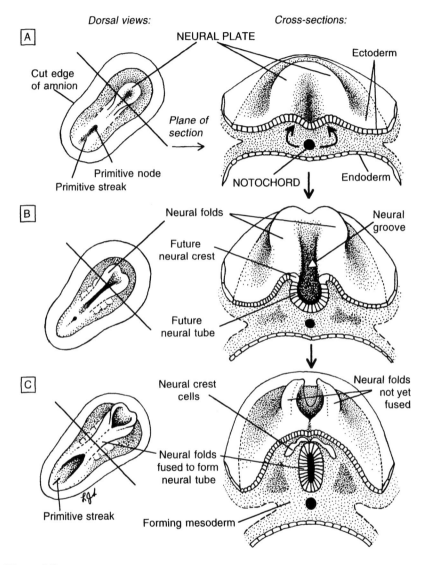

Figure 5-8
Neuroectoderm induction (A) and formation of neural tube and neural crest (B and C).
(A) and (B), late week 3; (C) early week 4.

arate to form groups of neural crest cells. The neural folds then grow toward each other until they meet and fuse along their length to form the neural tube. The neural tube separates from the surface ectoderm to form a self-contained tube.

• The neural tube and neural crest have different fates within the nervous system (see Fig. 5-9).

> The neural tube forms all the components of the brain and spinal cord. Together these constitute the central nervous system.

The cell types derived from the neural tube include (1) all nerve cells and (2) most central nervous system "support" cells, called *glial cells.* The glia perform many of the functions that connective tissues perform in other organ systems.

> The neural crest forms the peripheral nervous system and a whole bunch of other things.

These cells differentiate into a variety of neural and non-neural cell types. Crest cells become mesenchymal and migrate to a number of locations in the body before they differentiate. This partially accounts for the distribution of derivatives throughout the body.

The neuronal cell types all form components of the peripheral nervous system. This refers to neural tissue outside the central nervous system, or at the "periphery" of the body. The derivatives include nerve cells (clumped into ganglia) and support cells (which are sometimes referred to as glia). (These developments are covered in more detail in Chap. 9.)

The non-neural derivatives of the neural crest become several different cell types in several portions of the body: melanocytes (pigment cells) of the skin, endocrine secretory cells in the adrenal gland medulla, and some connective tissue elements in the head. These connective tissue derivatives, which include some cartilages and bones, are formed in a region of the embryonic head called the pharyngeal arches, which form most of the structures of the jaw and lower face. At this point, these non-neural derivatives are simply a list of unconnected items which you may be tempted to memorize. Don't! They are listed here just to give you a preview of coming attractions. They *are* going to be important to learn later, however, because congenital defects have been attributed to failure of development of neural crest components in their target organs. (These derivatives are covered in more detail in Chaps. 9 and 10.)

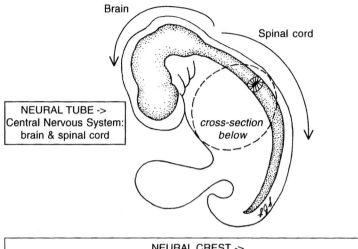

NEURAL TUBE ->
Central Nervous System:
brain & spinal cord

NEURAL CREST ->
Peripheral Nervous System ganglia and several nonneural tissue components:

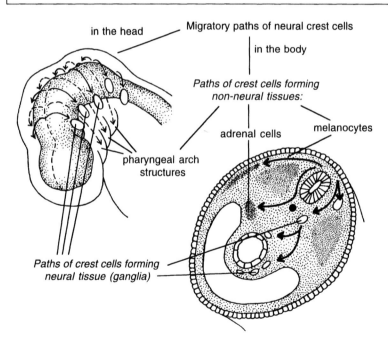

Figure 5-9
Overview of neural tube and neural crest derivatives.

Surface ectoderm forms the epidermis of the skin

The ectoderm that remains after the neuroectoderm is formed differentiates into a specific epithelium, the *epidermis,* or outermost layer of the skin (see Fig. 5-10). This boundary between the body and the outside environment is a textbook example of the protective function of epithelia.

> *Putting it all together:* The skin is an organ that is formed by the epidermis, its specializations, and underlying connective tissues.

The epidermis is anchored to the body by an underlying connective tissue layer called the *dermis,* and under it, a looser connective tissue layer called the *hypodermis.* These connective tissue components are derived from mesoderm. Together these tissue layers constitute the skin. It may seem strange to refer to the skin as an organ, but it is an important one. It protects the body against mechanical damage, invasion by infectious agents, and helps regulate body temperature, as well as water and ion secretion and retention.

The basic components of the skin are established during the embryonic period, but development continues throughout fetal life and after birth. First, the surface ectoderm begins to proliferate just after the neuroectoderm separates from it. It forms a multilayered (stratified) epithelium, the epidermis. Underlying mesoderm proliferates to form the dermis and hypodermis. As the dermis forms, it is invaded by developing sensory nerve endings and blood vessels. *Melanocytes* are neural crest derivatives that invade the epidermis as it forms. They produce the pigmentation of the skin and hair.

• **The epidermis layer also forms specialized structures such as hair, nails, and glands.**   It is not immediately obvious that surface specializations such as hair follicles, nails, sweat glands, and even mammary glands are also derived from the ectodermal layer. They are formed in specific locations by the ectoderm in response to inductive signals from the underlying mesoderm. Hair follicles and glands begin as downgrowths of surface ectoderm into underlying mesoderm. Ectoderm forms the hair shaft and its surrounding hair sheath, while mesoderm surrounds its terminal ending to form a connective tissue root sheath. Glands are formed by epithelial downgrowths, which retain a central lumen connected to the surface (ducts). Epithelial cells become the secretory glandular cells.

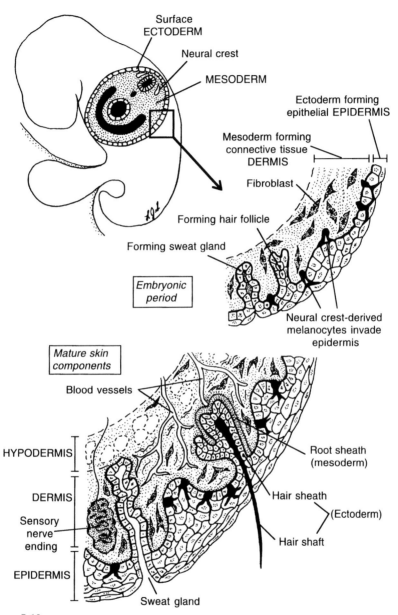

Figure 5-10
Formation of the epidermis, its specializations, and all the layers of the skin.

ENDODERM DERIVATIVES

Epithelial linings of many internal organs

During the body folding process, the endoderm is formed into an epithelial tube, which runs the length of the body. The derivatives of the endoderm tube are all epithelial tissues (see Fig. 5-11).

• **The epithelial lining of the gastrointestinal tract forms directly from the endoderm tube.** The epithelial lining of the lumen of the gastrointestinal (GI) tract extends from the mouth to the anus. To the uninitiated, this epithelial lining may seem like a trivial component of this system. However, the epithelial lining cells of the GI tract (and of many other organs) are usually its key "business" cells. These cells perform the major functions of each organ, such as manufacturing and secreting digestive enzymes and absorbing nutrients.

> *Putting it all together:* The organs that are lined by endodermal epithelium have their other tissues formed by mesoderm. These include connective tissue and smooth muscle layers.

The endoderm and mesoderm mutually induce each other to form derivatives appropriate to each specific part of the GI tract. Thus, for example, only the stomach epithelium forms acid-secreting cells.

• **Epithelial components of several other organs form by budding from the endoderm tube.** A wide range of organs are formed by a series of endoderm buds, or diverticula, which grow out into the surrounding mesoderm. The endoderm forms epithelial components, while the mesoderm forms the other tissues of these organs. Some endoderm buds later separate from the GI tube, so that their endoderm origins are obscured. Only some of these buds form components of the GI system.

Here's a preview presented in sequence from head to toe to get you oriented. Outgrowths of the cranial or pharyngeal endoderm form the epithelial components of several glands: the palatine tonsils, the thymus, the thyroid, and the parathyroids. These buds initially grow into the surrounding pharyngeal arches. (These derivatives are described in Chaps. 10, 16, and 17.) Just caudal to this, a lung bud forms the epithelial lining of the entire respiratory system, from the tra-

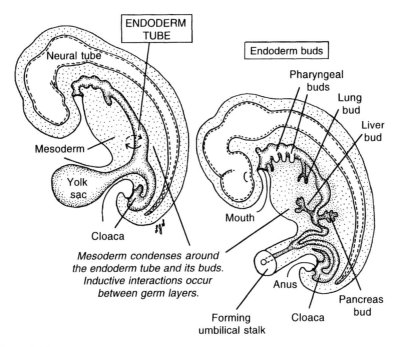

Figure 5-11
Endoderm derivatives.

chea to the smallest branches in the lungs where gaseous exchange occurs (Chap. 13). In the future abdominal region, several buds form just caudal to the stomach region, which give rise to the epithelial components of the liver, gallbladder, and pancreas (Chap. 12). (At last, organs that have some direct relevance to the digestive tract!) Finally, the most caudal portion of the endoderm tube expands, and a portion (called the *cloaca*) will line the terminal part of the urogenital system (Chaps. 14 and 15).

Only epithelia in these organs are formed by *endoderm*; most of the remaining tissues are derived from *mesoderm*.

MESODERM DERIVATIVES

• **Mesoderm contributes to most organs and structures in the body.**

Mesoderm gives rise to all muscle (skeletal, cardiac, and smooth) and all connective tissue in the body and limbs and most in the head. It also gives rise to *certain* epithelia.

This leaves only one tissue type which it doesn't form: nerve!

As you might suspect, the origins of each tissue are not random within the mesoderm layer. Shortly after the mesoderm layer is created, much of it condenses from a loose mesenchyme into distinct regions on each side of the body.

Each mesoderm region is committed to a specific fate as it forms. Subsequently, each gives rise to specific tissues. This is why all books on embryology, including this one, torture you with the details of these regions. The following overview is more detailed than those for other germ layers, because of the complexity of mesoderm subdivisions and their derivatives. As you read through, try to *understand,* not *memorize.* You can come back to this overview anytime as you study the development of specific organ systems.

Formation of mesoderm subdivisions

The mesoderm becomes subdivided into regions during the end of week 3 into week 4, as the body is folding (see Fig. 5-12). The regions of the mesoderm are named for their location on the transverse axis of the body.

The mesoderm regions are (from medial to lateral): axial, paraxial, intermediate, and lateral plate mesoderm.

Axial mesoderm forms along the midline of the cranial-caudal axis, while the other regions are formed bilaterally (i.e., on each side of the body). Embryonic folding and the formation of the body cavity affect the configuration of the lateral plate region dramatically while it is in the process of forming.

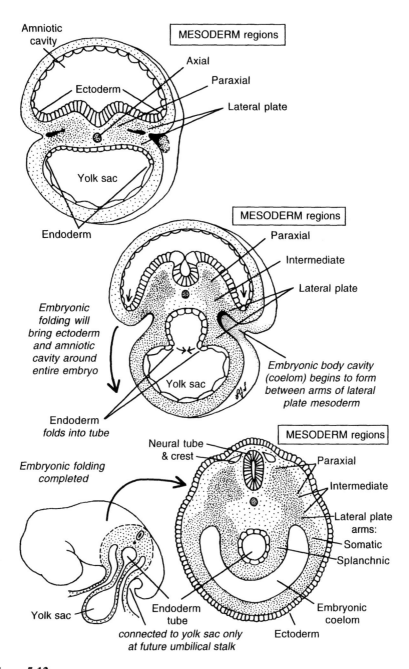

Figure 5-12
Regional divisions of mesoderm form as the body folds in late week 3 and early week 4
(cross-sections).

• OVERVIEW OF DERIVATIVES OF EACH SPECIFIC MESODERM REGION

• **Axial mesoderm forms the notochord (see Fig. 5-13).**   Since the notochord forms along the cranial-caudal axis, it is called the *axial* mesoderm. It has already been described as the dense cord of mesoderm that induces neuroectoderm commitment. Its only adult derivative is to be found in the center of the vertebrae (see Chap. 7).

• **Paraxial mesoderm forms into somites after passing through a somitomere stage.**   Paraxial mesoderm is formed next to (*para*) the axial mesoderm on each side of the body. It first partially condenses into an intermediate stage of organization called *somitomeres.* Sometime during this condensation, the cells become committed to their respective fates. During week 4, most somitomeres then compact further into a series of separate, segmented blocks called *somites.* Somites develop in a cranial-caudal sequence along the length of the body. Like everything else in the body, somites develop at the cranial end of the body first.

• **A specific number of somite pairs are formed bilaterally.**   A total of 42 to 44 pairs of somites are formed, although 6 to 8 pairs will degenerate without forming any derivatives (the most cranial pair, and most caudal 5 to 7 pairs). The timing of their formation can be used as a marker for staging embryonic development.

   The first 7 pairs of somitomeres (surrounding much of the developing brain) never go on to become organized as somites and are not numbered in the official somite count. Nevertheless, they cannot be ignored, since they make important contributions to the head. The reason for this annoying inconsistency is that the existence of the cranial somitomeres was not understood when somites were originally numbered. Somitomeres give rise to many of the same derivatives as somites, but without first forming recognizable subdivisions.

Each somite differentiates into three regions: *sclerotome, myotome,* and *dermatome.* Each region has a different fate.

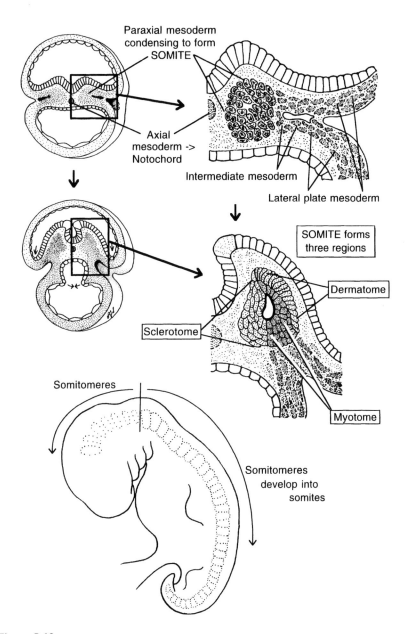

Figure 5-13
Development of somites from paraxial mesoderm (late week 3 to early week 4).

• SPECIFIC DERIVATIVES FORM FROM EACH SOMITE REGION

Somites (and somitomeres) are the specific portions of the mesoderm that give rise to all skeletal muscle, some specific bones of the body, and some connective tissue components of the skin. Each region of the somite forms specific tissues. Somites form sclerotome, dermatome, and myotome regions during weeks 4 and 5. These regions then begin to progressively separate from the somite and migrate to their final destinations where they differentiate (see Fig. 5-14).

• The somitic sclerotome forms the bones of the axial skeleton.
The sclerotome is the most medial region of the somite and the first to differentiate. Sclerotome cells from each side migrate medially to surround the neural tube and notochord. These cells form the bones of the axial skeleton: that is, the vertebrae and ribs in the body and some parts of the base of the skull in the head.

> *Putting it all together:* Cartilage and bones are formed by several mesoderm regions. The somitic sclerotome forms only the bones of the axial skeleton. All other cartilage and bones of the body and limbs, and many in the head, are formed by lateral plate mesoderm (as is covered in Chap. 7). In addition, some bones of the head originate from neural crest (as is covered in Chap. 10).

• The more lateral part of the somite forms the dermomyotome.
This then subdivides into the dermatome laterally and the myotome medially. Both regions become traveling cells.

• Myotomes form all skeletal muscles of the body, head, and limbs.
To do this, many of the myotome cells migrate far from their orgins into the limbs and throughout the head. (This is covered in detail in Chap. 8.)

• Dermatomes contribute to the dermis connective tissue of the skin.
The dermatome cells migrate underneath the ectoderm covering much of the body, head, and limbs to contribute to the dermis. These cells don't make it as far as the ventral body wall, so only the dorsal and lateral parts of the dermis are formed from somite derivatives.

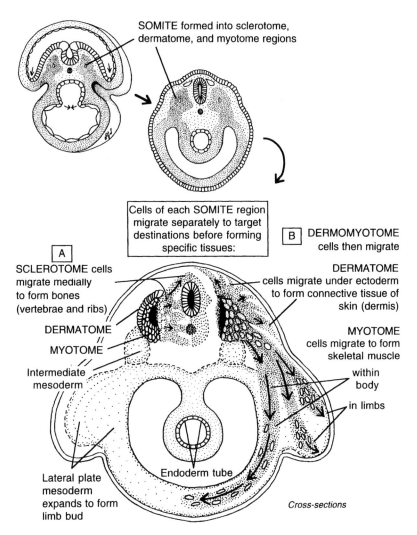

SOMITE formed into sclerotome, dermatome, and myotome regions

Cells of each SOMITE region migrate separately to target destinations before forming specific tissues:

B | DERMOMYOTOME cells then migrate

A | SCLEROTOME cells migrate medially to form bones (vertebrae and ribs)

DERMATOME

MYOTOME

Intermediate mesoderm

Lateral plate mesoderm expands to form limb bud

Endoderm tube

DERMATOME cells migrate under ectoderm to form connective tissue of skin (dermis)

MYOTOME cells migrate to form skeletal muscle

within body

in limbs

Cross-sections

Figure 5-14
Dermatome, myotome, and sclerotome derivatives.

Putting it all together: The connective tissue layers of the skin are formed from several mesoderm regions. The more dorsal parts of the dermis are formed by somitic dermatomes, while the remaining dermis and the deeper layer of the skin, the *hypodermis*, are formed by *lateral plate mesoderm*.

• INTERMEDIATE MESODERM DERIVATIVES

This germ layer is (cleverly) named for its intermediate position between paraxial and lateral plate mesoderm (see Fig. 5-15).

> Intermediate mesoderm forms all tissues of most organs in both the urinary and genital systems: this means connective tissues, smooth muscle, and epithelial linings. The endoderm provides the remaining epithelial linings of some organs. (Remember the cloacal enlargement of the endoderm described earlier in this chapter?)

These apparently simple origins in no way reflect a simple developmental story. (This story is covered in Chaps. 14 and 15.)

• LATERAL PLATE MESODERM DERIVATIVES

• Lateral plate mesoderm forms long somatic and splanchnic arms (see Fig. 5-15).   Lateral plate mesoderm is formed at the lateral extensions of the embryo. The lateral body folds change its configuration greatly, elongating it so that it comes to completely surround the endoderm tube laterally and ventrally. A cavity, or *coelom,* forms within it while the body is folding, splitting the lateral plate mesoderm into two plates, or arms, around this coelom: *somatic* and *splanchnic* (or *visceral*) *lateral plate mesoderm.* Somatic mesoderm lines the inside of the ectoderm, while splanchnic mesoderm covers the outside of the endoderm tube. (In the head, these arms—and the intervening coelom—do not form, so there is only lateral plate mesoderm to form derivatives.) *Somatic* refers to *body* or *soma,* while *splanchnic* or *visceral* refers to internal organs (or *viscera*). You should learn these terms, as they are important in both developmental and mature anatomy.

> Lateral plate mesoderm is the region of mesoderm that gives rise to most smooth muscle and connective tissues. This includes the majority of bones and cartilages. In addition, it forms some specific epithelia and all cardiac muscle.

• Each lateral plate mesoderm arm gives rise to a host of different derivatives related to its location.   Both arms form all the tissue components of blood vessels and connective tissues in their respective territories. In addition, the sur-

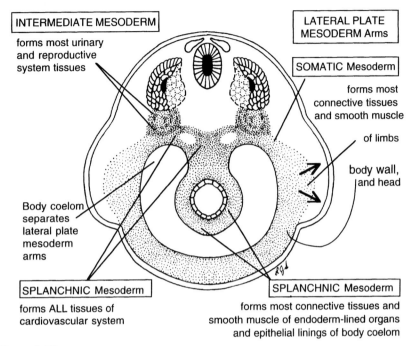

Figure 5-15
Derivatives of intermediate and lateral plate mesoderm begin to form during weeks 4–5.

face cells of both arms that face the body coelom form the epithelial linings of these cavities. Beyond this, it is helpful to distinguish which derivatives are formed by each lateral plate arm.

• **Somatic lateral plate mesoderm derivatives.** This arm gives rise to most connective tissue and smooth muscle components of the wall of the body. It is also the mesoderm region that forms the bulk of the tissues of the limbs, including the cartilage and bones of the limbs and limb "girdles" (bones that attach the limbs to the body).

• **Splanchnic mesoderm derivatives.** This arm forms the smooth muscle and connective tissue components of endoderm-lined organs. Near the cranial end of the body, splanchnic mesoderm gives rise to *all* the tissues of the cardiovascular system (cardiac muscle, connective tissues, and epithelial linings).

SUMMARY OF GERM LAYER DERIVATIVES

Table 5-1 should provide you with a handy reference as you proceed into the embryogenesis of specific organ systems.

TABLE 5-1
GERM LAYER DERIVATIVES

Ectoderm Derivatives	Epithelium of skin (superficial epidermis layer)	
	All nervous tissue: formed by neuroectoderm: Brain and spinal cord (neural tube) All peripheral nerve tissue (neural crest)	
Endoderm Derivatives	Epithelial linings of:	The gastrointestinal tract
		Organs that form as buds from the endoderm tube: Pharyngeal gland derivatives* Respiratory system Digestive organs (liver, pancreas) Terminal part of urogenital systems
	Hypoblast Endoderm: Gametes migrate to gonads	
Mesoderm Derivatives	All connective tissues**	General connective tissues
		Cartilage and bone
		Blood cells (red and white)
	All muscle types:	Cardiac, skeletal, smooth
	Epithelial linings of:	Body cavities
		Some organs: Cardiovascular system Reproductive and urinary systems (most parts)

*Pharyngeal derivatives: palatine tonsils, thymus, thyroid, parathyroids
**Some connective tissues in the head are derived from neural crest

· C H A P T E R · 6 ·

FORMATION OF EMBRYONIC REGIONS: TRUNK, LIMBS, AND HEAD

·

· · · · · · · · · · · ·

FORMATION OF THREE EMBRYONIC REGIONS

Body (or trunk), head, and limbs

The embryo develops three distinct regions as body folding progresses. Folding first creates distinct body (or trunk) and head regions, beginning in week 3. In week 5 limbs begin to bud from the body wall. The embryonic structure described in Chaps. 4 and 5 applies in its entirety only to the body proper, or trunk. The head and limbs have a somewhat different germ layer organization and composition. This chapter presents an overview of these differences. All of these points will come up again in relevant chapters on development of specific organ systems.

Development of the components of the body or trunk are covered throughout the remaining chapters on a system by system basis. This chapter briefly ties some of those developments together. It then introduces you to unique features of development of the head. These features are covered in more detail in Chap. 10. Most of the focus of attention in this chapter is on the development of the limbs, since there is no other chapter in which all the forces directing their development as a whole will be covered. The development of bones and muscles within the limbs are covered in more detail in Chaps. 7 and 8, respectively.

Embryonic features unique to the body or trunk

• **BODY COELOM**

• **The body proper is the only region of the embryo that contains a cavity or coelom (see Fig. 6-1).** The embryonic coelom is created within the lateral plate mesoderm. Thus, the lateral plate mesoderm is split into separate somatic and splanchnic arms only in the body proper. Initially the body cavity is continuous with an extraembryonic coelom that develops in the trophoblast support layers surrounding the embryo. Body folding rapidly causes the intraembryonic coelom to become a closed cavity as the arms of ectoderm, mesoderm, and endoderm all come together ventrally and fuse together everywhere except at the yolk stalk. This stalk then continues to narrow until the body cavity is completely sealed off from the outside. The body coelom and lateral plate mesoderm arms are important because they form the housing of the visceral organs in the body cavity.

• **LATERAL PLATE MESODERM SPLITS INTO TWO LAYERS**

• **The lateral plate mesoderm forms septa that divide the body coelom into several cavities.** The first septum to form is the *diaphragm*. It forms across the common coelom just cranial to the yolk sac stalk during month 2. The diaphragm divides the body cavity into thoracic and abdominal (or peritoneal) cavities. Both lateral plate mesoderm arms contribute to its formation. First, the ventral portion of the somatic lateral plate mesoderm proliferates to form the septum transversum, which grows toward the splanchnic mesoderm surrounding the endoderm tube to form the central part of the diaphragm. The more dorsal and lateral parts of the diaphragm are formed by more dorsal somatic lateral plate mesoderm (dubbed the pleuropericardial membrane), which also grows inward from the body wall to fuse with the splanchnic mesoderm.

The peritoneal cavity remains a single cavity which houses the bulk of the organs of the gastrointestinal, urinary, and reproductive systems. The thoracic cavity will be further subdivided into a pericardial cavity centrally and two pleural cavities laterally by other ingrowths of somatic lateral plate mesoderm. These cavities will contain the developing heart and lungs, respectively. (See also Fig. 6-2 and Chaps. 11 through 13.)

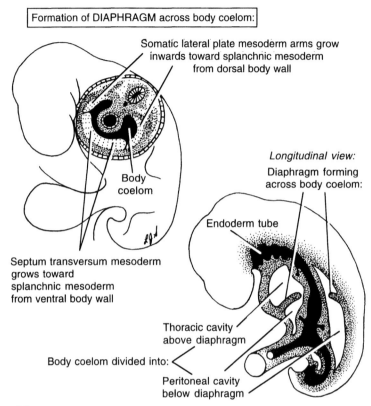

Formation of DIAPHRAGM across body coelom:

Somatic lateral plate mesoderm arms grow
inwards toward splanchnic mesoderm
from dorsal body wall

Body
coelom

Longitudinal view:
Diaphragm forming
across body coelom:

Endoderm tube

Septum transversum mesoderm
grows toward
splanchnic mesoderm
from ventral body wall

Thoracic cavity
above diaphragm

Body coelom divided into:

Peritoneal cavity
below diaphragm

Figure 6-1
Formation of the body coelom and initial steps in its division by the diaphragm (month 2).

• Lateral plate mesoderm forms serous membranes that line the body cavities. The entire body coelom becomes lined by an epithelium, referred to as a *serous* or *mesothelial membrane* (see Fig. 6-2). This lining also covers the outer surfaces of the internal organs where they face the coelom. The serous membranes are formed by the surface cells of the lateral plate mesoderm arms. In the peritoneal or abdominal cavity, the lining is called *peritoneum*. As the thoracic cavity is divided into pleural and pericardial cavities by lateral plate mesoderm, the surface of these cavities become lined by pleural and pericardial membranes.

• The internal organs are anchored within their cavities by derivatives of lateral plate mesoderm. Internal organs don't just hang out in free space within the body cavity. In the peritoneal cavity, many visceral organs become anchored to the body wall and to each other by membranous sheets called *mesenteries*. They are formed by the same splanchnic lateral plate mesoderm that surrounds the endoderm tube, and their surfaces are also covered by peritoneum. Mesenteries form during month 2 as the coelom expands and plasters the left and right splanchnic mesoderm arms together dorsal to the endoderm tube. These arms fuse to form a primitive dorsal mesentery along the length of the body cavity. (A ventral mesentery forms from splanchnic mesoderm that remains continuous across the ventral coelom, but it is limited to a short segment in the midgut region of the endoderm.) The final configuration of the mesenteries is covered in more detail in Chap. 12.

Mesenteries provide a framework for blood vessels, lymphatics, and nerves to enter and leave the organs in the peritoneal cavity.

• The internal organs are either in a retroperitoneal or intraperitoneal location. Peritoneal (or abdominal) organs that continue to hang out in the abdominal cavity suspended by mesenteries are referred to as intraperitoneal organs. Other organs that form or later become incorporated into the thick mesoderm of the dorsal body wall are then "behind" the peritoneal lining, or retroperitoneal. Understanding this difference is clinically relevant with regard to the surgical approaches to organs.

In the thoracic cavity, outgrowths of somatic lateral plate mesoderm form septa which divide this cavity into pericardial and pleural cavities. Here also, surface cells of the mesoderm arms form serous membranes lining the cavities. Extensions of these coverings are pushed ahead of the developing lungs and heart as they expand into their respective cavities to anchor the organs to the dorsal body wall.

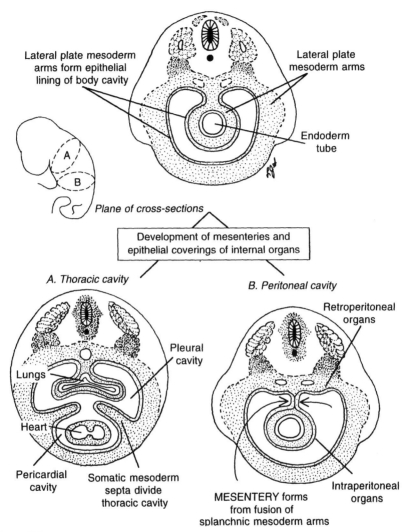

Figure 6-2
Further division of the coelom and formation of mesenteries during month 2.

Embryonic features unique to the head

As described in Chap. 5, an identifiable head region begins to form when the cranial end of the embryo begins to fold or curl toward the ventral surface of the body at the end of week 3 (see Fig. 6-3). The lateral folds in the cranial region curl the thick mesoderm layer around the cranial ends of both the endoderm tube and the more dorsal neural tube.

> The head mesoderm is a solid mass that never contains a coelom. Head mesoderm does not form several of the subdivisions formed in the body: there is no intermediate mesoderm and no subdivision of lateral plate mesoderm into splanchnic and somatic mesoderm layers.

• **Axial, paraxial, and lateral plate mesoderm form many (but not all) of the same derivatives that they form in the body.**   Axial mesoderm, or the notochord extends into the head, as would be expected if its presence is required to induce neuroectoderm to form. Paraxial mesoderm is also formed in the head, except for the most cranial end. However, it organizes only as far as the somitomere stage here. It nevertheless gives rise to the same types of derivatives in the head as in the rest of the body. The remaining mesoderm in the head does not become organized into distinct regions, but its fate makes it most directly comparable to lateral plate mesoderm.

• **There are differences in neuroectoderm derivatives formed in the head.**
The neural tube in the head expands both longitudinally and laterally, forming the future brain region of the central nervous system. This expansion also contributes to the formation of the head fold. By contrast, in the rest of the body, the neural tube remains a modest-sized tube with a small lumen as it differentiates into the spinal cord. The neural crest formed in the head migrates into many regions of the head and neck, where some of it differentiates into "typical" neural crest derivatives, such as ganglia of the peripheral nervous system.

> The neural crest in the head gives rise to atypical derivatives: connective tissue components, including many cartilages and bones.

• **Development of the head involves formation of a unique set of structures, the pharyngeal arches.**   The ventral part of the forming head expands into a series of five pairs of arches which bulge from the surface bilaterally. The arches form around the endoderm tube by rapid proliferation of the local mesoderm from

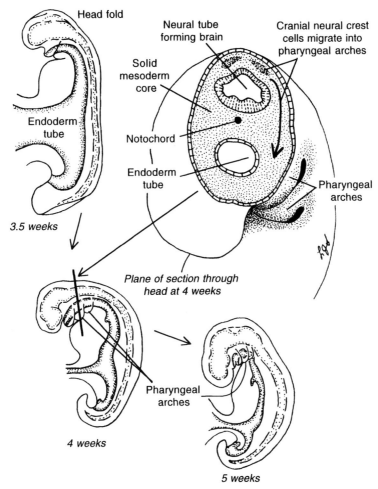

Figure 6-3
Formation of the head fold, organization of its germ layer components, and initial formation of pharyngeal arches.

the end of week 3 into week 5, supplemented by invading neural crest cells. This tissue is then partially separated into "arches" by growth of the endoderm and ectoderm toward each other.

• **The head can be subdivided into two regions, each defined by their bony elements: the neurocranium and viscerocranium (see Fig. 6-4).**   Each region consists of a "centerpiece" structure surrounded by bone and skeletal muscle, which join the regions together. Development of the structures of the head is covered in detail in Chaps. 9 and 10, but at this point you should understand a few basic points about developments in the head which alter the configuration of the embryo as a whole at the same time that other organ systems are beginning to form.

The centerpiece of the neurocranial region is the forming brain.

The brain becomes surrounded by the bones of the cranium. Outside that, a thin layer of skeletal muscle and connective tissue form. These derivatives come from typical mesoderm regions, as well as some unusual sources: neural crest cells form some of the connective tissues, including some bones.

The centerpiece of the viscerocranial region is the cranial (or pharyngeal) end of the endoderm tube. The visceral components of the head form around this tube.

These internal components include the structures of the mouth, nasal cavities, and pharynx. Externally, the structures of the face tie these two regions together.

• **Pharyngeal arches supply tissues to both regions of the head.**   The arch mesoderm forms the muscle and connective tissue components of the future mouth, nose, and pharynx, while the endoderm forms the epithelial lining of these structures. Internally, the cranial (or pharyngeal) end of the endoderm tube fuses with the surface ectoderm at the site of the future mouth opening (*stomodeum*) between the left and right portions of arch I. Both mesodermal and neural crest cells of the arches also undergo extensive migration over both the region of the future face and the region of the forming neurocranium, before forming muscle or connective tissue derivatives. Thus, the arches form structures in both regions of the head, tying them together in the process.

• **Formation of the face comes from both regions of the head.**   The structures that are referred to collectively as the face extend from chin to cheeks to forehead, including many internal and external components of the mouth, nose, eyes, and

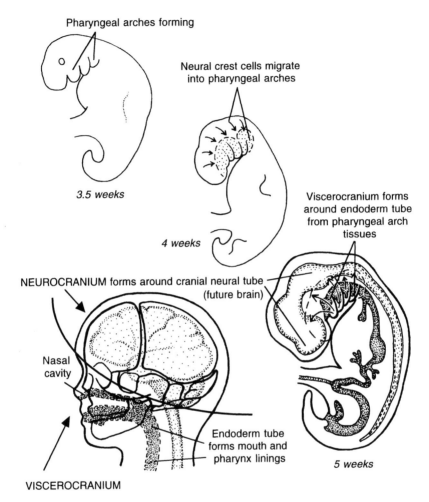

Figure 6-4
Formation of neurocranial and viscerocranial regions of the head.

ears. These structures (bone, skeletal muscle, and connective tissue framework) are formed by the first two pharyngeal arches on each side of the mouth in combination with a portion of the nonarch tissues of the frontal neurocranial portion of the head. The other arches form tissues of the neck and corresponding internal regions of the pharynx.

Embryonic features unique to the limbs

Limbs are the final body region to form (see Fig. 6-5). The limbs begin to form at the very end of week 4 after the basic plan of the body and head are established. All their basic components are in place by week 8, or the end of the embryonic period.

• **Limbs form by "budding" out from the ventrolateral body surface.** The first detectable event in limb development is the proliferation of specific regions of somatic lateral plate mesoderm. This "limb" mesoderm becomes mesenchymal and pushes out the covering ectoderm, forming limb buds. Arms (or forelimbs) are formed cranially, and legs (or hindlimbs) caudally.

Limbs are formed by ectoderm covering a solid mesoderm core, with no endoderm contributions. There is no coelom.

---

1. Somatic lateral plate mesoderm will form all cartilage and bone in the limbs, as well as all general connective tissues.
2. Surface ectoderm forms the epidermis of the skin and its specializations (hairs and nails).
3. Skeletal muscle is an "outsider," migrating in from the somites.
4. Nerves and blood vessels grow in from the body using connective tissue as a guide.

The specifics of formation of skeletal muscle and bone components are covered in Chaps. 7 and 8 on musculoskeletal system development.

• **Limb formation requires mutual induction between limb mesoderm and surface ectoderm.** First, the limb mesoderm induces the overlying surface ectoderm to form the aptly named *apical ectodermal ridge (AER)* during week 5. The AER is a thickened ridge of ectoderm at the apical tip of the forming limb. The AER in turn induces the mesoderm just under it to continue to proliferate, and to then commit to specific derivatives. These derivatives are left behind as the limb tip grows forward. The derivatives include bone models and clusters of general connective tissue precursors. These clusters may direct organization of skeletal muscle masses from muscle cell precursors that migrate separately from the somites. Limb mesoderm also induces the formation of limb-specific ectoderm specializations such as nails. Mesoderm and the AER *require* each other's signals: take either one away, and the other ceases to proliferate or commit to any fate.

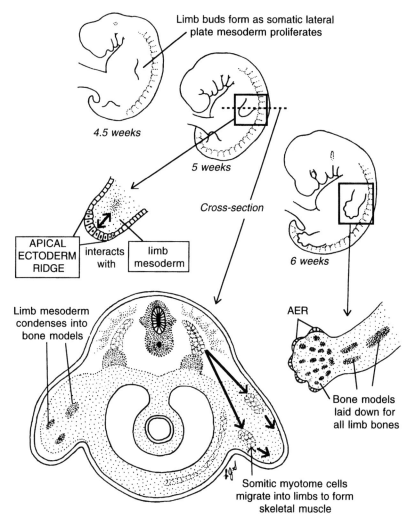

Figure 6-5
Germ layer contributions to development of the limbs.

• **Development of the limbs (and all other parts of the body) requires inducing specific patterns of polarity or axes.**   All parts of the body require directional information as they form, so that they "know" which end is up. With regard to limb development, patterning of structures must be directed along three axes: *proximal-distal, cranial-caudal,* and *dorsal-ventral* (see Fig. 6-6). Limb axes are named for their relationship to the body proper. (To understand the axes, extend your arms straight out sideways from your body, with your palms facing forward. Use this position for the following axis descriptions.)

• **Proximal-distal limb polarity is directed by the AER.**   The proximal-distal axis (or long axis) runs from the junction of the limb with the body *proximally* to the *distal* tips of the digits (fingers and toes). The AER directs the formation of structures with proper polarity along this axis. It does this by inducing the underlying mesoderm to deposit cells committed to form specific limb bones in a proximal-to-distal sequence. For example, the first deposit is programmed to form the most proximal bone of the limb (humerus in the arm), while the last deposits form the bones of the fingers (phalanges). Interruption of the AER signals can result in failure to lay down bone models for specific limb segments, which in turn results in missing limb segments.

• **The dorsal-ventral axis of the limbs is established early, as this axis is established for the whole body.**   The dorsal-ventral axis runs across the thickness of the limbs. The dorsal side is continuous with the dorsal (or "back") surface of the body, and the ventral side with the ventral (or "belly") surface of the body. Any factors involved in establishing the polarity of structures across this axis are not known currently.

• **Cranial-caudal limb polarity is established by a gradient of inducing signals released from cells of the "zone of polarizing activity" (ZPA).**   The cranial-caudal axis runs across the thickness of the limb from its cranial junction with the body to its more caudal junction. The specific *shape* of limb bones is directed by inducing signals that diffuse across this axis. Mesoderm cells along the caudal side of the limb (the ZPA cells) produce an inducing signal which diffuses across this axis, setting up a gradient. Those bone precursors closest to the ZPA are exposed to the highest concentration of inducer. Differences produced in bone shapes in the five digits are easiest to understand. The most caudal (or "pinky") finger bones form in response to exposure to a maximum of inducer, while those bone precursor cells exposed to the lowest concentration of this inducer form the most cranial digit, or thumb bones.

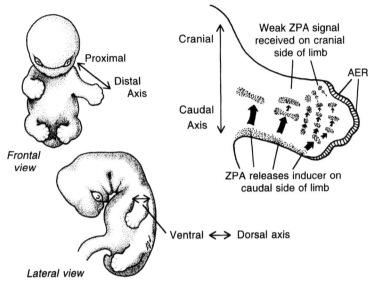

Figure 6-6
Development of axes of embryonic limbs.

• **For the cranial-caudal axis, the actual inducing signal and its method of action are beginning to be understood.** *Retinoic acid* may be the ZPA inducer, or an intermediary in that pathway. The inducer activates different complexes of homeobox genes along its concentration gradient. The homeobox genes then activate other genes which direct development. Retinoic acid directs axis polarity in the central nervous system and vertebral column bone development, where it acts by turning on complexes of homeobox genes.

A role for retinoic acid in development is clinically relevant, since excess retinoids introduced, for example, in acne medicines can cause abnormal development by activating the wrong complexes of homeobox genes, which in turn cause the "wrong" structures to form.

• **Limb buds appear at the end of week 4 and the beginning of week 5 and become externally constricted into regions by week 8.**   By week 6, the hand and footplates form at the tips of the limb buds, defined by circumferential constriction of the ectoderm covering (see Fig. 6-7). Finger and toe rays then form during weeks 7 and 8 by longitudinal constriction of the ectoderm. The rays are completely separated into digits by week 8. Also by week 8, a second, more proximal constriction forms, marking externally the division between the two more proximal segments of the limb.

These constrictions are directed by the AER. Finger and toe rays are formed when short stretches of the AER undergo programmed cell death (a common phenomenon in embryonic development). The absence of bits of AER results in regression of the underlying mesoderm, creating constrictions that define finger and toe rays. The active AER, meanwhile, continues to direct the formation of digit cartilage precursors from mesoderm underneath it.

• **Final feature of limb development: limbs rotate about their long axis in opposite directions.**   The limbs rotate about their long axes with the body during weeks 6 to 8. The arms rotate 90° dorsolaterally about their long axes, causing the elbows to point dorsally. The thumbs continue to point cranially and laterally. The legs rotate 90° ventromedially about their long axes, with more dramatic results. The knees now point ventrally, and the big toe now points medially.

Rotation of the limbs results in:

1. The final orientation of the joints.
2. The final location and orientation of muscle groups. (This occurs because muscles form their connections to the limb bones prior to rotation and are stretched and twisted along with the rotation of bones.)
3. The mature patterns of sensory innervation of the skin, called *dermatome patterns*. (This occurs because nerve fibers also connect with the connective tissue or dermis layer of skin prior to rotation and are pulled along with the rotating dermis.)

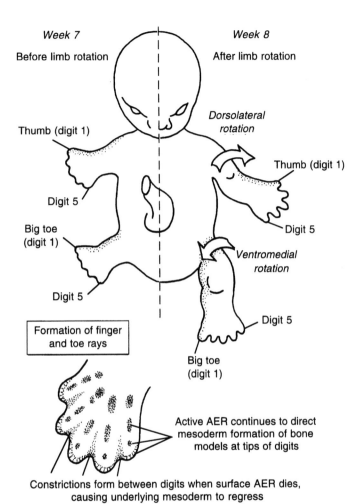

Week 7
Before limb rotation

Week 8
After limb rotation

Dorsolateral rotation

Thumb (digit 1)

Thumb (digit 1)

Digit 5

Digit 5

Big toe
(digit 1)

Ventromedial rotation

Digit 5

Digit 5

Formation of finger
and toe rays

Big toe
(digit 1)

Active AER continues to direct
mesoderm formation of bone
models at tips of digits

Constrictions form between digits when surface AER dies,
causing underlying mesoderm to regress

Figure 6-7
Formation of limb regions and limb rotation.

EXTERNALLY VISIBLE CHANGES IN BODY FORM

• **Externally visible features distinguish embryos from the first three weeks of development.**   The *morula*, *blastula*, and *gastrula* stage embryos can all be distinguished from each other by the shape of the embryo, and by the presence of externally visible bulges such as the primitive streak and neural plate. More dramatic changes occur in body form from weeks 4 to 8, as the body folds and the head and limbs form (see Fig. 6-8).

• **Forming somites are externally visible.**   Since somites are formed from the mesoderm close to the surface on each side of the body, they cause visible bulges in the surface ectoderm to either side of the dorsal midline. Their visibility makes them valuable for staging embryos from the earliest period of body folding. Somites form in a cranial-to-caudal sequence at the approximate rate of three pairs a day. Their number reveals the stage of development from the end of week 3 through week 5, when the maximum of 42 to 44 pairs is reached. During week 4, the number of pairs of somites constitutes the main externally visible feature of the body.

• **Body folding curves the embryo into a C-shape beginning in week 5.** Body folding results in the first clinically detectable measure of age, termed the *crown-rump (C-R)* length. This measures the maximum length of the embryo in its curved shape, extending from the apex of the forming head (top of the skull) to the apex of the forming caudal region (otherwise known as the butt!). This measure works into the early fetal period (third month) and can be detected by noninvasive techniques such as ultrasound.

• **Pharyngeal arches form on the ventral surface of the forming head during weeks 4 and 5, and their reconfiguration is largely responsible for creating the mature form of the face.**   Throughout the second month, the shape and size of the head changes greatly. The internal and external structures of the face, including the ears, nose, and eyes, form between weeks 5 and 8. The expanding brain enlarges the neurocranial region of the head. During the fetal period, these features assume their mature shapes.

• **Limb buds appear at the end of week 4 and the beginning of week 5 and become externally constricted into regions by week 8.**

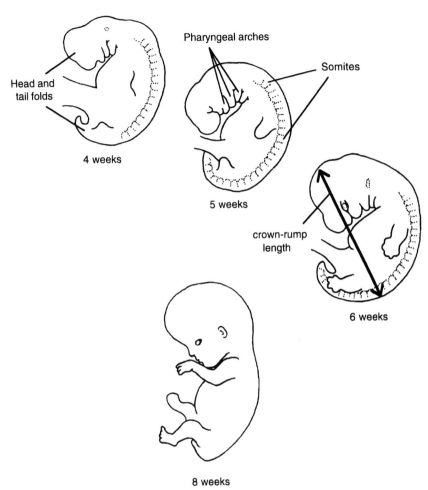

Figure 6-8
Changes in external body form during the embryonic period (through week 8).

· C H A P T E R · 7 ·

SKELETAL SYSTEM

·

·   ·   ·   ·   ·   ·   ·   ·   ·   ·   ·   ·

The skeletal system provides a framework that supports the body, protects internal organs, and coordinates movement via connections with skeletal muscle. The skeleton consists of rigid bones and more pliable cartilage. Bones form the majority of the skeleton. Cartilages can occur both as independent structures (such as the thyroid cartilage and tracheal cartilage rings) or as pliable connectors of bones (such as the ribs to sternum). While most cartilage and bone are derived from *mesoderm*, the story of their development is not a simple one because different subdivisions of the mesoderm germ layer give rise to the cartilages and bones of the different regions of the body: the trunk, the limbs, and the head. Embryonic development of the skeleton is thus best studied by focusing on each of these regions in turn. Since many bones develop from preexisting cartilage models, a brief description of the histogenesis of cartilage and bone is included so that the importance of proper formation of these early cartilage models can be fully appreciated.

GERM LAYER ORIGINS OF SKELETAL TISSUE

• **Mesoderm forms all connective tissues of the body and limbs.** This includes all cartilage and bones (see Fig. 7-1). Several mesoderm regions are involved in forming skeletal tissues. As was described in Chap. 4, the mesoderm layer condenses into three distinct regions: *paraxial, intermediate,* and *lateral plate mesoderm.* Specific subdivisons of paraxial and lateral plate mesoderm form skeletal structures. Paraxial mesoderm condenses to form somites, which further divide into sclerotomes, myotomes, and dermatomes.

> The sclerotome regions of the somites form all cartilages and bones of the *axial skeleton* in the body and many in the head.

The axial skeleton runs along the midline longitudinal axis of the body. In the body, it consists of the vertebrae and ribs. In the head, it consists of the skull.

> Somatic lateral plate mesoderm forms all cartilages and bones of the limbs, or the *appendicular skeleton.*

The appendicular skeleton includes the limb bones and the limb "girdles," which connect the limbs to the body. Be alert to the difference between somitic mesoderm and somatic mesoderm. *Somitic* refers to somites. *Somatic* refers to *soma,* or body. Here, it refers to the layer of lateral plate mesoderm that forms the body wall, or soma.

> Mesoderm and neural crest both give rise to connective tissues in the head, including the cartilages and bones of the skull.

The skull is quite complex. It can be divided into bones that surround the brain, the *neurocranium,* and those that surround the pharyngeal end of the endoderm tube, the *viscerocranium.* Both somitic sclerotomes and somitomere derivatives give rise to some bones of the skull. (The most cranial somitomeres never form somites, but give rise directly to many of the same derivatives as somites.) Lateral plate mesoderm gives rise to other skull bones. (Remember that there is no coelom in the head, and thus no division into lateral plate layers.) Finally, the neural crest gives rise to a number of bones in the head as well.

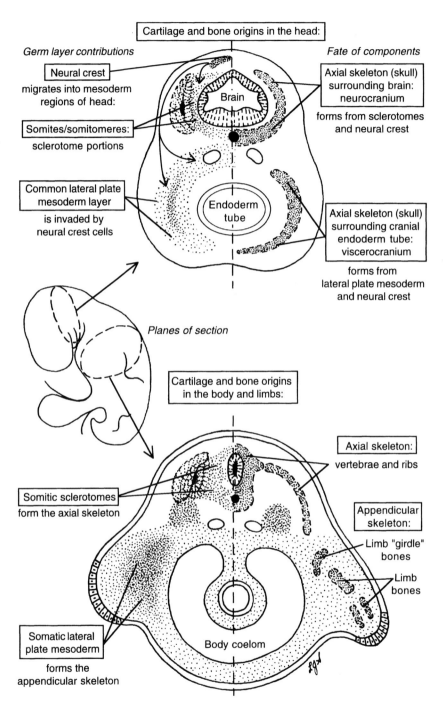

Cartilage and bone origins in the head:

Germer layer contributions

Neural crest

migrates into mesoderm regions of head:

Somites/somitomeres:

sclerotome portions

Common lateral plate mesoderm layer

is invaded by neural crest cells

Brain

Endoderm tube

Fate of components

Axial skeleton (skull) surrounding brain: neurocranium

forms from sclerotomes and neural crest

Axial skeleton (skull) surrounding cranial endoderm tube: viscerocranium

forms from lateral plate mesoderm and neural crest

Planes of section

Cartilage and bone origins in the body and limbs:

Axial skeleton:

vertebrae and ribs

Somitic sclerotomes

form the axial skeleton

Appendicular skeleton:

Limb "girdle" bones

Limb bones

Somatic lateral plate mesoderm

forms the appendicular skeleton

Body coelom

Figure 7-1
Germ layer origins of cartilage and bone.

HISTOGENESIS OF CARTILAGE AND BONE

• **A primer of the histogenesis of cartilage and bone.**   Cartilage and bone are specific forms of connective tissue in which cells are widely separated by an extensive *extracellular matrix*, which they secrete. The firm consistency of the extracellular matrix allows the tissues to bear mechanical stress and absorb shock without distortion. The major difference between the matrix of cartilage and that of the bone is that bone matrix becomes hardened (or mineralized) by deposits of calcium. The skeletal framework created by bone and cartilage provides protection for visceral organs internally and support for skeletal muscle externally. Cartilage forms the support tissue in many places where a more flexible and resilient support is desired, such as the joints between long bones, and the cartilage rings around the trachea. Most histology texts cover the histogenesis of both cartilage and bone in detail as part of their description of those tissues. This book concentrates on features which are relevant to embryonic development.

Keep in mind that the terms *bone* and *cartilage* refer not only to the tissues of those names, but also to the individual organs of the same name. Thus, for example, the humerus bone in the arm is one organ of the skeletal system. It is composed of bone tissue covered by general connective tissues.

Cartilage formation (chondrogenesis)

Cartilage forms when committed progenitor (stem) cells called *chondroblasts* condense, proliferate, and begin to differentiate into *chondrocytes* (see Fig. 7-2). The earliest cartilage begins to form in embryonic week 5. As part of the initial differentiation, cartilage cells deposit a gelatinous matrix around themselves, which separates chondrocytes from each other, and blood vessels regress in the target region. Cartilage forms as an avascular tissue (that is, without interior blood vessels), since nutrients and oxygen can diffuse through its matrix to interior cells. However, this same avascularity limits the maximum size of cartilages.

    As development proceeds, chondrocytes divide, creating nests (called *isogenous groups*) surrounded by a matrix. Cartilage continues to grow by adding cells from its external surface (called the *perichondrium*), where stem cells reside throughout life.

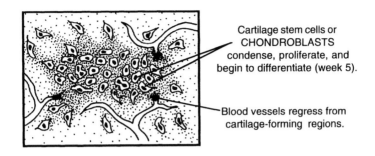

Cartilage stem cells or CHONDROBLASTS condense, proliferate, and begin to differentiate (week 5).

Blood vessels regress from cartilage-forming regions.

CHONDROBLASTS in center transform into CHONDROCYTES as they begin to secrete cartilage MATRIX.

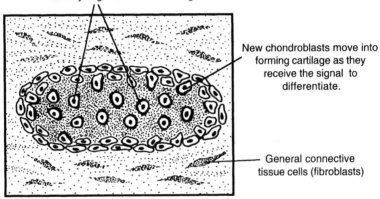

New chondroblasts move into forming cartilage as they receive the signal to differentiate.

General connective tissue cells (fibroblasts)

Chondrocytes multiply, creating isogenous groups of cells widely separated by cartilage matrix.

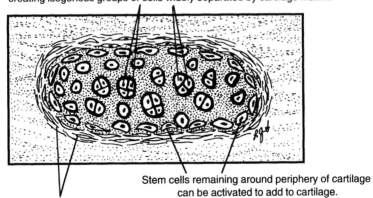

Stem cells remaining around periphery of cartilage can be activated to add to cartilage.

Outer connective tissue covering called perichondrium forms around cartilage.

Figure 7-2
Steps in formation of cartilage.

Bone formation (ossification)

All bone formation begins with condensation of progenitor osteoblasts (see Fig. 7-3). As they begin to differentiate into *osteocytes*, they secrete a calcified extracellular matrix. Formation of bone tissue, unlike cartilage, is accompanied by extensive vascularization, since this matrix prevents diffusion of nutrients and oxygen. Vascularization permits bone tissue to form larger structures than cartilage. Fetal bone formation places a large demand on the maternal circulation for calcium from the time bone tissue begins to form in month 3. Calcium will be withdrawn from maternal bones and teeth if insufficient quantities are ingested.

The rigid mineralized matrix forms spicules of bone, which form a network of *spongy bone*. This may later be remodelled into denser *compact bone*, containing parallel layers of matrix. Compact bone forms the shafts (diaphyses) of long bones. Spongy bone persists in most smaller and flat bones and at the ends (epiphyses) of long bones. At the center of many bones is a bone marrow cavity, in which many cells of the hematopoietic system develop (covered in Chap. 17).

Bone is formed by two methods: endochondral ossification and intramembranous ossification.

The histogenesis of bone is complicated. What you need to concern yourself with to understand embryonic development is simply that there are two types of bone formation and the key differences between them.

• **Most bones form by endochondral ossification of cartilage models.**   Cartilage formation is the first step in endochondral ossification: ossification inside (*endo*) cartilage (*chondral*). This is why description of most embryonic bone formation begins with a description of the formation of cartilage models, which are then transformed into bone. Ossification of cartilage models begins at the start of the fetal period (month 3). Cartilage cells die, leaving spaces into which osteoblasts and blood vessels penetrate. Osteoblasts begin to differentiate and form bone matrix. The initial random arrangement of matrix is soon remodelled into more parallel arrays. Bone marrow cavities form as spaces coalesce. At birth, the shafts of long bones are all ossified, but some smaller bones don't begin to ossify until early childhood. Ossification is completed in the early 20s. Bone growth and repair continue throughout life, using stem cells that persist in bone, as they do in cartilage.

• **Intramembranous ossification forms a small number of important bones, which are mostly superficial flat bones in the head.**   Bones are formed directly within (*intra*) mesenchymal condensations of osteoprogenitor cells. These cells initially form membranous sheets which secrete bone matrix directly.

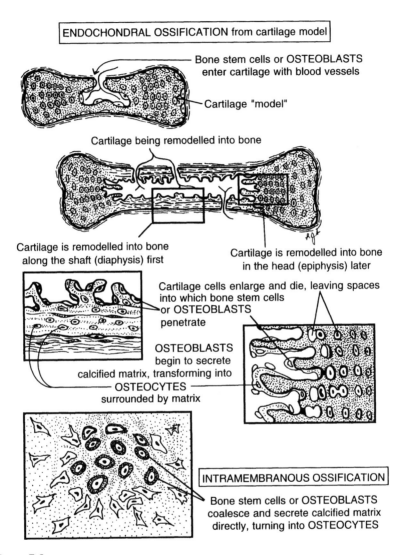

Figure 7-3
Methods of formation of bone.

ANATOMIC REGIONS OF THE MATURE SKELETON

It is useful to divide the study of the development of the skeleton into its separate anatomic regions, since each of these regions has somewhat different origins (see Fig. 7-4).

• **The axial skeleton consists of the bones of the long axis of the body and head.**

1. The vertebrae and ribs in the body.
2. The skull in the head.

• **The appendicular skeleton consists of the bones of the appendages.**

1. The intrinsic bones of the limbs:
   a. Bones contained entirely within the limbs.
2. The bones of the appendicular girdles connect the limbs to the body:
   a. The shoulder girdle connects the arms to the body.
   b. The pelvic girdle connects the legs to the body.

Rather than clutter up this chapter with all the names of individual bones, they are described in groups wherever possible. These groupings will allow you to learn the overall picture. The specific bones in each category should be easily found in any anatomy textbook. Only the major bones in each group are named, except in cases where origins can be a source of confusion. More bones in the head are identified by name for this reason. If it is not important for your purposes to learn the anatomy of the mature skeletal system, you should stick with the major groupings of bones provided earlier to learn the origins of each part of the skeleton. The development of the axial skeleton of the body is covered first, then that of the appendages. Development of the axial skeleton of the head is covered last, since that is the most complex portion of the skeleton.

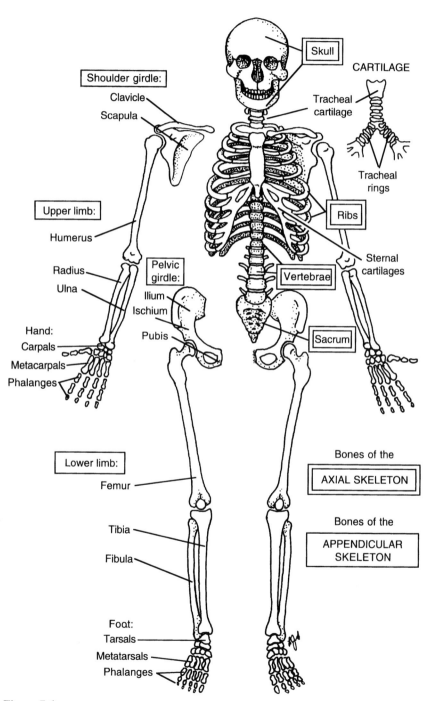

Figure 7-4
Regions of the skeleton.

FORMATION OF REGIONS OF THE SKELETON

Axial skeleton of the body: the vertebrae and ribs

• **Vertebrae and ribs are formed by endochondral ossification of the sclero-tome regions of somites (see Fig. 7-5).** Vertebrae are formed by sclerotome cells from somites on each side of the body. They form cartilage models first, which are transformed into bone by endochondral ossification. Beginning in week 4, the sclerotome cells surround the developing neural tube (future spinal cord) and notochord. The ventral portion of each vertebra, called the *body*, or *centrum*, forms around the notochord. The dorsal portion of each vertebra forms costal processes laterally and the vertebral arch dorsally. In the 12 thoracic level vertebrae, these processes articulate with ribs. Intervertebral disks are formed between vertebrae by condensations of other sclerotome cells. The notochord remains at the center of each fibrous disk as the *nucleus pulposus*, while it degenerates within the bodies of the vertebrae.

• **All somites contribute to the formation of the axial skeleton of the body and head.** The 42 to 44 pairs of somites develop in a cranial-caudal sequence: 4 occipital (1 degenerates), 8 cervical, 12 thoracic, 5 lumbar, 5 sacral, 8 to 10 coccygeal (last 5–7 degenerate). The sclerotomes from somites at each end fuse to form larger bones. Caudally, the *sacrum* is formed by fusion of all the sacral somitic sclerotomes, and the *coccyx* is formed by fusion of all the coccygeal somitic sclerotomes. Cranially, the sclerotomes of the first cervical somite and the occipital somites cranial to them fuse to form the base of the skull. This is described in more detail later in this chapter.

   The segmented nature of somites is retained only in their vertebral derivatives. Vertebrae are formed from 7 cervical, 12 thoracic, and 5 lumbar vertebrae during the first half of month 2. Each vertebra is formed by sclerotome cells from *two* somite levels: the caudal and cranial halves of sequential sclerotomes fuse with each other. Thus, for example, the first vertebra, designated cervical vertebra 1 or C1, is formed by the caudal half of sclerotome C1 plus the cranial half of sclerotome C2 from each side of the body. Each vertebra has a unique morphology.

• **Ribs develop as outgrowths of the lateral (costal) processes of thoracic level vertebrae.** Twelve pairs of ribs form normally. They develop during month 2 after the basic form of the vertebrae have been established. They grow around the curvature of the body wall toward the ventral body surface within the somatic lateral plate mesoderm layer. Here the first seven pairs of ribs are united ventrally by the *sternum*, which is also formed from migrating sclerotome cells. The ribs are joined to the sternum by costal cartilages.

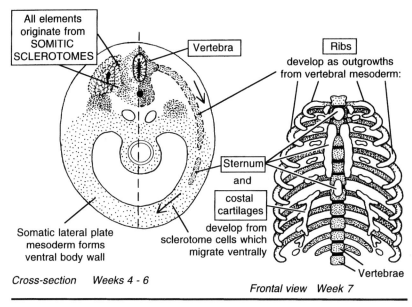

All elements originate from SOMITIC SCLEROTOMES

Vertebra

Ribs
develop as outgrowths from vertebral mesoderm:

Sternum
and
costal cartilages
develop from sclerotome cells which migrate ventrally

Somatic lateral plate mesoderm forms ventral body wall

Vertebrae

Cross-section   Weeks 4 - 6

Frontal view   Week 7

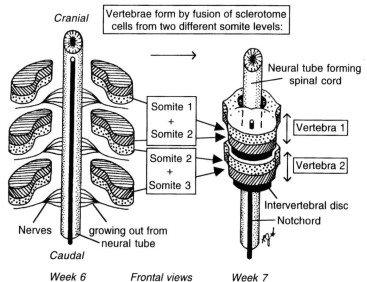

Cranial

Vertebrae form by fusion of sclerotome cells from two different somite levels:

Neural tube forming spinal cord

Somite 1
+
Somite 2

Vertebra 1

Somite 2
+
Somite 3

Vertebra 2

Intervertebral disc
Notchord

Nerves   growing out from neural tube

Caudal

Week 6   Frontal views   Week 7

Figure 7-5
Formation of bones and cartilages of the axial skeleton.

• CONGENITAL DEFECTS OF VERTEBRAE AND RIBS
• Congenital defects of the axial skeleton are often the result of faulty induction along one or more axes of the skeleton. Abnormalities are produced by both genetic abnormalities and teratogenic factors. These can include metabolic disturbances such as excess insulin or high glucose levels encountered in maternal diabetes, or excess retinoic acid (RA) taken in multivitamins or antiacne medicines. The mechanism of action of RA is rapidly being elucidated.

As first described in Chap. 6, all regions of the embryo are exposed to positional cues that direct formation of appropriate structures along three-dimensional axes. Induction of the axial skeleton along its cranial-caudal axis defines the number and unique morphology of vertebrae at each level, as well as the base of the skull and the tailbones at each end. Appropriate structures are induced to form along this axis by exposure to a cranial-caudal gradient of RA, which activates different combinations of *homeobox* (Hox) genes at each sclerotome level. This effect closely parallels the induction of bones along the cranial-caudal axis of the limb, as detailed in Chap. 6. However, the evidence for direct involvement of RA is stronger in the axial skeleton. Excess levels of RA shift the type of vertebrae formed to an inappropriately more caudal type by causing cranial-caudal shifts in the level of homeotic gene expression. One example of this shift is *Brevicollis*, or *Klippel-Feil syndrome*, which includes a severely shortened neck caused by a reduced number of cervical vertebrae.

Inducing signals released across the transverse axes (dorsal-ventral and medial-lateral) direct the formation of specific regions of the vertebrae (centrum, arch, and costal processes). These as yet unidentified signals come from the notochord, neural tube, and ganglia derived from neural crest just lateral to the vertebrae. A spectrum of serious congenital defects can occur in development of the transverse axes of vertebrae (see Fig. 7-6). This spectrum of defects is termed *spina bifida* (split spine). Incomplete development of the dorsal arches causes failure of the left and right halves of the arches to fuse. The primary cause of this defect can be failure of normal vertebral induction. Alternatively, vertebral defects can be a secondary consequence of failure of the neural tube to close dorsally. In either case, the opening in the vertebral arch can allow the spinal cord and/or its connective tissue coverings (meninges) to herniate between these defects. Failure is most common at either end of the vertebral column. Caudal lumbar vertebral defects are usually small, confined to a single vertebra, and don't involve the spinal cord or meninges. Cranially, defective formation of the somite-derived base of the skull is more severe, since it is usually secondary to failure of the cranial neural tube to close, which means the brain fails to develop (*anencephaly*). (See Chap. 9.)

Scoliosis, or curvature of the spine, is another transverse axis defect in which the vertebral column bends laterally. It can be a congenital defect caused by defective formation of one side of the vertebral centrum. In severe cases, only half a vertebra forms (*hemivertebra*).

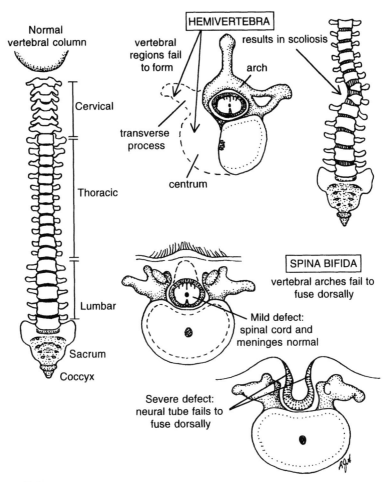

Figure 7-6
Congenital defects in the formation of the axial skeleton of the body.

The appendicular skeleton

• **Somatic lateral plate mesoderm forms the skeleton of the appendages—the limb bones and appendicular girdles (see Fig. 7-7).** The limb bones are intrinsic to the limb: that is, they are entirely contained within it. The appendicular girdles are the bones tying the limbs to the body. The shoulder girdles consist of the *scapula* and *clavicle*, which tie the arms to the body, while the pelvic girdles consist of the *coxa* or hip bone, which is composed of three parts: the *ilium*, *ischium*, and *pubis*. They tie the legs to the body.

> It is important to realize that these connecting "girdle" bones originate with the other limb bones and then reposition to the trunk.

As you will see in Chap. 8, "big ticket" muscles of the body are the ones that connect the limbs to the body via attachment to these bones.

Both limbs contain a single long bone in their proximal segment (*humerus* in the arm, *femur* in the thigh), and two in the distal segment (*radius* and *ulna* in the forearm, *tibia* and *fibula* in the leg). The arm continues into a wrist made of eight carpals, a hand made of five *metacarpals*, and digits with three *phalanges* in the fingers and two in the toes. The leg continues into an ankle made of seven *tarsals*, a foot made of five *metatarsals*, and digits with three *phalanges* in all toes except two in the big toe.

• **The appendicular skeleton is formed by endochondral ossification of cartilage models.** The only exception is the clavicle, which forms by intramembranous ossification. All other bones begin to form by condensation of cartilage mesenchyme in week 5. Cartilage models begin to form in week 6, and by week 8, all cartilage models are completed. Ossification begins in the third month in many bones, but others do not begin to ossify until well after birth.

• **Factors involved in induction of limb bones are partly known.** The limb, like the body, has three axes. Factors directing deposits of proper patterns of cartilage models for limb bones have been partly identified for two of the three axes. Formation of bones along the long axis (proximal-distal axis) is directed by signals from the apical ectodermal ridge (or AER) at the tip of the limb bud. These signals induce the underlying mesoderm to deposit cells programmed to form specific limb bones in a specific sequence. Proper bone morphology is determined by signals from the zone of polarizing activity (ZPA) along the caudal border of the limb. These signals diffuse across the thickness of the limb, exposing bone models to graded levels of this inducer (highest caudally, lowest cranially).

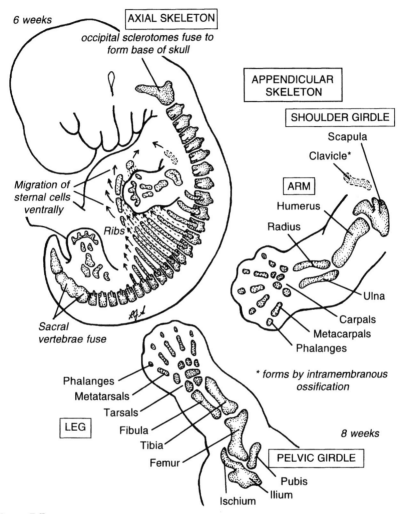

Figure 7-7
Formation of bones of the limbs and appendicular girdles.

Whether or not this inducer is RA, as in the vertebral column, it activates different complexes of homeobox genes in a caudal-cranial pattern across the limb, just as occurs in vertebral formation. (See Chap. 6 for details.)

• CONGENITAL DEFECTS OF THE LIMBS

• **Causes of congenital defects of the limbs.**   Most defects in limb formation are rare. Most are caused by genetic abnormalities. However, environmental factors can cause these defects. The critical period for susceptibility to teratogenic insults is between 3.5 to 6 weeks of development, during which the structures of the limbs form. Known environmental factors include hyperthermia, some drugs including aspirin and the anticonvulsant dimethadione, and excess RA. The broad range of defects that follow, however rare, underscore the reason for the current research focus on uncovering mechanisms directing limb development and on discovering how they may affect development of the body axes. Since most defects of the limbs begin with defects in formation of bones, they are covered in this chapter. Many defects can be classified as duplications or reductions (eliminations) of bony elements.

• **Reduction defects or missing elements (see Fig. 7-8).**   All of these defects are rare when caused by genetic factors. However, they can also be caused by teratogens. *Amelia* refers to the complete absence of limb(s): development is suppressed entirely during the fourth week. *Meromelia* refers to absence of segment(s) of the limb. *Phocomelia* is a form of meromelia in which proximal structures (the long bones) are small or absent, but the distal portions are normally formed, so that a hand or foot is attached directly to the body. These defects may be set in motion by factors that damage the blood vessels in the proximal limb segments during weeks 5 and 6 after all bone models are formed. *Hemimelias* are defects in which pre- or postaxial compartments of limbs are missing. *Preaxial* refers to the first (cranial) three digits and carpal bones and the radius of the forearm, whereas *postaxial* refers to the two caudal digits and carpal bones and the ulna of the forearm.

• **Defects in digit formation are usually genetic in causation.**   *Polydactyly* refers to extra digits (fingers or toes), often incompletely formed and useless. This is the most prominent example of a duplication defect. *Syndactyly* refers to fused or webbed digits. (Some forms are unfortunately referred to as "lobster claw.") This defect is due to tissue between the digits failing to break down during development. This probably reflects a failure of the AER to regress between digits.

• **Achondroplasia (or "dwarfism").**   This defect results from premature ossification of the ends (epiphyseal plates) of long bones. This prevents the long bones of the limbs from growing to their normal lengths. Other bones are of normal size.

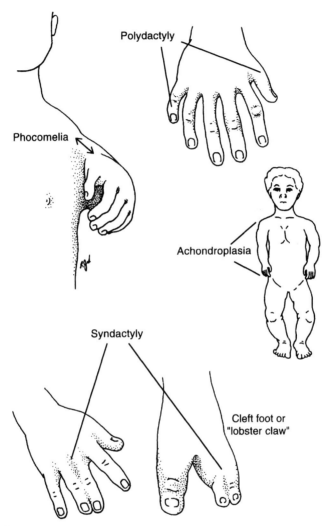

Figure 7-8
Limb defects.

• **Mechanical factors can also cause defects in limb formation.** *Intrauterine amputations* can result from bands of amniotic membrane wrapping around digits. *Club foot* (or talipes equinovarus) can result from excess mechanical pressure from the uterine wall.

The skeleton of the head

The skull is the cranial extension of the axial skeleton. It can be divided into two regions (see Fig. 7-9). The *neurocranium* surrounds and encases the brain and forms capsules surrounding the sense organs. The *viscerocranium* forms the internal structures of the face and surrounds the visceral structures of the mouth leading into the pharynx. If you don't need to learn the anatomy of the cranial skeleton, this division should be sufficient. If you do need to learn the mature anatomy, the following details of the embryogenesis should help in this process.

• **Each region of the skull can be subdivided according to whether bone forms by endochondral or intramembranous ossification.** The superficial flat bones covering both face and brain are formed directly by intramembranous ossification. The rest are formed by endochondral ossification of cartilage models. The factor that makes studying difficult is that each region has multiple germ layer origins.

• **Bones and cartilages of the head are derived from several sources.** Many are derived from mesoderm, as in the rest of the body. This includes sclerotomes of cranial (occipital) somites and similar regions of cranial somitomeres. (Again, while the first somitomeres in the head never progress to the somite stage of organization, they give rise to the same types of tissue derivatives.) Lateral plate mesoderm forms many other bones. Finally, cranial neural crest forms a number of bones.

• **THE NEUROCRANIUM (OR BRAIN SKELETON)** The neurocranium is divided into the base underlying the brain (*chondrocranium*) and the vault covering the brain (*membranous neurocranium*). Its formation relies on signals from underlying brain tissue, just as the formation of vertebrae relies on spinal cord signals.

• **The vault encasing the brain (membranous neurocranium) is formed directly by intramembranous ossification.** These bones are superficial flat bones. Collectively called the *calvaria*, they include one *frontal* and two *parietal* bones, as well as a part of the *occipital* bone (interparietal). They probably originate from neural crest, although there is some evidence they may originate from mesoderm. Soft connective tissue sutures develop between the calverial bones, permitting the skull to expand as it (and the brain) develop, to deform as it goes through the birth canal, and to grow through infancy.

Sources of bone and cartilage in the head

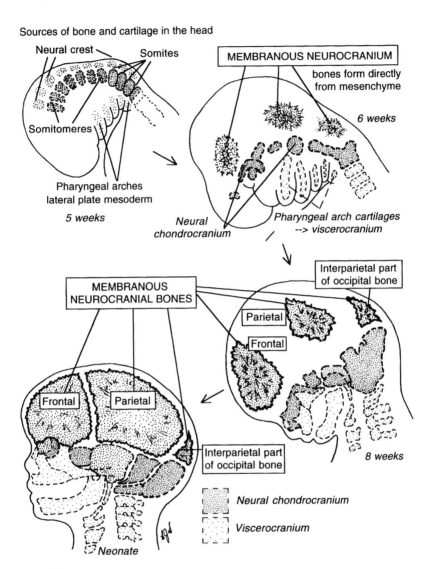

Figure 7-9
Regions of the skull and formation of intramembranous neurocranium.

• **The base of the skull (chondrocranium) is formed by endochondral ossification (see Fig. 7-10).**   The base of the skull is a midline structure that supports the brain. Its more lateral components form capsules surrounding and protecting the sensory organs (nasal cavities, eyes, and inner ears). It consists of five major bones. The midline *ethmoid* and *sphenoid bones* form the most cranial portion of the floor of the brain case, as well as the lateral walls of the nose (ethmoid), and the orbits encasing the eyes (ethmoid and sphenoid). The *petromastoid parts* of both *temporal bones* form the more lateral walls of the brain case and encase the components of the ears. The *occipital bone* forms the caudal portion of the floor supporting the brain and contains the opening through which the spinal cord leaves the skull (*foramen magnum*).

These bones are designated as the chondrocranium because they form by endochondral ossification from three pairs of midline cartilage models and three more lateral sensory capsules (olfactory, optic, and otic). These cartilages, and the bones derived from them, have a complex germ layer origin. The two most cranial pairs of midline cartilages are derived from both neural crest and somitomeric mesoderm, whereas the caudal pair is derived from only mesoderm: the sclerotomes of the three first (occipital) somites and the cranial half of the first cervical somite. (Did you notice that part of somite 1 was unaccounted for when the formation of the vertebrae was covered?) The sensory capsules are derived either from sclerotome cells of cranial somitomeres and occipital somites or from cranial neural crest cells.

The first pair of midline cartilages forms the ethmoid bone, which fuses with the olfactory capsule to form internal structures of the nose. The second midline cartilage pair forms the body of the sphenoid bone, while the optic capsules merge with it to form the sphenoid wings which encase the eyes. The occipital bone is formed by the third pair of midline cartilages. (Its origin from the most cranial somites makes it essentially a fusion of vertebral elements.) The otic capsules form around the developing structures of the inner ear, and form the petromastoid part of the temporal bones.

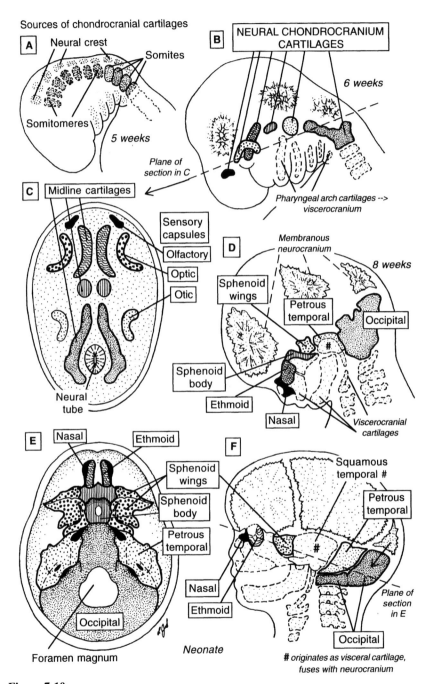

Figure 7-10
Formation of the neural chondrocranium.

- **THE VISCEROCRANIUM (OR SKELETON OF THE FACE)** The viscerocranial cartilages and bones form the major components of the jaw, which surround the visceral tissues of the mouth, and separate it from the nasal cavities. They also form the supporting structures surrounding the beginning of the pharynx and respiratory tree in the neck. Some of them are tied to the neurocranium by fusion with those bones. The origins and fates of these bones are very complex, because the structures of the viscerocranium begin their development within the pharyngeal arches (see Fig. 7-11).

- **How the cartilages and bones of the viscerocranium form within the embryonic pharyngeal arches.** The arches form bilaterally along the ventral side of the head fold region beginning late in week 4. The core of each arch is formed by lateral plate mesoderm, which condenses around the most cranial portion of the endoderm tube—the pharyngeal endoderm. Neural crest cells migrate into each arch, where they make significant contributions to both the mass and connective tissue derivatives of the arches. Separate bands or arches are created when the outer ectodermal covering and inner endodermal lining of this region form a series of constrictions that almost separate the mesodermal core into five regions on each side. In the core of each arch, connective tissue, cartilage, bone, and skeletal muscle components will form. Many of these derivatives subsequently migrate some distance to their final destinations, obscuring their origins.

- **Specific arch derivatives.** The arch pairs are numbered in cranial-caudal sequence 1, 2, 3, 4, and 6. (Arch 5, if it ever exists, is a transitory structure with no derivatives.) Arches 1 and 2 form structures of the face, arch 3 forms structures of both the face and neck, and arches 4 and 6 form neck structures. Neural crest cells form most of the general connective tissue derived from all the arches. In addition, neural crest forms all cartilage and most bones in arches 1 to 3. The cartilages formed in arches 4 and 6 are derived from lateral plate mesoderm. These distinctions are important because of the number of congenital defects that are due to abnormalities in formation of neural crest components. (For more detail on the origins and specific fates of bones of the head, see Chap. 10.)

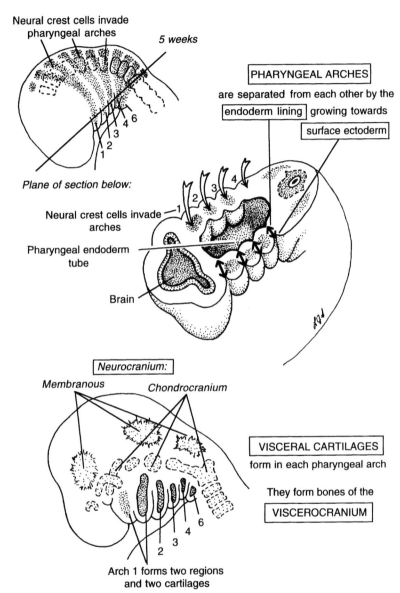

Figure 7-11
Pharyngeal arch formation.

• **Viscerocranial bones form many components of the face and jaw.** The viscerocranial bones all originate in the pharyngeal arches (see Fig. 7-12). However, some of them migrate considerable distances to their destinations, and some even become incorporated into neurocranial bones, obscuring their origins. The jaw bones that surround the mouth are the *maxillae, palatine bones*, and the *mandible*. Long *zygomatic bones* connect the maxillae to the temporal bones of the neurocranium on each side. Arch tissues give rise to the flat squamous portions and long styloid processes of these temporal bones, which then become merged. Small but important arch derivatives contribute to the walls surrounding the eyes (*lacrimal*) and nasal cavities (*nasal* and *vomer*), which are largely formed by neurocranial bones. Three small but very important visceral bones become key components of the middle ear: *incus, malleus*, and *stapes*. Finally, arch bones and cartilages contribute to formation of the neck: the *hyoid* bone surrounds the pharynx and the *laryngeal cartilages* surround the opening to the trachea.

Viscerocranial bones are formed by both endochondral and intramembranous ossification.

• **Most of the major viscerocranial bones of the face are formed by membranous ossification (the membranous viscerocranium).** The major bones of the face form around the start of the pharyngeal endoderm tube, which becomes the mouth. They are all formed in arch 1 directly by membranous ossification from neural crest. The maxilla, palate, zygomatic, and squamous temporal bones form cranial to the endoderm tube, while the mandible forms caudal to it. It may be surprising that these bones are formed by membranous ossification in an arch in which two major cartilages are formed. These cartilages, however, largely regress. Only small portions become transformed by endochondral ossification into bones.

• **Endochondral ossification forms small but important viscerocranial bones from cartilages in all of the first three arches.** The malleus, incus, and stapes of the middle ear are formed by endochondral ossification of cartilage derived from the major cartilage models formed in arches 1 and 2. In addition, the styloid processes of the temporal bone form initially from arch 1 cartilage and later fuse with it. Arches 2 and 3 together form the hyoid bone, which supports the tongue and anchors it to the neck. All the cartilage models and their bone replacements are derived from neural crest.

• **Laryngeal cartilages form in the neck from arches 4 and 6.** These cartilages, which include the *thyroid* and *cricoid* cartilages, are the only skeletal deriv-

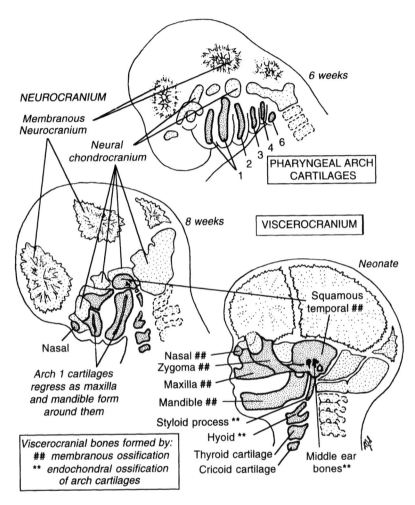

Figure 7-12
Formation of the viscerocranium from arches.

atives of these arches. They surround the origin of the endoderm tube near the point of outgrowth of the respiratory tract lining from the endoderm tube. They form from lateral plate mesoderm, while neural crest cells form the other connective tissue elements derived from these arches.

• **CONGENITAL DEFECTS OF THE SKULL**   Defects in early induction of the face and skull, as well as the nervous system, can be caused by the teratogenic effects of alcohol, drugs, or excess levels of RA; by high blood glucose levels in diabetic mothers; by mechanical factors; and by genetic syndromes (see Fig. 7-13). Defects of the skull can be secondary to maldevelopment of the brain or vice versa.

> Both genetic and environmental factors can create many of these defects by disturbing normal neural crest migration into and/or proliferation within the pharyngeal arches, which creates a deficit of connective tissue mesenchyme in the arches. This is not a factor in development of the axial skeleton of the trunk, or that of the limbs, since neural crest does not form any connective tissues in the body.

Anencephaly refers to failure of development of the brain and skull, whereas *microcephaly* refers to their underdevelopment. Both usually start with defective neural tube closure in the cephalic region during the first month. When this happens, brain tissue doesn't differentiate, and an abnormal or incomplete skull forms around it. These defects are often due to excess alcohol consumption.

Craniosynostosis (or premature closure of sutures between the bones of the vault of the skull) can produce a small skull and constrict development of the brain, resulting in brain defects.

• **A spectrum of facial defects occurs when defects in pharyngeal arch development affects viscerocranial bone development.**   Most pharyngeal arch defects include defective bone development, or *dysostosis*. *Craniofacial dysostosis* refers to a range of defects in development of the viscerocranial bony elements derived from the first two arches. Defects can involve underdevelopment of the jaw, as well as the bony supports for the eyes, ears, and nose. *Mandibulofacial dysostosis* refers to a specific spectrum of defects in underdevelopment of the lower face, primarily affecting the maxillae, palate and mandible. *First arch syndrome* is an alternative term for these defects, since most of them are due to maldevelopment of first arch structures. Underdevelopment of the jaw only is termed *micrognathia*.

DiGeorge syndrome refers to craniofacial defects that affect all arches, the range of defects depending on the severity and timing of the teratogenic insult. Defects include some of the craniofacial abnormalities described earlier, as well as defects in other tissue derivatives of these and other arches, including internal viscera. (These are covered in Chap. 10 on the head.)

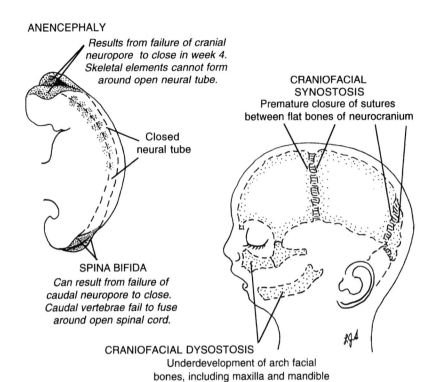

ANENCEPHALY

Results from failure of cranial neuropore to close in week 4. Skeletal elements cannot form around open neural tube.

Closed neural tube

CRANIOFACIAL SYNOSTOSIS
Premature closure of sutures between flat bones of neurocranium

SPINA BIFIDA

Can result from failure of caudal neuropore to close. Caudal vertebrae fail to fuse around open spinal cord.

CRANIOFACIAL DYSOSTOSIS
Underdevelopment of arch facial bones, including maxilla and mandible

Figure 7-13
Congenital defects of the skull.

MUSCULAR SYSTEM

·

·   ·   ·   ·   ·   ·   ·   ·   ·   ·   ·

Skeletal muscles work in concert with the skeletal system to generate the movements of the body. When they contract, they move the skeletal elements to which they are attached. Skeletal muscles are *organs* which consist not just of skeletal muscle tissue, but also of connective tissue wrappings which carry nerves and blood vessels throughout the muscles, and which attach the muscles to cartilages and bones. Thus, skeletal muscle development is more than simply the story of the germ layer origins of muscle cells. This chapter divides the story of muscle development into the same regions as were used to examine development of the skeleton in the last chapter: the trunk, limbs, and head. While skeletal muscle is formed from a single region of mesoderm, the *myotome* portions of somites all along the length of the embryonic body, there are significant regional differences in what happens to those myotome cells on their way to becoming skeletal muscles.

Even though the axial skeleton is also formed from the somites, the induction and initial formation of these two tissues are directed independently of each other. Later fetal growth and maturation of skeletal muscle is, however, closely intertwined with development of the skeletal system and, also, with nervous innervation. It is hard to learn about muscles without reference to the bones on which they originate and insert, so you may want to review the material in Chap. 7 while reading the details in this chapter.

SKELETAL MUSCLE TISSUE FORMATION

Histologic structure of skeletal muscle (see Fig. 8-1)

Skeletal muscle is different from most other tissues, as well as other muscle types, in that it is composed of *multinucleated* cells. The cells are called *fibers* because of their long, tapered, spindle shape. Each skeletal muscle fiber runs the entire length of its muscle, which can be more than a foot, and often contains hundreds of nuclei. Skeletal muscle also develops several different fiber types, which are named for the fast, slow, and intermediate speeds at which they contract. Most skeletal muscles contain a mixture of these types, and the specific patterns are characteristic for each muscle.

It is important to realize that the organs called *skeletal muscles* are built from skeletal muscle tissue, as well as from connective tissues.

The connective tissues participate in several ways. First, loose connective tissue bundles the individual skeletal muscle fibers into larger and larger bundles, until they form individual skeletal muscles such as the biceps or deltoid, which are organs. These connective tissue wrappings also provide the path through which blood vessels and nerves enter and leave the muscle. Second, these connective tissues transmit the pull of contraction of the muscle by merging into dense connective tissue tendons which attach the muscles to bones at either end.

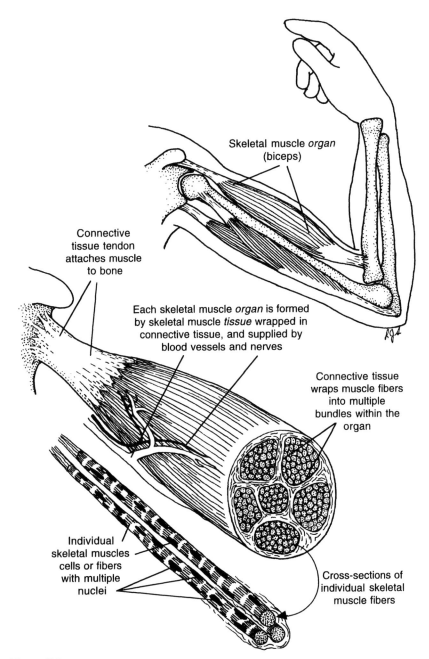

Figure 8-1
Structure of skeletal muscle fibers and skeletal muscle organ.

Germg layer origins: All skeletal muscle is derived from somitic myotomes

As first described in Chap. 5, the mesoderm layer condenses into three distinct regions: paraxial, intermediate, and lateral plate mesoderm. *Paraxial mesoderm* condenses to form *somites*, which further divide into sclerotomes, myotomes, and dermatomes. *Myotomes* differentiate into all skeletal muscle of the body, head, and limbs (see Fig. 8-2). (Just for reference, remember that the other two types of muscle, cardiac and smooth muscle, are formed from lateral plate mesoderm.)

The connective tissue components of skeletal muscles are derived from a different region of mesoderm than skeletal muscle tissue, *somatic lateral plate mesoderm*. In addition, some connective tissues of muscles in the head are derived from *neural crest*.

Histogenesis of skeletal muscle

Skeletal muscle precursor cells, which are called *myoblasts* or *myogenic* cells, are committed to their *myogenic* fate during their stay in the somite. The factors directing this initial commitment have not been identified, although signals from the neural tube play a role. Recent research has shown that a number of genes are activated in committed myoblasts, which are collectively called myogenic determination factors. Their products trigger differentiation by activating the transcription of a battery of muscle-specific genes.

Muscles of the limbs, head, and neck are formed by myotome cells which must first migrate some distance to their target destinations, where they reaggregate into *pre-muscle masses*. The trunk muscles are formed by myoblasts which remain in the somite and merely stretch out around the body wall. Myoblasts begin to differentiate only after they have arrived at their destinations.

• **Connective tissue directs muscle mass formation.** Evidence suggests that connective tissue elements lay down "tracks" before myoblasts migrate. These tracks somehow direct the migration of myoblasts, as well as their formation into specific pre-muscle masses.

• **Formation of multinucleated skeletal muscle cells occurs by fusion of myoblasts with each other.** The first step in the differentiation of skeletal muscle is the fusion of myoblasts to form multinucleated myotubes, which begins during week 5. The forming myotubes rapidly begin to express the proteins that make up their contractile machinery while myoblasts continue to be incorporated into them. Different fiber types are established as myotubes form, although their

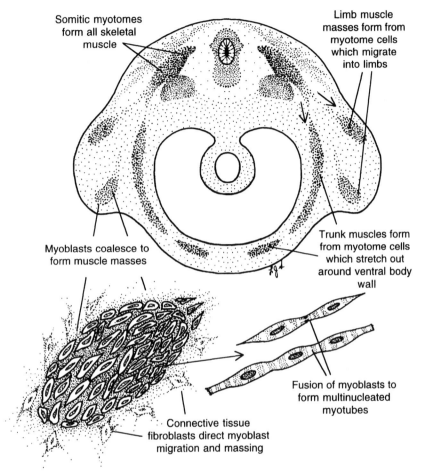

Somitic myotomes form all skeletal muscle

Limb muscle masses form from myotome cells which migrate into limbs

Trunk muscles form from myotome cells which stretch out around ventral body wall

Myoblasts coalesce to form muscle masses

Fusion of myoblasts to form multinucleated myotubes

Connective tissue fibroblasts direct myoblast migration and massing

Figure 8-2
Development of skeletal muscle.

contractile properties do not completely mature until after birth. Again, the connective tissue "housing" of each forming muscle contains the instructions for fiber type commitment. Myotubes mature into long muscle *fibers* during the fetal period.

During postnatal growth, skeletal muscles grow by hypertrophy of existing fibers. This occurs by continued incorporation of mononucleated myoblasts, now called *satellite cells*, into fibers.

• **Skeletal muscle cell fusion, formation of contractile machinery, and specific fiber types do not require nerve input.**   Considering that mature skeletal muscle fibers require motor nerve innervation to contract, it may surprise you to learn that these events in skeletal muscle development occur without input from nerve. However, muscle development and maturation through the fetal period require nerve contact. In return, nerve cells must synapse with muscle to survive. Motor axons enter muscle masses during week 5, before these masses split into individual muscle primordia (see Fig. 8-3). Once again connective tissue appears to be responsible for the capacity of nerve to find the right muscle masses, since branching patterns (or projections) of nerve processes to muscle masses are correct even without muscle tissue present. Sensory nerve processes enter later, after individual muscle masses are established. Sensory innervation to skeletal muscle, as well as all internal organs, is necessary to provide feedback to the central nervous system about the state of contraction of the muscle. This is referred to as proprioceptive sensory input.

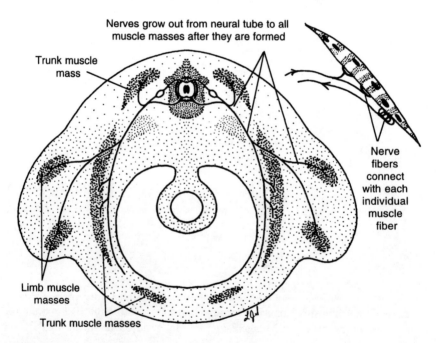

Figure 8-3
Innervation of skeletal muscle.

Terminology of muscle actions

In order to understand the major muscle groupings, it helps to learn them by their collective actions (see Fig. 8-4). The following definitions of muscle action should permit you to do this.

Flex/extend: bend (decrease angle)/straighten (increase angle) of joint
Adduct/abduct: move structure closer to/farther from midline
Rotate: move bone around its long axis
Dorsiflex/plantarflex: raise toes/lower foot
Pronate/suppinate: turn palm down/up

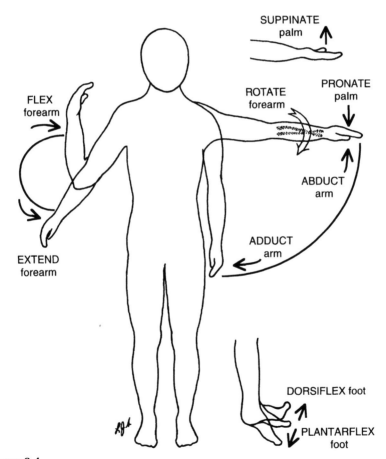

Figure 8-4
Terminology of muscle actions.

FORMATION OF REGIONS OF SKELETAL MUSCULATURE

As with the skeletal system, skeletal muscles are described in groups so that you can learn about their origins without having to already know all the skeletal muscles (see Fig. 8-5). Some of the better known skeletal muscles are used as examples to orient you to each group. In some cases, muscle groups are classified according to major actions. However, many muscles have multiple functions whose descriptions are beyond the scope of this book. You can find individual muscles in each group in any anatomy text.

• **Distinguishing between skeletal muscles that originate in the trunk (axial muscles), head (pharyngeal arch muscles), and limbs.**   Trunk (axial) muscles form directly from myoblasts remaining in the myotomes after many of their fellow myoblasts have left on their journey to the limbs. The cells that migrate to the limbs will form not only the intrinsic limb muscles, but also the muscles of the shoulder and pelvic girdles which connect the limbs to the body. Cells from the most cranial myotomes form many head and neck muscles only after they migrate into the pharyngeal arches.

• **Innervation patterns hold the key to the origins of skeletal muscles.** Skeletal muscles become innervated as they form within muscles masses. Thus, however much their origins may be disguised by their subsequent growth or migration, skeletal muscle origins can be discovered if you pay attention to their innervation. First, are they innervated by cranial or spinal nerves? Muscles formed in the pharyngeal arches from cranial somites are all innervated by cranial nerves, which, as their name suggests, originate from the brain. This is a whole different kettle of fish from the spinal nerves, which originate from the spinal cord. Spinal nerves innervate all the other skeletal muscles from the neck on down through the body, as well as those of the limbs. If muscles are innervated by spinal nerves, then pay attention to whether they are innervated by dorsal or ventral primary rami (branches) of these nerves. These distinctions will become clear as you read about the origins of the musculature of each region of the body.

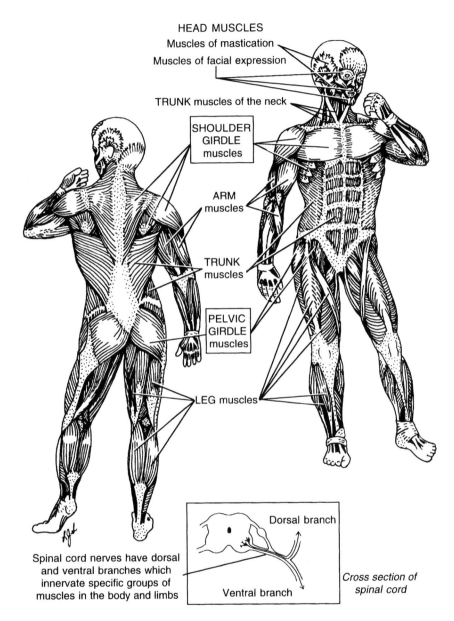

HEAD MUSCLES
Muscles of mastication
Muscles of facial expression

TRUNK muscles of the neck

SHOULDER
GIRDLE
muscles

ARM
muscles

TRUNK
muscles

PELVIC
GIRDLE
muscles

LEG muscles

Dorsal branch

Ventral branch

Cross section of
spinal cord

Spinal cord nerves have dorsal
and ventral branches which
innervate specific groups of
muscles in the body and limbs

Figure 8-5
Muscle regions of the body, head, and limbs.

Axial muscles of the body or trunk

• **Trunk (axial) muscles form directly from myotomes.**   After the limb muscle precursors leave the myotomes on their journey to the limbs, the remaining myotome cells in the somites break into two major series of muscle masses which extend for most of the length of the body (see Fig. 8-6). The dorsal portions of the myotomes form the *epimeres*, which combine to become the *epaxial*, or deep back muscles of the vertebral column. They extend (or straighten) the vertebral column; when muscles on only one side contract, they produce lateral bending. These muscles consist of the *erector spinae* and deeper *transversospinalis* muscle groups. In addition, the cervical level epimeres form the *suboccipital triangle muscles* at the back of the neck. They connect the head and neck dorsally, by connecting the first two vertebrae to the occipital bone, and extend and rotate the head.

The larger ventral portions of the myotomes form the *hypomeres*, which combine to become the more substantial *hypaxial* muscles of the lateral and ventral body wall. These muscles flex the body. The deeper muscles flex or rotate the vertebral column directly, while the more superficial ventral muscles flex the body by connecting to bones such as the ribs and sternum. When the muscles on only one side contract, they bend the body laterally.

Each somite level forms different groups of muscles. The cervical level hypomeres form the "strap" muscles of the ventral neck. These muscles originate on the vertebrae and insert on the ribs. Some cervical level myotome cells migrate farther to form the skeletal muscle component of the diaphragm. The thoracic and lumbar hypomeres form the bulk of the ventral body wall muscles, which flex the ventral body wall (*intercostals*, *external* and *internal obliques*, *transversus abdominis*, and midline *rectus abdominis*).

In addition, cells from the thoracic, abdominal, and sacral hypomeres move deeper into the body wall to form muscles that flex the vertebral column or bend it ventrally. These include the *psoas* muscles, which flex the pelvic portion of the vertebral column and the quadratus lumborum, which flexes the thigh against the body. The sacral and coccygeal myotomes largely degenerate, although connective tissue ligaments take their place.

• **Innervation provides information as to origins.**   All trunk muscles are supplied by spinal nerves.

All epimere derivatives are innervated by the *dorsal primary rami* of the spinal nerves, whereas all hypomere derivatives are innervated by the *ventral primary rami*.

TRUNK MYOTOMES DIVIDE INTO EPIMERES AND HYPOMERES

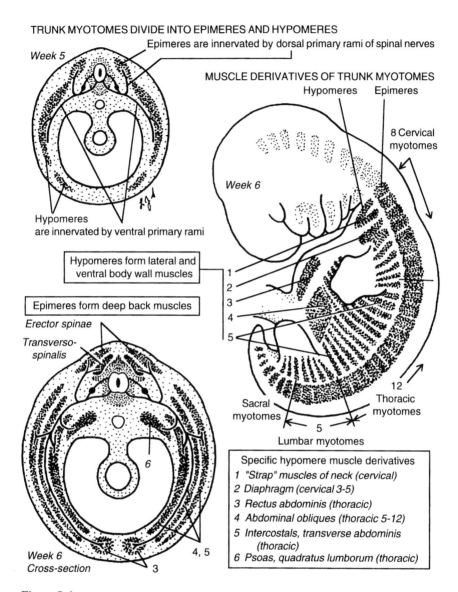

Figure 8-6
Development of muscles of the body and differences in their patterns of innervation.

Appendage muscles: limbs and appendicular girdles

• **Limb muscles and appendicular girdle muscles all originate from myo-tomal cells that migrate into the limbs.** Limb muscles and the muscles of the shoulder and pelvic girdles form from myoblasts that first migrate out of specific myotomes into the developing limb buds. The last five cervical and first thoracic myotomes form the arm muscles, while the lumbar and first two sacral myotomes form the leg muscles. These cells condense into two muscle masses in each limb, the *dorsal* and *ventral limb bud masses* (see Fig. 8-7). These masses subsequently split into specific muscles. The muscles that originate and insert entirely within the limb are called *intrinsic limb muscles*. The muscles of the shoulder and pelvic girdles are called the *extrinsic limb muscles* because they cross the joints between the limbs and the body and, thus, are contained partly within the limbs and partly within the trunk.

• **The intrinsic limb muscles are formed from both limb muscle masses.** The dorsal limb bud masses form all the *extensors* of the limbs, as well as the *suppinators* of the upper limb and *abductors* of the lower limb. In the upper limb, these muscles form the posterior compartment of the arm and forearm and the lateral compartment of the forearm and hand. In the lower limb, these muscles form the anterior compartment of the thigh and leg, the lateral compartment of the leg, and the muscles of the dorsum of the foot. (These compartments are useful groupings in learning the anatomy of individual muscles. Remember that individual muscles migrate away from the original position of their muscle masses and that whole muscle groups are moved by the rotation of the limbs about their axes as described in Chap. 6.)

    The ventral limb bud masses form all the *flexors* of the limbs, as well as the *pronators* of the upper limb and *adductors* of the lower limb. In the upper limb, these muscles form the anterior compartment of the arm and forearm and muscles of the palmar surface of the hand. In the lower limb, these muscles form the medial and posterior compartments of the thigh, the posterior compartment of the leg, and all plantar surface muscles of the foot.

> All the appendage muscles are supplied by the ventral rami of the spinal nerves. All muscles derived from the dorsal muscle mass are innervated by the dorsal branches of the ventral primary rami, while all muscles derived from the ventral muscle mass are innervated by the ventral branches of the ventral primary rami.

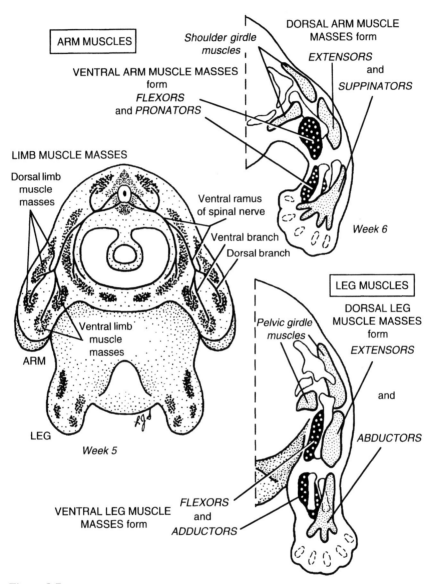

ARM MUSCLES

Shoulder girdle
muscles

DORSAL ARM MUSCLE
MASSES form

EXTENSORS
and
SUPPINATORS

VENTRAL ARM MUSCLE MASSES
form
FLEXORS
and PRONATORS

LIMB MUSCLE MASSES

Dorsal limb
muscle
masses

Ventral ramus
of spinal nerve

Ventral branch

Dorsal branch

Week 6

Ventral limb
muscle
masses

ARM

LEG

Week 5

LEG MUSCLES

DORSAL LEG
MUSCLE MASSES
form
EXTENSORS

and

ABDUCTORS

Pelvic girdle
muscles

VENTRAL LEG MUSCLE
MASSES form

FLEXORS
and
ADDUCTORS

Figure 8-7
Development of muscles of the limbs.

• **Limb muscle masses form all appendage girdle muscles.**   It is important to distinguish between extrinsic limb muscles, which originate from limb muscle masses, and intrinsic muscles of the trunk, which arise directly from the myotomes within the body. Muscles that cross the shoulder joint or the hip joint are extrinsic limb muscles. Many of these muscles insert or originate on the appendicular girdle bones (see Fig. 8-8). The bones of the shoulder girdle are the *clavicle* and the *scapula*, while the pelvic girdle is composed of the hip bone, or *coxa*.

All muscles of the appendicular girdles are derived from the dorsal limb muscle masses.

The major muscles of the shoulder girdle that link the humerus of the arm to the bones of the ventral body wall are the *pectoralis major* and *minor*, while the *serratus anterior* connects the scapula to the ventral body wall. The major muscles that link the humerus to the bones of the dorsal body wall are the *trapezius*, *latissimus dorsi*, *rhomboids*, *teres major*, and *sit* muscles (*s*upraspinatus, *i*nfraspinatus, *t*eres minor) which run from the scapula to "sit" on the head of the humerus. And of course we cannot overlook that major shoulder muscle, the *deltoid*, which links the humerus all around the joint to both scapula and clavicle. In general, the ventral muscles adduct and flex the arm, while the dorsal muscles extend and abduct the arm. However, many of their actions depend on the position of the arm at the time the action is initiated.

The major muscles of the pelvic girdle are the dorsal *gluteal group* muscles and the *adductor magnus* which link the *femur* of the thigh to the dorsal body; and the ventral *iliopsoas group* and *quadriceps femoris group*, which link the thigh to the ventral body. The ventral muscles flex the thigh towards the abdomen, while the dorsal muscles extend (straighten) and abduct the thigh away from the midline. Some also act at the knee joint to flex or extend the (lower) leg.

• **Innervation again provides information as to origins.**

All appendage muscles are supplied by the ventral rami of the spinal nerves. Since all extrinsic limb muscles are derived from the dorsal muscle mass, they are innervated by the dorsal branches of the ventral primary rami of the spinal nerves.

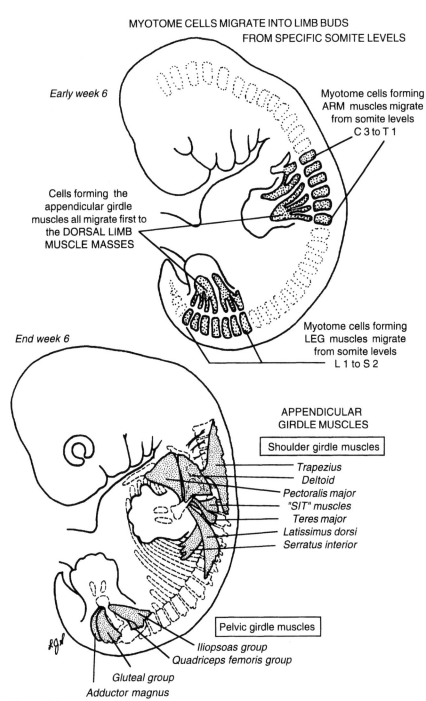

MYOTOME CELLS MIGRATE INTO LIMB BUDS
FROM SPECIFIC SOMITE LEVELS

Early week 6

Myotome cells forming
ARM muscles migrate
from somite levels
C 3 to T 1

Cells forming the
appendicular girdle
muscles all migrate first to
the DORSAL LIMB
MUSCLE MASSES

End week 6

Myotome cells forming
LEG muscles migrate
from somite levels
L 1 to S 2

APPENDICULAR
GIRDLE MUSCLES

Shoulder girdle muscles

Trapezius
Deltoid
Pectoralis major
"SIT" muscles
Teres major
Latissimus dorsi
Serratus interior

Pelvic girdle muscles

Iliopsoas group
Quadriceps femoris group
Gluteal group
Adductor magnus

Figure 8-8
Development of muscles of the shoulder and pelvic girdles.

Muscles of the head and neck

• **Precursors of most skeletal muscles of the head migrate into pharyngeal arches before forming muscles.**   The development of the pharyngeal arches on the ventral side of the forming head has already been described in Chap. 6, and is described in greater detail in Chap. 10. Most skeletal muscles of the head and deep neck are classified as *pharyngeal arch muscles* since they form within the arches (see Fig. 8-9). It should be remembered, however, that the myogenic cells are generated in the cranial somites and somitomeres, and become committed there before migrating into the arches. As in the rest of the body, the myoblasts use the connective tissue (formed in the arches by neural crest, not mesoderm) as guides to migrate into the arches. Here, the ingrowing cranial nerves connect with the forming muscle cells, and receive their marching orders to their final destinations.

• **Innervation helps to distinguish the origins of muscles of the head and neck as it does in the rest of the body and limbs.**   Muscles that form in the arches are innervated by cranial nerves, not the spinal nerves which innervate all other skeletal muscles. Nerves establish contact with muscles as they form in the arches and then remain connected to the muscles as they migrate. Innervation is useful in determining which muscles are derived from arches. It is also useful in determining their *specific* arch derivations. This is because

---

Each arch is innervated by a separate cranial nerve.
Arch 1: cranial nerve 5 (trigeminal, mandibular division)
Arch 2: cranial nerve 7 (facial)
Arch 3: cranial nerve 9 (glossopharyngeal)
Arch 4 and 6: cranial nerve 10 (vagus)

In addition, a few muscles form in the head from myotome cells which differentiate outside the arches. These include the extrinsic muscles of the eyes, which move the eyeball. They are innervated by cranial nerves 3, 4, and 6. They also include the muscles of the tongue, which initially develop outside the arches, become innervated by cranial nerve 12, and then migrate (with their innervation) into the most ventral portions of the arches.

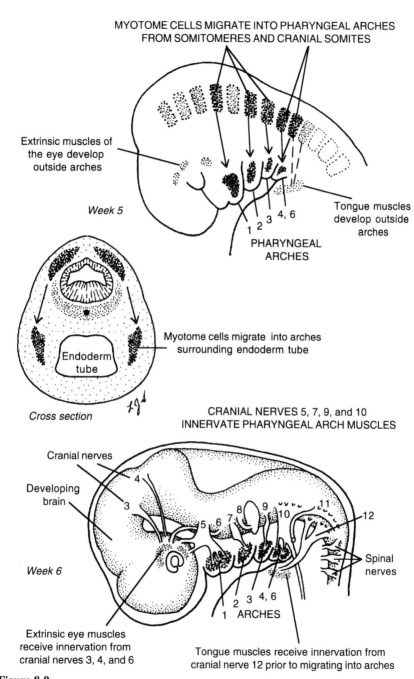

Figure 8-9
Development of muscles from the pharyngeal arches and their innervation by cranial nerves.

• **Pharyngeal arch-derived muscles include most of the muscles of the head (see Fig. 8-10).**   The major muscle groups formed in the first two arches include the muscles of mastication, which close the jaw to permit chewing (arch 1), and the muscles of facial expression, whose function is self-explanatory (arch 2). The developing muscles of facial expression migrate over the surface of the face and head, obscuring the original boundaries of the arches. Most attach to the connective tissue layer of the skin and not to bones. In addition, a few muscles from arches 1 and 2 help to open the jaw and move the tongue by their attachment at one end to the mandible, and at the other to either the hyoid bone at the base of the tongue, the thyroid cartilage, or the styloid process of the temporal bone of the skull. You might at first confuse some of these muscles with ventral neck muscles which are derived from trunk myotomes. Innervation helps distinguish their origins: if the muscles are arch derived, they are innervated by cranial nerves; if they are derived from trunk myotomes, they are innervated by spinal nerves of the cervical or thoracic levels. Arches 1 and 2 also give rise to the small muscles of the middle ear which transmit vibrations of the eardrum to the middle ear bones.

Arch 3 gives rise to only a single muscle, the stylopharyngeus, which helps to raise the pharynx during swallowing.

Arches 4 and 6 give rise to the internal muscles of the soft palate (which raise the palate during swallowing), the pharynx (pharyngeal constrictors which carry the swallowing action down toward the esophagus), and the larynx (which move the voice box).

Arches 1–4 form the structures of the tongue. The intrinsic skeletal muscles of the tongue are derived from the 3 occipital somites whose myotome cells migrate into these arches, carrying their motor innervation from cranial nerve 12 with them.

The major muscles in the head which don't ever "do time" in the pharyngeal arches are the *extrinsic eye muscles*: the skeletal muscles that move the eyeball. The eye muscles develop from the myogenic cells of three of the first five somitomeres, often called *preotic somites*, and are innervated by cranial nerves 3, 4, and 6.

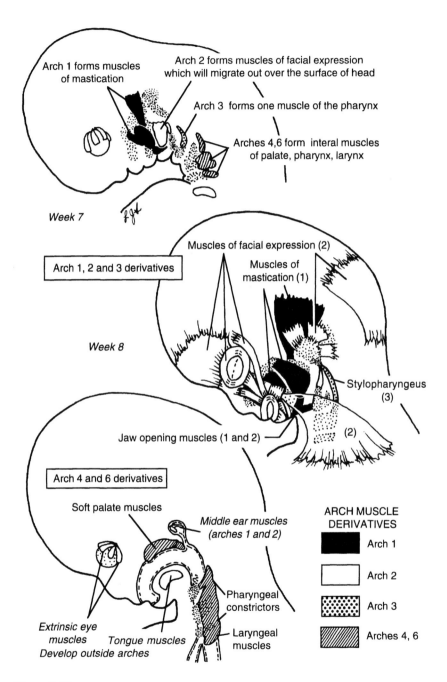

Figure 8-10
Head and neck muscles are formed in the pharyngeal arches.

Congenital defects

The range of defects already described in the skeletal system does not occur in formation of skeletal muscle. The most significant muscle defects are actually disease processes that affect skeletal muscle once it is formed. Most defects are caused by genetic abnormalities. *Muscular dystrophy* refers to a family of genetic diseases in which there is postnatal degeneration of various muscle groups. *Duchenne muscular dystrophy* has been shown to be caused by a lack of a protein in skeletal muscle fibers called *dystrophin*. It is an actin-binding protein (part of the large spectrin supergene family of actin-binding proteins). It links the actin within the cell to the cell membrane; without it, muscle fibers are more susceptible to damage when stressed.

• **ABSENT OR UNDERDEVELOPED MUSCLE GROUPS**   Rarely, individual muscles or groups may be absent (*atretic*) or underdeveloped (*hypoplastic*). This is usually secondary to underdevelopment or atresia of the bones to which they attach. This is seen most frequently in the limbs and in the face and neck muscles formed from pharyngeal arches.

A few major defects are unassociated with bone defects. *Prune belly syndrome* refers to hypoplastic or absent abdominal muscles. It may include an absent or hypoplastic diaphragm. In Poland syndrome, the pectoralis major muscle may be absent.

NERVOUS SYSTEM

·

•   •   •   •   •   •   •   •   •   •   •   •

The nervous system is a complex system whose embryonic origins hold the key to learning its components. Anatomically, it is divided into the central nervous system and the peripheral nervous system, each of which have many subdivisions. Histologically, the nervous system contains a variety of different types of nerve cells and supporting cells which are essential for nerve cell function. In spite of its complexity, virtually the entire nervous system originates from one part of the embryonic ectoderm, the neuroectoderm.

The beginning of the chapter presents an overview of development of the nervous system sufficient for learning the origins of the major tissue components and the major regions of the nervous system. The bulk of the chapter then covers the development of each region of the central and peripheral nervous system in more detail. Even in these portions of the chapter, each section begins with an overview which can be read on its own.

• **Alert: concentrate on just what you need to know.**   This may be more of a challenge in this chapter than in others. It shouldn't surprise you that this chapter is the longest in the book, since the mature nervous system is so complex it usually requires a separate course in the medical curriculum just to learn its salient features. Pay attention to the details in each section only if you need to learn them. The detail is there primarily to help you learn the mature anatomy of the nervous system.

NERVE TISSUE FORMATION

Germ layer origins: neuroectoderm forms all neural tissue

The following description of the early events in the formation of neural tissue summarizes events first introduced in Chap. 5. Neural tissue is the first tissue type to be committed to its fate. The events described below occur in week 3, while the embryo is still forming the third germ layer and folding into its three-dimensional shape.

Ectoderm in the midline of the cranial-caudal axis is induced to form *neuroectoderm* by the underlying notochord. The neuroectoderm thickens into a neural plate, which rises up into neural folds along its length on each side (see Fig. 9-1). The cells at the crest of each neural fold separate to form groups of cells called the *neural crest*, which migrate to a variety of destinations in the body before beginning to differentiate into nervous system components.

The neural folds fuse together along their length and then separate from the surface ectoderm to form the self-contained *neural tube*. Fusion of the neural folds begins in the midsection of the tube first, temporarily leaving openings called *neuropores* at either end of the neural tube. The neuropores close early in week 4. While the neural tube is closing, it also begins curving ventrally at both ends. This curvature is partly responsible for body folding.

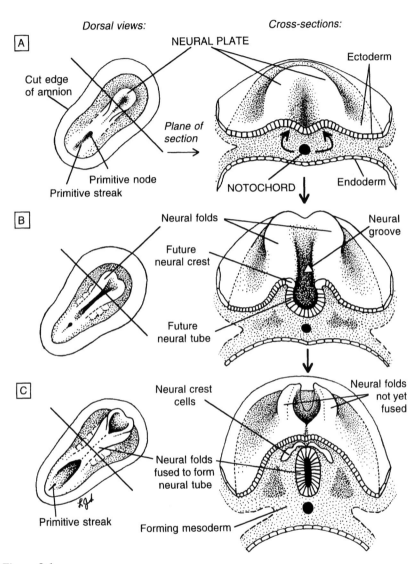

Figure 9-1
Neuroectoderm forms the neural tube and neural crest in late week 3 (A and B) and early
week 4 (C).

The neural tube and neural crest form different parts of the nervous system

The different nervous system components formed by neural tube and neural crest derivatives are an important reason for learning the distinction between these two neuroectoderm derivatives (see Fig. 9-2).

> The neural tube forms all the components of the brain and spinal cord, which together form the central nervous system (CNS).

The neural tube forms the brain and spinal cord by extensive growth, which "morphs" the simple tube into a variety of shapes and thicknesses along its length. These changes are most dramatic in the formation of the brain. The cells within this tube proliferate to form both types of cells formed in the nervous system: nerve cells, or *neurons*, and support cells called *glia*. Support cells are essential for the differentiation, survival, and function of neurons.

> Neural crest forms most components of the peripheral nervous system (PNS).

The crest consists of the neural tissue outside the CNS, or at the "periphery" of the body. It is a widespread network of nerve cell groupings (called *ganglia*) and nerve cell processes bound together to form *peripheral nerves*.

Neural crest cells migrate to their many target destinations in the body before they differentiate into components of the PNS. Some crest cells clump together to form the nerve cells and support cells of ganglia. Peripheral nerves are formed by collections of processes (or fibers) that grow out together to innervate targets throughout the body. The nerve cell bodies of these peripheral nerve fibers are located in both PNS ganglia and in the CNS. Some support cells in the PNS are formed by neural crest, whereas others are formed by surrounding mesoderm.

> Some neural crest forms the non-neural components in the body and head.

These derivatives are covered in more detail in Chap. 10.

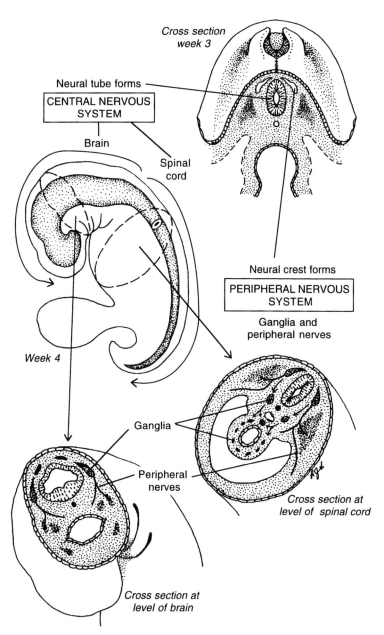

Cross section
week 3

Neural tube forms

CENTRAL NERVOUS
SYSTEM

Brain

Spinal
cord

Neural crest forms

PERIPHERAL NERVOUS
SYSTEM

Ganglia and
peripheral nerves

Week 4

Ganglia

Peripheral
nerves

Cross section at
level of spinal cord

Cross section at
level of brain

Figure 9-2
Components of the CNS and PNS.

Histogenesis of nerve and support tissues

• **CELL TYPES FORMED IN THE NERVOUS SYSTEM**   Two major cell lineages form in the nervous system: the nerve cell lineage (*neuroblasts*) and supporting cell lineage (see Fig. 9-3). Once neuroblasts are committed to their lineage, they undergo no more division. Support cells, on the other hand, continue to divide as needed throughout life.

• **Neuroblasts differentiate into nerve cells, or neurons.**   Neurons have the largest cell bodies of any cell type in the body. They form long processes that grow out to synapse with target cells. *Synapses* are specialized sites of membrane contact which permit nerve impulses to be transmitted between cells. Neurons form only one outgoing process, or axon, to carry signals to targets, but they can have multiple incoming processes, or dendrites, to receive input. Target cells include other nerve cells, as well as all types of muscle.

> Neurons need to "reach out and touch" each other by forming synapses to survive.

A unique question in nerve development not faced by other tissues is the question of how nerve cells correctly extend processes over long distances to their proper targets. In the CNS, how do they find their correct targets in the midst of all the other neurons? In the PNS, how do they find correct nerve or muscle targets that are distributed throughout the body? The answers that are emerging involve a complicated interaction of factors. Initial pathfinding may utilize physical pathways established by support cells in both regions. Specific cell adhesion molecules placed on nerve and support glial cell membranes provide recognition along the way and initial adhesion between cells. *Chemoattractant growth factor molecules* attract specific subsets of neurons once they arrive in the vicinity.

• **Neurons come in several functional types.**   *Sensory*, or *afferent*, neurons receive input from the body. *Motor*, or *efferent*, neurons transmit signals to target effector cells. *Interneurons*, or *association neurons*, integrate input from several sources and transmit it to selected neurons. Sensory and motor nerves are formed in both the CNS and PNS, while interneurons are confined to the CNS.

• **Different support cell types form in the CNS and PNS.**   The term *glia* refers to all support cell types formed in the CNS. The PNS has no collective term, and *glia* is often applied here too. Even though support cells in the CNS and PNS are derived from different sources and form different cell types, they perform the same range of protective, supporting, and metabolic functions.

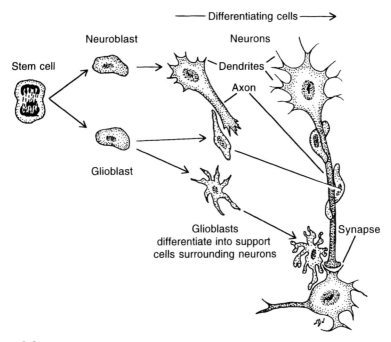

Figure 9-3
Development of nervous system components.

• **Differentiation of nervous system components extends throughout the embryonic and fetal periods into neonatal life.** The major structural regions in the nervous system are established during the embryonic period. Most proliferation and commitment occurs during this period. Differentiation begins in the embryonic period, but continues through the fetal period. Major synaptic connections form from the embryonic period into the neonatal period. Most myelination of processes occurs in late fetal or neonatal life.

> The fact that nervous system development extends from the embryonic period into neonatal life means that it is more vulnerable to teratogenic insults or inadequate nutrition throughout fetal life than are other organ systems.

CENTRAL NERVOUS SYSTEM DEVELOPMENT
Early brain and spinal cord development

• **The initial cell divisions of neural tube cells create both neuronal and glial progenitors.** The single cell layer of the early neural tube gives rise to the two major cell lineages in the nervous system, neuroblasts and glioblasts (see Fig. 9-4). Evidence suggests that neuroblasts are produced by the first divisions and only then are glial progenitors produced.

Neuroblasts elongate and begin to migrate toward the outer surface of the neural tube, forming multiple cell layers in the process. Only when they reach their destinations do they begin to differentiate into neurons. Glioblasts are important partners in the process of neuronal migration: they not only accompany the neuroblasts on their migration, but in many regions facilitate that migration.

• **Three types of glia are formed by the neural tube: astrocytes, oligodendrocytes, and ependyma.** *Astrocytes* wrap around both capillaries and neurons. From this position they provide structural support, perform repair processes, facilitate metabolic exchange between the blood vessels and neurons, and help to form the blood-brain barrier, although the walls of the capillaries do most of this work.

Oligodendrocytes surround and insulate nerve processes in the CNS. In addition, oligodendrocytes myelinate many processes within the CNS. Myelination is a process in which the glia wrap around each nerve process many times, forming myelin sheaths from multiple layers of glial cell membrane. Myelination increases the speed of impulse transmission and further protects the processes. It is a complex process which begins in the fetal period and continues into neonatal life. Only specific types of neurons become myelinated.

The *ependyma* is an epithelium that lines the central lumen of the brain and spinal cord. It is formed from the cells that remain as the inner layer of the neural tube after all other cell types are generated.

• **A fourth type of glial cell enters the CNS from outside.** *Microglia* are small scavenger cells that gobble up debris. They are an exception to the neural tube monopoly on CNS derivatives: they are produced by mesoderm cells that invade the CNS early in its embryonic development. They form from the same lineage as that of the monocyte-macrophage system of scavenger cells in the rest of the body.

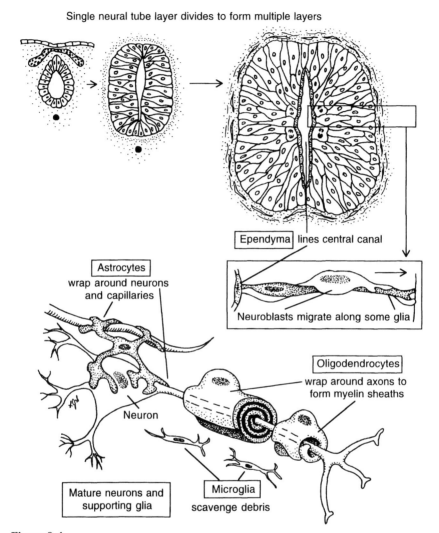

Single neural tube layer divides to form multiple layers

Ependyma lines central canal

Neuroblasts migrate along some glia

Astrocytes
wrap around neurons
and capillaries

Oligodendrocytes
wrap around axons to
form myelin sheaths

Neuron

Mature neurons and
supporting glia

Microglia
scavenge debris

Figure 9-4
Neural tissue histogenesis within the CNS.

• Neural tube development involves formation of separate regions along its length. While neuroblasts and glioblasts are generated, anatomic regions of the CNS are also established in the neural tube (see Fig. 9-5). The cranial end of the tube, which will form the brain, begins to expand laterally as the neural tube fuses. Furthermore, two bends, or *flexures*, then form in the region, causing the brain to fold ventrally under the rest of the neural tube during week 4. The lateral expansion of parts of the developing brain causes it to become demarcated into first three and, then, five distinct regions along its length.

The more caudal end of the tube, which will form the spinal cord, remains a relatively constant width and shape. The spinal cord does not become longitudinally divided into regions. However, both the brain and spinal cord give rise to segmental nerves, which emerge along their length at discrete points.

• The neural tube is induced to form different regions along its length by retinoic acid. Researchers are currently hot on the trail of this story. One important inducing agent is vitamin A. It is essential for normal development, and yet excess intake can cause neural tube defects. As you have already learned in Chap. 6, vitamin A is a member of the retinoic acid (RA) family. Retinoids have been shown to activate *hox* (homeobox, or homeodomain) genes in several places in the body, including the neural tube. It has been shown that the neural tube is normally exposed to a gradient of RA (highest caudally), that this gradient is essential for induction of proper regions, and that this is due to induction of expression of different combinations of hox genes in each of these regions by the gradients of RA.

Excesses of RA upset development by inappropriately "caudalizing" regions of the neural tube (i.e., by inducing the future forebrain region to form incorrect hindbrain structures). Teratogenic excesses can result from several sources, including the use of antiacne medications containing vitamin A while pregnant.

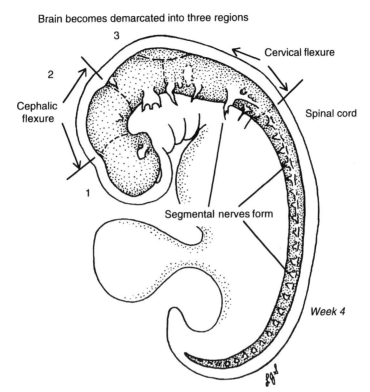

Figure 9-5
Distinctions along the length of the neural tube develop during week 4.

• **Neural tube development also involves development of separate regions, or zones, across the thickness of the neural tube.**   As the neural tube develops multiple cell layers, they form separate cellular zones. Cells are "born" in the innermost layer and move to the peripheral layers in stages (see Fig. 9-6).

1.   The inner *ventricular (ependymal) zone* lines the central canal. It remains a "germinal" mitotic layer which gives rise to the other layers. The cells that remain eventually form the ependyma (the epithelium lining the central canal).
2.   The *intermediate (mantle) zone* is formed by neuroblast cells. It becomes the "gray matter" of the CNS. All the nerve cell bodies impart a gray appearance under the microscope.
3.   The outer *marginal zone* is formed by neuronal processes. It becomes "white matter." All the myelin sheaths surrounding the processes impart a white appearance.

• **In some regions of the brain, more layers will form.**   These three layers are retained in the spinal cord and in the portion of the brain called the *brainstem*. In the "higher centers" of the brain (the cerebellum and cerebrum), these three layers are expanded to five by further cell migration.

• **The dorsal and ventral portions of the neural tube develop distinct regions called *horns* or *plates*.**

1.   The dorsal portion of the tube is the *dorsal horn*, or *alar plate*. Functionally, the dorsal horn will contain sensory nerve components.
2.   The ventral portion is the *ventral horn*, or *basal plate*. Functionally, the ventral horn will contain motor nerve components.

These regional differences are maintained throughout differentiation of both the brain and spinal cord, although development of the brain obscures some origins because of their movement or regression.

• **Induction of dorsal-ventral specialization across the neural tube involves signals from the notochord.**   The notochord's job is not done when it induces the neuroectoderm. It also induces ventral horn cells to become motor neurons. In addition, researchers are discovering patterns of expression of several gene families within the neural tube across its dorsal-ventral axis. These families may be involved in inducing regional specificity, since their products, like hox gene products, can direct expression of a range of other target genes.

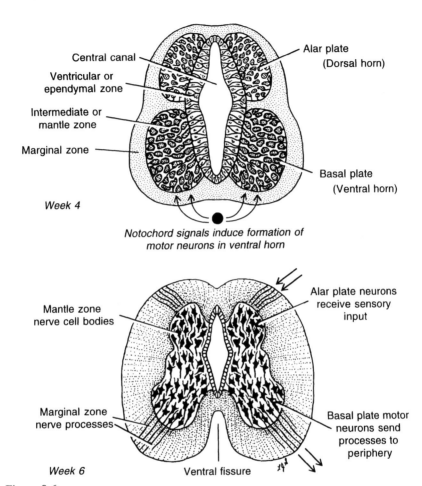

Figure 9-6
Development of regional specialization across the neural tube.

Spinal cord formation

• **The basic plan of the early neural tube is largely preserved in the spinal cord.** The spinal cord preserves both the cross-sectional organization of the neural tube stage, as well as a fairly uniform thickness and narrow central lumen, which becomes the *central canal* (see Fig. 9-7). The collections of nerve cells that differentiate in its mantle zone (gray matter) form an H-shape around the central canal. The peripheral marginal zone comes to contain mostly myelinated nerve processes (white matter). The right and left sides of the cord remain connected across the midline by dorsal roof and ventral floor plates, which will become the site of nerve processes crossing in bundles called *commissures*. A deep external groove, or *fissure*, forms in the midline of the ventral surface, while only a slight depression, or *sulcus*, develops in the dorsal midline. In addition, neuronal processes will enter and exit the lateral surfaces of the spinal cord in spinal nerve roots all along its length. They will join to form segmented spinal nerves just outside the spinal cord.

Cross-sections of the spinal cord at different levels vary somewhat in size and shape because of different sizes of neuronal masses (gray mantle zone) and fiber tracts (white marginal zone). The volume of gray matter is greater at levels where neurons to and from the limbs are located (at cervical and lumbosacral levels). The cord diminishes in overall thickness toward its caudal end, as the number of processes in the white matter diminishes.

• **The vertebral column extends caudally beyond the spinal cord.** The spinal cord and vertebral column initially form in concert with each other, with the cord extending the full length of the vertebral column and all spinal nerves forming in line with the intervertebral spaces through which they exit. (You can review these relationships in Chap. 7 on skeletal system development.) However, during the fetal period, the vertebral column continues to lengthen more than the forming spinal cord. By birth, the spinal cord terminates at the L2-3 vertebral level. The most caudal spinal nerves must therefore lengthen during the fetal period to accommodate the ever increasing distance to their point of exit between vertebrae. These nerves form a flowing *cauda equina* ("horse's tail") leading away from the end of the spinal cord.

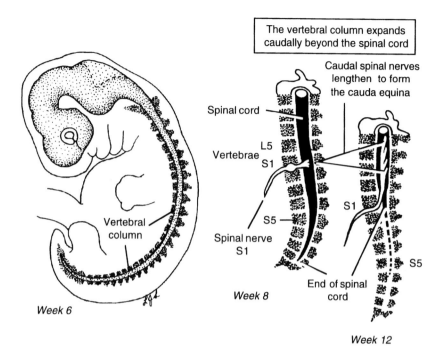

The vertebral column expands caudally beyond the spinal cord

Spinal cord

Caudal spinal nerves lengthen to form the cauda equina

Vertebrae L5 S1

Vertebral column

S5

S1

Spinal nerve S1

S1

Week 8

End of spinal cord

Week 6

S5

Week 12

The basic plan of the neural tube is preserved in the mature spinal cord

Dorsal roof plate

Central canal

Mantle zone

Marginal zone

Ventral fissure

Ventral floor plate

Cross sections of the mature spinal cord at different levels

Cervical

Thoracic

Lumbar

Sacral

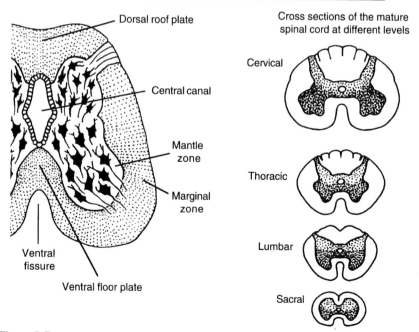

Figure 9-7
Formation of the spinal cord.

159

• **Specialized regions develop in the mantle and marginal zones of each horn in the spinal cord (see Fig. 9-8).**

The *dorsal alar plate* is the sensory horn of the spinal cord.

Nerve cell bodies in the dorsal mantle zone differentiate into *interneurons*, or *association neurons*, which receive the first input from sensory neurons located in the PNS. The white matter of the marginal zone is formed by the processes of these PNS afferent, or sensory nerves, as they enter the dorsal side of the spinal cord, and by the processes of interneurons as they grow up the spinal cord to synapse with higher level interneurons. The afferent association neurons are classified into two functional categories: *general somatic afferents (GSA)* from the soma, or body, and *general visceral afferents (GVA)* from internal viscera.

The *ventral basal plate* is the motor horn of the spinal cord.

The ventral mantle zone contains nerve cell bodies that differentiate into efferent or motor neurons. These are voluntary motor neurons to skeletal muscle, classified as *general somatic efferents (GSE)*. In addition, at most levels in the spinal cord, a group of ventral horn motor neurons form a small region of their own between the dorsal and ventral horns called the *intermediolateral plate*, or *lateral horn*. These cells become autonomic, or involuntary, motor neurons to internal viscera, classified as *general visceral efferents (GVE)*. The ventral marginal zone becomes filled with processes of those motor neurons as they leave the spinal cord ventrally, as well as processes of nerves that originate in the higher centers of the brain, and grow down to synapse with these motor neurons. The association interneurons also extend processes to synapse with the motor neurons to form a simple reflex arc.

• **Spinal nerves form along the length of the spinal cord.**   Spinal nerves are formed by the merger of the *dorsal sensory nerve roots* and the *ventral motor nerve roots* just outside the spinal cord. Thus, they all contain a mixture of sensory and motor nerve processes. The nerve roots enter and exit continuously along the cord; they clump into segmented spinal roots due to signals from the surrounding segmented sclerotomal mesoderm.

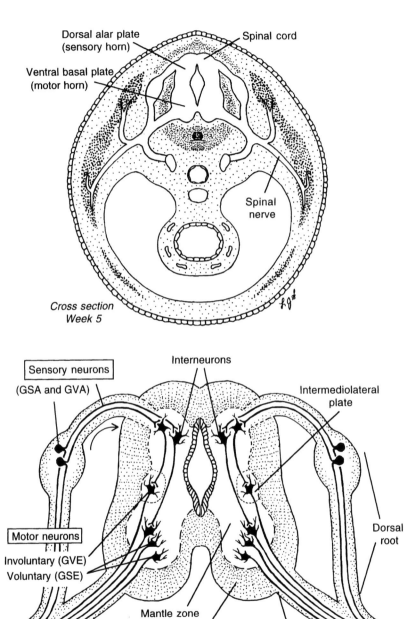

Figure 9-8
Formation of regions of the spinal cord.

Brain formation

• **The original organization of the neural tube is altered in the formation of many regions of the brain.**   The three basic layers formed across the width of the neural tube become altered in many parts of the brain (see Fig. 9-9). The alar plates are moved almost lateral to the basal plates in many regions. In some regions the basal plates largely disappear. In addition, extra layers of neurons are formed in "higher centers" of the brain, adding a gray matter cortex outside the white matter of the marginal layer.

• **Nerve cells form concentrated collections called nuclei in the brain.**   Just as in the spinal cord, sensory (association) nerves develop in the alar plates and motor nerves develop in the basal plates. Some coalesce to form nuclei for *cranial nerves*. Special functional categories of neurons form in the brain in addition to those also formed in the spinal cord. Special cranial categories include *special somatic afferents (SSA)* to receive input from the "special" body senses of sight and sound, *special visceral afferents (SVA)* to receive input from "special" visceral senses of smell and taste, and *special visceral efferents (SVE)*, which innervate the "special" skeletal muscles formed in the pharyngeal arches (at one time thought to be derived from special visceral mesodermal sources).

In addition to these cranial nerve nuclei, a number of nuclei form within the brain which serve as synaptic relay stations between different regions. You will need to know many of these nuclei for neuroanatomy; only some of the most important are mentioned in the following sections. If this is a level of detail you do not need, don't worry about it.

• **Dilations of the central lumen form ventricles in the brain.**   The central lumen of the neural tube assumes several different shapes in the brain. Where the lumen becomes expanded, it forms ventricles. The ventricles are connected to each other by narrow interventricular channels. Unfortunately, you must learn a different name for each of these regions.

• **The central lumen of the CNS become filled with cerebrospinal fluid secreted by choroid plexuses formed in the brain.**   Choroid plexuses are formed in the walls of all the ventricles, in regions where the wall consists only of the ependymal lining. Overlying blood vessels proliferate and push the ependyma ahead of them into the ventricular cavities, forming choroid plexuses. The plexuses produce and release cerebrospinal fluid into the ventricles.

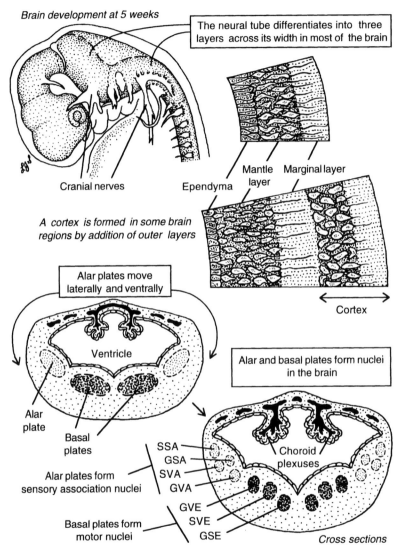

Brain development at 5 weeks

The neural tube differentiates into three layers across its width in most of the brain

Cranial nerves   Ependyma   Mantle   Marginal layer
                                                 layer

A cortex is formed in some brain regions by addition of outer layers

Alar plates move laterally and ventrally

Cortex

Ventricle

Alar and basal plates form nuclei in the brain

Alar plate

Basal plates

Alar plates form sensory association nuclei

Basal plates form motor nuclei

SSA
GSA
SVA
GVA
GVE
SVE
GSE

Choroid plexuses

Cross sections

Figure 9-9
Development of specializations within the brain.

• BRAIN SUBDIVISIONS BEGIN TO APPEAR WEEK 5
• Formation of brain flexures is the first sign of subdivision (see Fig. 9-10).
The brain region bends, or flexes, at three points. Beginning in week 4, it flexes
ventrally at two points, curling the forming brain under the rest of the neural tube
to form an exaggerated C shape. The *cranial*, or *cephalic*, *flexure* extends
throughout the length of the future midbrain region. The *cervical flexure* forms
caudal to it, at the junction of the brain with the spinal cord. In week 5, the *pontine flexure* begins between the other two flexures. It is actually a reverse, or dorsal, flexure, folding the brain back on itself.

**• Five separate regions become distinguishable in the brain as the neural
tube expands to form five vesicles along its length.**   Three primary brain vesicles form initially. Two of these vesicles become further subdivided, to form a
total of five secondary brain vesicles. Each vesicle gives rise to specific regions
of the mature brain (see Table 9-1).

• All regions of the central lumen have different names.   The lumen within
the forebrain telencephalon on each side dilates to form the *lateral ventricles*
(which can be considered the first and second ventricles). Narrow *interventricular foramina of Monro* lead into the single *third ventricle* in the diencephalon
region of the forebrain. This leads into the narrow lumen of the midbrain, called
the *aqueduct of Sylvius*, which leads into the *fourth ventricle* in the hindbrain.
This, in turn, leads into the *central canal* of the spinal cord.

• The brain vesicles develop into brainstem and higher centers.   The central
"stem" of the neural tube is retained through the length of the brain. Its deriva-

TABLE 9-1
BRAIN SUBDIVISIONS

PRIMARY BRAIN VESICLES	SECONDARY BRAIN VESICLES	MATURE BRAIN REGIONS
Forebrain prosencephalon	Diencephalon	Thalamus, hypothalamus pituitary, etc.
	Telencephalon	Cerebrum
Midbrain mesencephalon		Colliculi, etc.
Hindbrain rhombencephalon	Myelencephalon Metencephalon	Medulla oblongata Pons, cerebellum

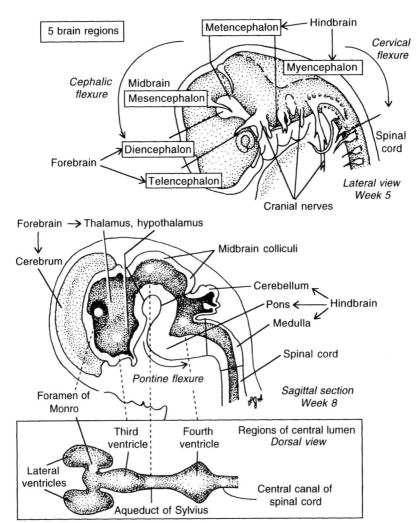

Figure 9-10
Formation of the first brain regions.

tives form the brainstem, which retains an organization similar to the spinal cord—the hindbrain *medulla* and *pons*, the *midbrain*, and the forebrain *diencephalon*. By contrast, two of the secondary vesicles form outgrowths from the brainstem, which become "higher centers" of the brain—the hindbrain *cerebellum* and forebrain *cerebrum*. They each produce an outer, neuron-rich *cortex*, which integrates and coordinates functions of the brain.

Formation of specific brain regions

The following sections contain a number of specifics, under the assumption that you will need to know these details to correlate the embryogenesis of the brain with its mature anatomy. If this is not the case, concentrate simply on learning the different regions of the brain that form from each of its embryonic subdivisions. The following regions are described from caudal to cranial ends of the brain.

• **The hindbrain (rhombencephalon) becomes divided into two regions: myelencephalon and metencephalon (see Fig. 9-11).** Differentiation of the neural tube begins in the hindbrain region. Its more caudal myelencephalon region forms the brainstem medulla, while its more cranial metencephalon region forms the brainstem pons and the cerebellar higher brain center. The pontine flexure folds the length of the pons back on itself dorsally. Another important feature of the hindbrain is that most of the cranial nerve nuclei (4 to 12) are formed here, although a few (4 and part of 5) later migrate to the midbrain. (See the end of this chapter for a detailed description of cranial nerves.)

> The hindbrain myelencephalon forms the medulla oblongata.

The medulla oblongata is the transition from the spinal cord and retains a functional and structural organization similar to that of the spinal cord. The major alteration is that its walls and central lumen expand laterally, creating the fourth ventricle. The dorsal roof overlying the ventricle becomes stretched out into a broad thin alar roof plate. This lateral expansion causes the forming alar nuclei and tracts of nerve processes to be displaced, so they come to lie almost lateral to the basal plate and ventral to the ventricle. These nuclei include special categories (SVA and SVE) found only in the brain. In addition, cells of the alar plate migrate into the ventral plate to form a series of nuclei (collectively called the *olivary nuclei*), which serve as synaptic relay stations to the cerebellum from above and below. Finally, choroid plexuses form in the roof of the fourth ventricle, as they do in all ventricles.

> The medulla oblongata is a relay center for fiber tracts running in both directions between the spinal cord and brain. It contains nuclei that relay sensory input to the cerebellum (particularly hearing) and regulate autonomic (involuntary) motor regulation of heart rate and respiration. Four cranial nerve nuclei are formed here (9 to 12).

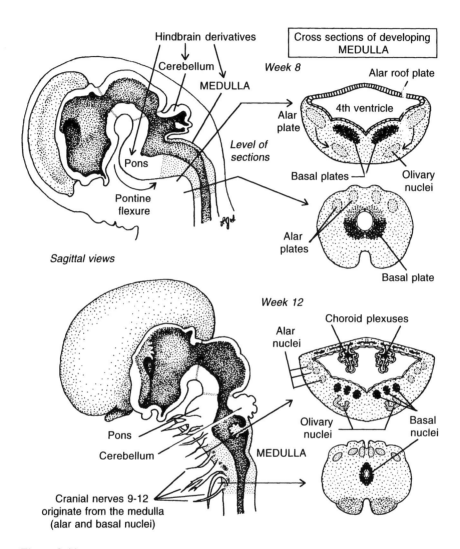

Figure 9-11
The myelencephalon forms the medulla oblongata.

The hindbrain metencephalon forms the pons and cerebellum (see Fig. 9-12).

The pons (or "bridge") forms as the cranial extension of the myelencephalon. The pons contains a number of nerve fiber tracts organized like the more caudal myelencephalon and spinal cord. Most tracts form in the basal plate. In addition, several important relay nuclei (pontine) are formed in the alar plate and migrate into the ventral plate during development. The fourth ventricle continues through the pons. The morphology of this region is dramatically changed by the pontine flexure, which flexes the pons back on itself. The roof of the caudal part of the pons expands to form a broad thin roof plate like that of the medulla.

The pons contains fiber tracts that relay input between the higher cortical centers of the cerebrum and cerebellum and then relays input between these centers and the spinal cord. It also contains pontine nuclei that serve as relay stations for some of these fiber tracts. Cranial nerve nuclei are located here for nerves 5 to 8.

The cranial end of the hindbrain metencephalon expands outwards to form the cerebellum.

The cerebellum is formed as a dorsal outgrowth from the cranial end of the pons by adding more cell layers and by elaborate remodeling of the basic neural tube organization. Along with the cerebrum, it becomes a higher center of the brain. Development in the fetal period includes the generation and differentiation of many cortical neuron layers, but development continues even after birth.

The cerebellum is formed by specialization of the widely separated dorsal alar plates. In the future cerebellar region, these alar plates thicken and bend internally to form dorsal "*rhombic lips.*" They form two cerebellar hemispheres, which overhang the pons and medulla. The hemispheres remain connected across the midline by the *vermis* of the cerebellum.

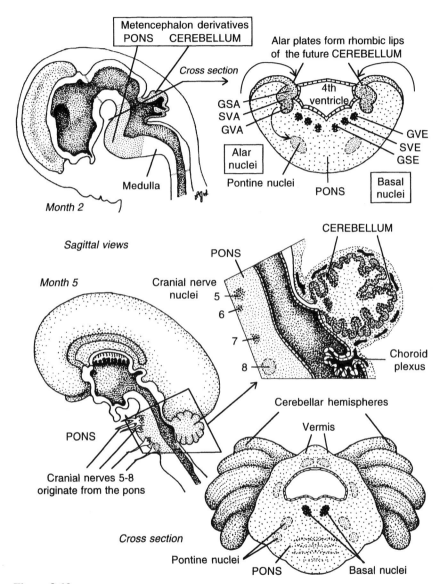

Figure 9-12
Formation of pons and cerebellum from the metencephalon.

• **Formation of the cerebellum (and cerebrum) involves formation of multiple neuronal layers in the cortex.** Initially these higher centers of the brain consist of the typical ventricular, mantle, and marginal zones, but then something different happens: there is a second wave of proliferation from the inner ventricular layer, turning it into the inner germinal layer (see Fig. 9-13). Some cells of the internal germinal layer migrate to form four deep cerebellar nuclei in each hemisphere. These nuclei relay input to and from the cerebellar cortex. Other cells migrate through the marginal layer to form the *external granular*, or *germinal*, *layer*, which will give rise to several superficial layers of neurons that will form the *cerebellar cortex*. As some of these neurons migrate, they leave an axon connected with the deep cerebellar nuclei.

• **Glia play a prominent role in migration of cortical neurons.** Glia are produced from both the inner and outer germinal layers, as are neurons. *Radial* glia are necessary for guidance of the majority of neurons to their destinations. They extend their processes from their origins in the inner germinal layer through the thickness of the neural tube to the periphery. Postmitotic neuroblasts then wrap around these glial processes and migrate out along them to their target layers of the brain.

• **The external cortical neurons become arranged in layers.** The neurons differentiate in the cortex to form several layers: the innermost granule layer (containing Golgi, granule, and stellate neurons), the intermediate Purkinje layer (containing Purkinje neurons), and the closely associated outermost molecular layer (containing basket and stellate neurons).

• **The cerebellar hemispheres undergo extensive folding.** Primary fissures form cranial and caudal lobes. Secondary fissures divided them into *lobules*. The surfaces of the lobules are thrown into transverse gyri called *folia*. This process increases the surface area of the cerebellar cortex.

The cerebellum is one of two higher centers in the brain. It is a coordination center for posture, movement, balance, and hearing. Its interior contains deep cerebellar nuclei that relay signals. Its outermost layers, or cortex, contain many interneurons which coordinate these signals.

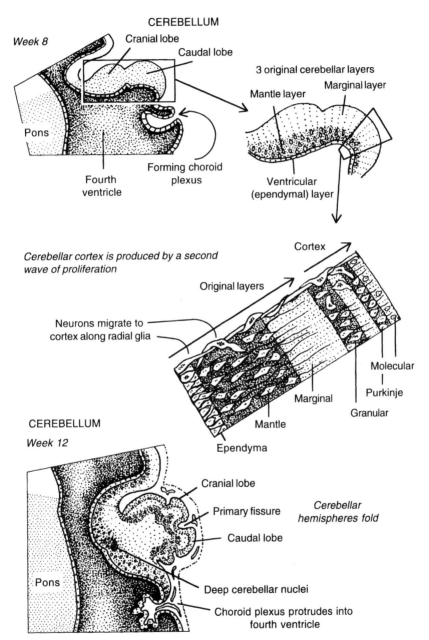

Figure 9-13
Formation of lobes and layers in the cerebellum.

> The midbrain, or mesencephalon, forms a number of brainstem derivatives (see Fig. 9-14).

The midbrain retains the simple undivided organization of the neural tube, with basal and alar regions preserved. It also retains a narrow central lumen, which is called the cerebral aqueduct (of Sylvius). The cephalic flexure extends through the whole midbrain, curving it ventrally.

• **The alar region forms four swellings called the *corpora quadrigemina*.** These dorsal swellings form the inferior (caudal) and superior (cranial) colliculi. Nuclei form within the colliculi, providing a synaptic relay station for sensory input to the cerebral cortex. Cells of the alar plate migrate into the ventral basal region to form several relay nuclei.

• **The ventral basal region forms gray matter in the tegmentum and white matter in the cerebral peduncles.** The cerebral peduncles contain fiber tracts that descend from the cerebral cortex to the cerebellum and spinal cord. The tegmentum contains the motor nuclei of cranial nerves 3 and 4. Only the motor nuclei of cranial nerves 3 originate there; the nuclei of nerves 4 migrate forward into the midbrain from their metencephalic origins. In addition, a sensory nucleus for cranial nerve 5 migrates into the basal region from its origin in the metencephalon. The basal region also contains two prominent relay nuclei. The *red nucleus* is formed there, while the *substantia nigra* migrates to the basal region from its origins in the alar region.

> The midbrain forms part of the brainstem. It is primarily a relay center that contains large numbers of fiber tracts, as well as many relay nuclei for auditory and visual systems in the colliculi of the alar region (which send input to the cerebral cortex). Cranial nerve motor nuclei for nerves 3 and 4 and sensory nuclei for nerve 5 are located here.

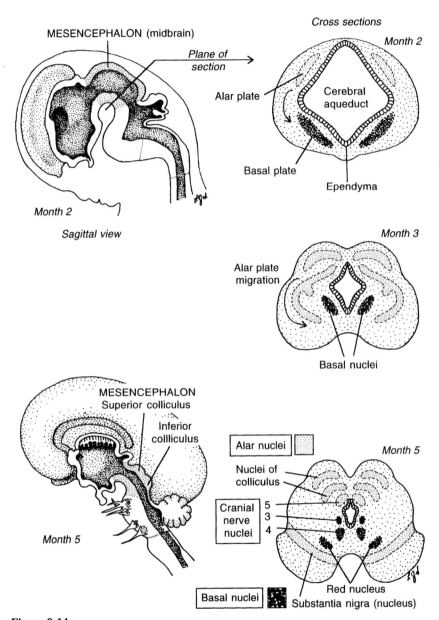

Figure 9-14
The many brainstem derivatives of the mesencephalon.

• **The forebrain subdivides into the diencephalon and telencephalon (see Fig. 9-15).**   The complex morphology of the mature derivatives of the forebrain is believed to originate from the same alar and basal plate configuration found throughout the rest of the neural tube. However, *in the forebrain, alar plates remain prominent, but the basal plates regress.* Bear this basic fact in mind as you read through the following details of the forebrain derivatives.

The diencephalon forms the midline brainstem portion of the forebrain, which connects the midbrain to the telencephalon. The telencephalon forms bilateral outgrowths from the diencephelon, which become the cerebral hemispheres.

The diencephalon forms a number of important brainstem regions from its alar plates, which contain relay nuclei.

The alar plates are displaced laterally by the expansion of the third ventricle. A number of regions are formed in the alar plates whose nuclei serve as relay stations between the cerebral hemispheres and all the lower parts of the nervous system (and they all have their own names). The *thalamus* and *epithalamus* form from the dorsal region of the alar plates. A midline diverticulum of the roof of the epithalamus then forms the *epiphysis*, or pineal body. The *hypothalamus* forms from the more ventral region of the alar plates. The *pituitary gland* is formed by a downgrowth of the hypothalamus fusing with an upgrowth of pharyngeal ectoderm.

The central lumen of the diencephalon dilates to form the third ventricle. In addition to a choroid plexus, the ependyma of this region also forms secretory structures called *circumventricular organs*, which add neuropeptides to the cerebrospinal fluid.

• **The only cranial nerves formed in the diencephalon are the optic nerves (cranial nerves 2).**   The optic nerves are the only cranial nerves that are formed completely from an extension of part of the neural tube wall—lateral outpocketings of the diencephalon called *optic vesicles*. (The formation of all components of the eye is covered more fully in Chap. 10.)

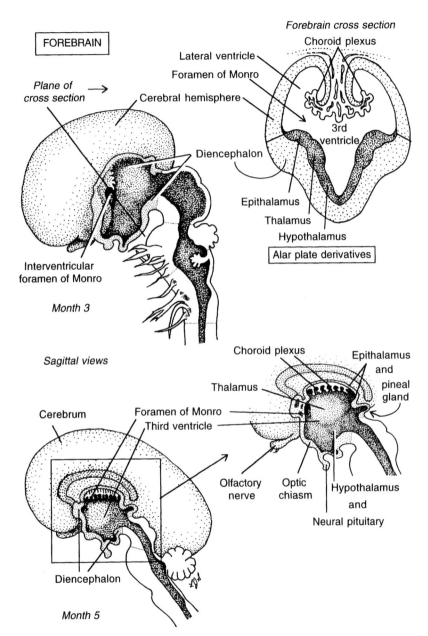

Figure 9-15
Diencephalon derivatives.

> The pituitary forms as an extension of the hypothalamus (see Fig. 9-16).

The pituitary or hypophysis is a neuroendocrine organ, formed by neural and endocrine gland contributions derived from two separate germ layers. A downgrowth of the forming hypothalamus, called the *infundibulum* (neuroectoderm) meets an upgrowth of the lining of the pharyngeal gut tube (ectoderm). Hypothalamic neurons send processes into the infundibulum to form the neural lobe of the pituitary, variously called the *neurohypophysis*, *posterior lobe*, or *pars nervosa*.

The endocrine portion is formed by an upgrowth of the ectoderm from the roof of the forming mouth, called *Rathke's pouch*. It partially cups around the neural infundibulum, and then loses its connection to the mouth. The endocrine or glandular portion of the pituitary is the *adenohypophysis*, or *anterior lobe*. The origins of the pituitary gland are covered in more detail in Chapter 16.

• Functions of mature derivatives of the diencephalon.

> The thalamus is the largest derivative of the diencephalon. It is the relay center for the cerebral cortex. It receives all input projecting to the cortex from below in its many nuclei, and relays it to appropriate cortical areas.
>
> The epithalamus contains nuclei which relay olfactory input to cerebral centers.
>
> The pineal body, which forms as an extension of the epithalamus, contains neurosecretory cells which regulate daily (circadian) rhythms by secreting melatonin.
>
> The hypothalamus contains many nuclei receiving input from many CNS areas. It regulates autonomic visceral functions (including sleep, body temperature, digestion). It also regulates endocrine secretions of the pituitary gland, which forms in part as a diverticulum of the hypothalamus.
>
> The optic nerves (cranial nerves 2) form entirely as a direct outgrowth of the diencephalon.

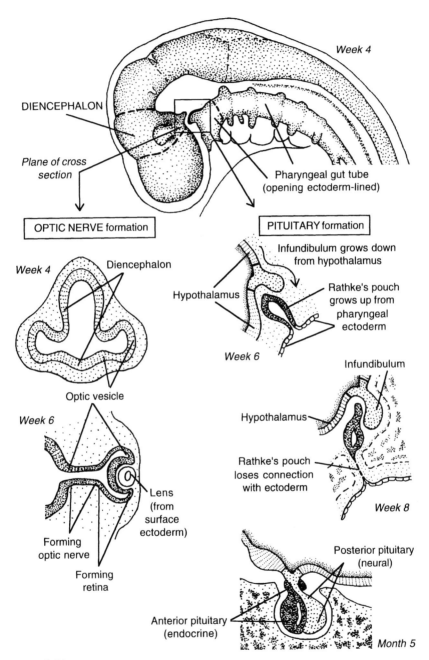

Figure 9-16
Pituitary and optic nerve development from diencephalon.

> The telencephalon forms the cerebral hemispheres by bilateral expansions (see Fig. 9-17).

The telencephalic vesicles grow in thickness and bulge into the lumen of the third ventricle lateral to the thalamus. The floor of each telencephalic vesicle thickens to form the *corpus striatum*. The corpus striatum will contain important groups of nerve cells, or nuclei, called *basal ganglia*, which serve as synaptic relay stations to and from the cerebral cortex. As the hemispheres grow, they press against the diencephalon internally. Meninges between the two disappear, so the thalamus becomes continuous with the floor of each cerebral hemisphere. This border is eventually crossed by a prominent fiber bundle called the *internal capsule*, which carries fibers between the thalamus and the cerebral cortex. Eventually the hemispheres hang over the diencephalon and mesencephalon.

• **Commissures develop that connect the two hemispheres.**   The two hemispheres remain connected to each other across the midline during their development. This connection becomes invaded by nerve fibers that cross-connect the two hemispheres, forming commissures. They include the long *corpus callosum* and the more compact *anterior* and *posterior commissures.*

• **Functions of the mature cerebral derivatives of the telencephalon include the following.**

> Nerve cell nuclei serve as synaptic relay stations between cerebral neurons and other parts of the nervous system. The fibers of these cerebral neurons then contribute to the fiber tracts of the brain.
>
> Projection fibers connect cerebral cortical neurons with neurons from other portions of the brain and spinal cord.
>
> Association fibers interconnect cortical neurons of the same hemisphere.
>
> Commissural fibers interconnect corresponding cortical regions of the two hemispheres.

Collectively, these interconnections integrate the information relayed by projection fibers, forming the basis for intelligence and memory.

• **Lateral ventricles form within each cerebral hemisphere.**   These ventricles open into the third ventricle via narrow interventricular *foramina (of Monro)*. A choroid plexus forms in each lateral ventricle.

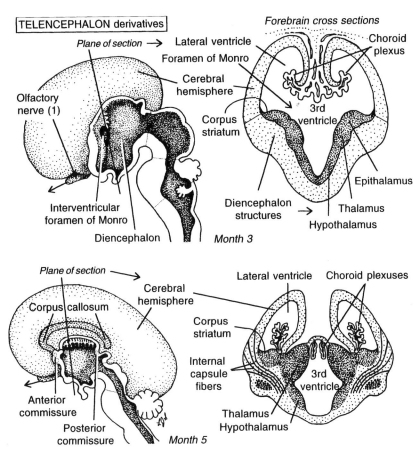

Figure 9-17
The telencephalon forms the cerebral hemispheres.

• **The only cranial nerves associated with the telencephalon are the olfactory nerves (cranial nerve 1).** The olfactory nerves form in a unique way from a combination of ingrowths from *nasal placodes* meeting outgrowths from the telencephalon (olfactory bulbs). Nasal placodes are formed by ectoderm, which generate primary sensory neuroblasts which extend axons into the olfactory bulbs on each side to synapse with secondary (or association) olfactory sensory neurons formed in these bulbs.

• **The cerebral cortex forms from the addition of multiple neuronal layers as in the cerebellum.** The inner germinal (ventricular) layer of the telencephalon generates cells that migrate in waves to form the cortex in a similar fashion to that already described for the formation of the cerebellar cortex (see Fig. 9-18). The waves of neuroblast migration from the ventricular zone form several layers between it and the superficial marginal zone. These layers, or zones, are, from deep to superficial, the *subventricular zone*, the *intermediate zone*, the *subplate zone*, and the *cortical plate zone*. The subventricular zone transiently serves as a staging ground to generate more neuroblasts, which migrate to form the cortical plate. The intermediate zone becomes a white layer (nerve fibers), as does the outer marginal zone, which becomes the molecular layer. The submarginal zones (the cortical plate plus the subplate) give rise to the cerebral cortex neuronal layers, which are now called the *neocortex*. It contains as many as six neuronal layers.

• **Forming multiple synaptic connections is important to the development of the brain.** Proper development of the nervous system involves the establishment of proper synapses between neurons. This is particularly relevant in the formation of the cortical areas of the brain, since thousands of synapses form on a single neuron in these cortical areas. These multiple synapses are necessary to form all the associations between functions, which are processed by the higher centers of the brain. The formation of synapses continues throughout the fetal period into the neonatal period.

• **The cerebral hemispheres fold into lobes and gyri.** As each hemisphere grows through the fetal period, it subdivides into *temporal*, *frontal*, and *parietal lobes*. Deep clefts called *sulci* separate some lobes. Hemisphere folding begins at 14 weeks. Convolutions called *gyri* appear between 6 and 8 months, massively increasing cortical surface area. Most of the substantial growth of the brain that occurs after birth is due to the myelination of its many processes. Nerve processes that require myelination do not function until it is completed, so delay or interference in myelination can delay (or stop) onset of function.

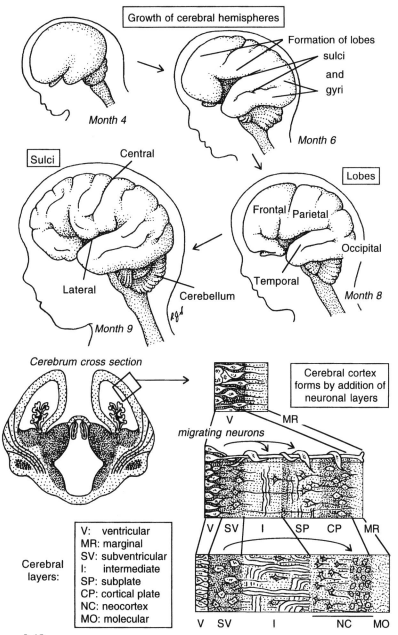

Figure 9-18
Cerebral cortex formation.

> Meninges form a protective coating around the entire CNS.

The CNS is protected by three layers of connective tissue which cover the outer surface of the brain and spinal cord. Collectively, they are referred to as the meninges (see Fig. 9-19). The tough outer coat is called the *dura mater*. It is separated by a subdural space from the middle layer, the *arachnoid*. This layer is configured like Swiss cheese: a continuous outer layer gives rise to a series of trabeculae, or branches, which extend across the subarachnoid space to contact the innermost pia mater layer. The *pia* is a thin layer, containing many blood vessels, which is closely applied to the outer surface of the whole CNS. The pia also surrounds all blood vessels as they enter or leave the CNS, down to the point at which they branch to form capillaries.

The subarachnoid space is filled with cerebrospinal fluid, forming a protective cushion for the brain. The fluid continuously enters from several points of contact with ventricular lumens and exits into the venous drainage system at specific points of contact.

> *Hydrocephalus* ("water brain") develops when blockages cause excess cerebrospinal fluid to build up within the developing brain ventricles. When this happens during embryonic development, the excess fluid pressure inhibits further forebrain tissue development, while the ventricles expand the brain enormously. Blockages can occur in the narrow channels between ventricles (most commonly the cerebral aqueduct) or at the points of fluid entrance or exit from the subarachnoid space.

• **The meninges originate from two sources: neural crest and mesoderm.** The outer dura is derived exclusively from the mesoderm surrounding the forming neural tube. The arachnoid and pia are also derived from the same mesoderm around the spinal cord and the more caudal portions of the brain. However, neural crest cells form the most cranial portions of arachnoid and pia, just as they form other connective tissues in the head. These layers merge into the connective tissue coat around the PNS components at each point where a nerve leaves or enters the CNS.

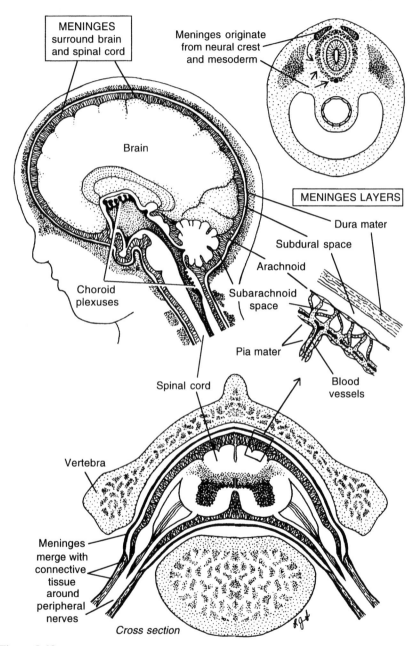

MENINGES
surround brain
and spinal cord

Meninges originate
from neural crest
and mesoderm

Brain

MENINGES LAYERS

Dura mater

Subdural space

Arachnoid

Choroid
plexuses

Subarachnoid
space

Pia mater

Blood
vessels

Spinal cord

Vertebra

Meninges
merge with
connective
tissue
around
peripheral
nerves

Cross section

Figure 9-19
Origin and structure of meninges.

Congenital defects of the central nervous system

• **Mental retardation may occur without any morphologically detectable brain abnormalities.** Retardation can be caused by factors that interfere with neuronal proliferation, synapse formation, or myelination. Many infectious agents have been implicated, but a primary cause of retardation is maternal alcohol abuse, resulting in a spectrum of defects called *fetal alcohol syndrome*.

• **Gross morphologic defects in formation of the CNS.** Defects in formation of the spinal cord and brain often involve defects in vertebral or skull formation (see Fig. 9-20). Many defects are initiated at the ends of the neural tube in the regions where it closes (neuropores). These defects can be caused by many teratogenic factors, including exposure to excess vitamin A, hyperthermia (as a result of maternal infection and fever), or excess glucose levels (as a result of maternal diabetes).

• **Defects in the region of the posterior or caudal neuropore.** *Spina bifida* refers to a spectrum of defects in which the left and right portions of one or more vertebrae fail to fuse dorsally with each other, leaving the spinal cord and its covering meninges exposed. *Spina bifida occulta* is the mildest defect in this spectrum: only vertebrae are involved. *Spina bifida cystica* collectively covers the more severe forms of this defect, in which the neural tube and/or meninges protrude through the vertebral defect(s) to form cystlike sacs, or *celes*. Cysts containing meninges only are called *meningoceles*. Cysts also containing portions of the spinal cord are called *meningomyeloceles*. This usually results in neurological deficits. The most serious deficit occurs if this same stretch of the neural folds fails to fuse into a tube (*rachischisis*), since the neural tissue fails to differentiate from here caudally.

• **Defects in the region of the anterior, or cranial, neuropore.** The same spectrum of defects can occur at the cranial end of the neural tube, with generally more devastating consequences since the brain and skull are involved. *Meningoencephalocele* occurs when brain tissue is herniated into cysts, usually protruding through defects in the occipital bone, near the base of the skull. *Meningohydroencephalocele* occurs when brain tissue and its ventricular lumen are herniated. These herniated regions do not develop normally. *Anencephaly* ("lack of brain") occurs when the forebrain neural folds fail to fuse. Neural tissue fails to differentiate, and the vault of the skull does not close over it.

• **Cerebellar defects.** Cerebellar underdevelopment (*hypoplasia*) or abnormal development (*dysplasia*) may produce no clinical signs or may cause *cerebellar ataxias*—abnormal coordination of movement, speech, etc. Many of these defects are caused by chromosomal anomalies, particularly trisomies (three copies) of chromosomes 13, 18, or 21.

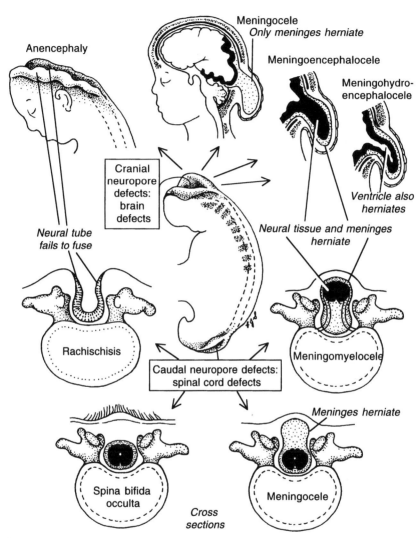

Figure 9-20
Congenital defects of the CNS.

PERIPHERAL NERVOUS SYSTEM DEVELOPMENT

Events in early formation

The PNS consists of the neural tissue outside the CNS, or at the "periphery" of the body (see Fig. 9-21). It contains nerve cell groupings, which, along with their support cells, are called *ganglia*. It also contains nerve cell processes bound together by support cells to form *peripheral nerves*. The ganglia are part of the sensory and autonomic motor arms of the nervous system.

Neural crest forms most of the PNS.

Neural crest migrates to target locations before differentiating. Commitment to its fate usually occurs during or after migration as a result of signals received along the way or at the target. In the head, however, neural crest appears to be committed to its specific fate as it is generated. Neural crest differentiates into all nerve cells in the PNS, and most of their support cells.

Two major functional types of ganglia form in the PNS: sensory and autonomic (or involuntary) motor ganglia.

Sensory neurons receive input from all parts of the body and transmit it to the CNS. Autonomic motor neurons transmit output from the CNS to internal viscera over which the individual has no voluntary control. Ganglia are formed at most levels along the neural tube.

The support cells of the PNS are derived from both neural crest and mesoderm.

The support cells of the PNS have functions that parallel those performed by the glial cells in the CNS. However, they are different cell types, which means you need to learn more names. The support cells formed by neural crest include *satellite cells* and *Schwann cells*. Satellite cells encircle the nerve cell bodies in all peripheral ganglia. Schwann cells wrap around all nerve processes in the PNS and myelinate any processes which require it. Thus, the nerve process of a single neuron can be surrounded by oligodendrocytes in the CNS and Schwann cells in the PNS. Schwann cells also play a role in the embryonic outgrowth of nerve cell

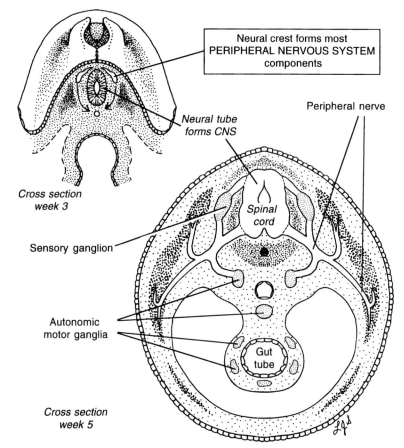

Neural crest forms most
PERIPHERAL NERVOUS SYSTEM
components

Neural tube
forms CNS

Peripheral nerve

Cross section
week 3

Spinal
cord

Sensory ganglion

Autonomic
motor ganglia

Gut
tube

Cross section
week 5

Figure 9-21
Origins of components of the PNS.

processes, much as radial glia do in the CNS. All other PNS support cells are connective tissue fibroblasts formed by invading lateral plate mesoderm.

Peripheral nerves are formed by collections of nerve cell processes and their
surrounding support cells.

The peripheral nerves contain processes of nerve cells housed in the PNS
ganglia, as well as processes of many CNS neurons, chief among them those of
the voluntary motor neurons. Peripheral nerves contain no nerve cell bodies, only
those of support cells.

Autonomic nervous system components in the peripheral nervous system

The autonomic nervous system is the motor component that regulates involuntary functions of internal, or visceral, organs. Regulation of autonomic functions in the brain is largely in the hypothalamus, as part of its oversight of most vegetative functions (see Fig. 9-22). Autonomic input regulates the rate of contraction of three types of muscle to maximize their performance: smooth muscle, cardiac muscle, and myoepithelial muscle components. These muscle types use neural input to modulate their rate of contraction. Smooth muscle controls functions such as motility in the gastrointestinal tract and blood vessel diameter. Cardiac muscle contraction controls heart rate. Myoepithelial cells surround glandular epithelial cells; their contraction causes glandular secretion.

• **The autonomic system consists of two arms: the sympathetic and the parasympathetic.** These two arms of the system generally have antagonistic functions to each other. In general, sympathetic components increase functions involved in the "flight or fight" response, while parasympathetic components promote relaxation and "basal metabolism" functions. Most viscera have a dual innervation. The exceptions are the smooth muscle of blood vessels and the myoepithelia of sweat glands and arrector pili, which receive sympathetic innervation alone.

• **The autonomic system consists of a two-neuron pathway that starts in the CNS and terminates in the PNS.** The first, or *preganglionic*, nerve cell is in the intermediolateral part of the ventral horn in the CNS. This nerve cell's axonal process leaves the CNS with axons of voluntary motor neurons, where they become incorporated into the forming peripheral nerves. The autonomic fiber leaves the nerve to grow toward its developing target—the second, or ganglionic, nerve cell—which is clumped with others in autonomic ganglia in the PNS. These ganglia are all formed by neural crest cells. The axons of these second cells, called *postganglionic* processes, grow out to their target muscle tissues (smooth, cardiac, or myoepithelia).

• **Contrast the two-neuron pathway of the autonomic system with the one-neuron pathway of the voluntary motor system.** Axonal processes of voluntary motor neurons in the ventral horn of the CNS grow out into the PNS to synapse *directly* with their skeletal muscle targets. Both systems are directed from higher neuronal centers in the brain, which send processes down to synapse with these "lower motor neurons."

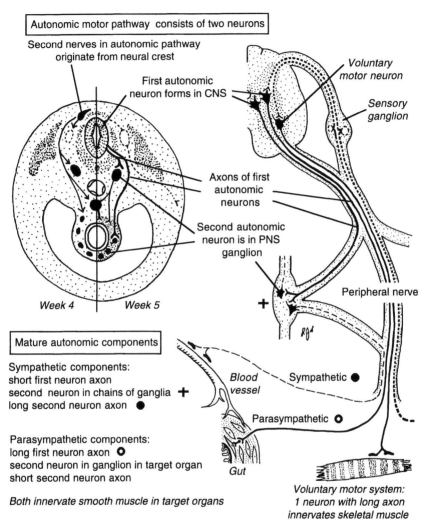

Autonomic motor pathway consists of two neurons

Second nerves in autonomic pathway originate from neural crest

First autonomic neuron forms in CNS

Voluntary motor neuron

Sensory ganglion

Axons of first autonomic neurons

Second autonomic neuron is in PNS ganglion

Peripheral nerve

Week 4   Week 5

Mature autonomic components

Sympathetic components:
short first neuron axon
second neuron in chains of ganglia +
long second neuron axon ●

Parasympathetic components:
long first neuron axon O
second neuron in ganglion in target organ
short second neuron axon

Both innervate smooth muscle in target organs

Blood vessel

Gut

Sympathetic ●

Parasympathetic O

*Voluntary motor system:
1 neuron with long axon
innervates skeletal muscle*

Figure 9-22
Origins of the autonomic motor system.

> Formation of the sympathetic component in the PNS involves formation of chain ganglia close to the vertebral column.

The primary nerves in the sympathetic system reside exclusively at the thoracic through lumbar levels of the spinal cord (from T1 to L3) (see Fig. 9-23). The secondary neurons with which they synapse are in sympathetic ganglia formed from the neural crest generated at cervical to coccygeal levels along the neural tube. Most of these ganglia are called *chain ganglia* because they form bilateral chains to either side of the vertebrae. A few ganglia that supply parts of the gut (prevertebral ganglia) are formed more ventrally; preganglionic fibers reach them via splanchnic nerves.

The secondary ganglia neurons form long postganglionic processes to cover the great distances to their targets. Many grow out along forming blood vessels, while others reenter spinal nerves for distribution. Since no primary sympathetic neurons originate in the brain, the source of sympathetic innervation in the head is the thoracic level of the spinal cord, which sends fibers to cervical ganglia in the neck, from which long fibers grow into the head.

> The parasympathetic component of the autonomic system has a widely split origin at opposite ends of the CNS.

The primary parasympathetic neurons are located only at cranial and caudal levels of the CNS (see Fig. 9-23). This anatomical separation does not mean that portions of the body go "uncovered" by parasympathetic innervation. Instead, a few long nerves carrying the primary (preganglionic) nerve fibers grow out great distances to a number of small, widely scattered ganglia containing secondary neurons. The ganglia form close to, or within, the walls of the target organs. They are formed from cranial (hindbrain) and caudal (sacral) levels of neural crest which migrate these long distances during development to invade or surround internal viscera.

The cranial primary parasympathetic nerves originate in midbrain and hindbrain nuclei and contribute fibers to four cranial nerves (3, 7, 9, and 10). These nerves innervate structures in the head. In addition, cranial nerve 10 is particularly important because it extends all the way into the body cavity, innervating internal viscera as far as the hindgut. The caudal nerves originate from sacral spinal cord segments 2 to 4. They innervate ganglia in all remaining internal viscera via pelvic splanchnic nerves.

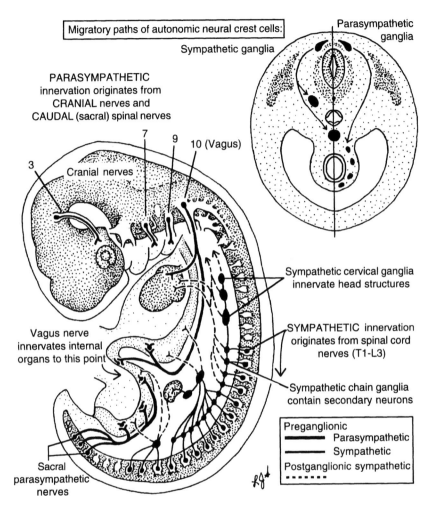

Figure 9-23
Sympathetic and parasympathetic systems.

An often fatal congenital defect called *Hirschsprung's disease* (or *aganglionic colon*) occurs when sacral neural crest fails to migrate to, or invade, part of the colon wall. The resulting absence of parasympathetic innervation of the colon causes an absence of peristalsis in those sections, often leading to fatal obstruction. Only this terminal colon portion of the gastrointestinal tract is affected.

Sensory components in the peripheral nervous system: ganglia

> Spinal, or dorsal root, ganglia are formed by neural crest.

Sensory input to the CNS begins with the sensory nerves whose nerve cell bodies reside in PNS sensory ganglia (see Fig. 9-24). They are called *dorsal root ganglia*, or *spinal ganglia*, because they form toward the dorsal sides of the forming vertebrae, and their axonal processes form the dorsal spinal roots which enter the spinal cord. They synapse with association interneurons in the dorsal horn of the spinal cord. The association nerves will transmit these signals to higher level relay stations in the brain. In addition, the axons of some primary sensory neurons and association neurons will synapse directly with motor neurons to form a simple reflex arc: the basis of the "knee jerk" reflex. The sensory ganglia neurons receive input by extending long dendritic processes to peripheral organs. These sensory processes grow out more slowly and later than do motor neuronal processes and often take advantage of this by growing along the motor processes. This bundles the fibers together to form peripheral nerves, coming and going to the same targets.

> Cranial ganglia neurons have a dual origin from neural crest and ectodermal placodes.

Sensory ganglia are associated with six cranial nerves: 1, 5, and 7 through 10. Most cranial sensory ganglia neurons are derived from a combination of cranial level neural crest and from ectodermal placodes (a unique source). Placodes are derived from cranial ectoderm. They separate from the ectoderm and migrate, often as self-contained vesicles. The factors involved in their induction are not clear. Only nerve 5 is totally crest-derived; only nerves 1 and 8 are totally placode-derived. Okay, you may be wondering, what about the optic nerve (cranial nerve 2)? That nerve is formed entirely by an extension of the forebrain, without any help from PNS ganglia.

The association neurons with which these primary sensory neurons synapse in the brain belong to the "usual suspects" found in the spinal cord levels (GSA and GVA), as well as uniquely cranial types—SVA to the special visceral structures in the head (taste buds) and SSA to the somatic sense organs of smell and hearing.

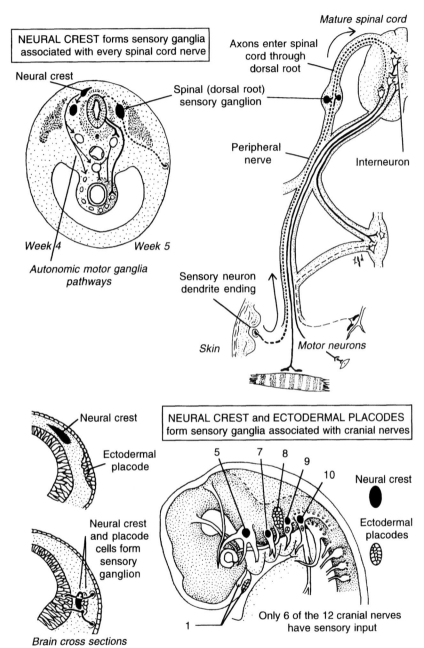

Figure 9-24
Sensory innervation.

Peripheral nerves: collections of nerve fibers and support cells

Peripheral nerves carry the processes of neurons located in the PNS, as well as processes of neurons located in the CNS (see Fig. 9-25). The formation of specific peripheral nerves is not covered here, since they all form by basically the same process. The bundling of fibers into specific nerves is in large part accomplished during the process of outgrowth of those processes toward their targets. The presence of "target" tissues is actually not required at this stage. Instead, the extracellular matrix laid down by both mesodermal cells and some neural crest cells appears to direct the initial outgrowth of "pioneer" neuronal processes. Schwann cell precursors are essential partners in the outgrowth of all neuronal processes. Motor nerve processes grow out first, and then sensory fibers grow out later, along the motor fibers, thus bundling sensory and motor fibers together. Subsequently, peripheral nerves from several levels may clump together into larger nerves. This is particularly prominent in the formation of the *brachial plexus* of nerves growing into the arms and the *lumbosacral plexus* of nerves growing into the legs.

• **Nerves are formed by combination of dorsal and ventral roots.** Dorsal roots are composed of axons of sensory neurons coming into the CNS loaded with information. Ventral roots are composed of axons of motor nerves leaving the CNS for the periphery. The dorsal and ventral roots join together to form a peripheral nerve just outside the spinal cord.

• **Peripheral nerves are formed at spinal and cranial levels.** The nerves that enter or leave the spinal cord are referred to as spinal nerves, while the nerves which enter or leave the brain are referred to as cranial nerves. The 31 spinal nerves are named according to the vertebrae between which they exit or enter: 8 cervical, 12 thoracic, 5 lumbar, 5 sacral, and 1 coccygeal. The 12 cranial nerves are named for the major targets with which they connect.

• **Voluntary motor neurons are represented in the PNS only by nerve fibers.** Unlike the other systems, the voluntary motor system is not represented in the PNS by nerve cells, because the axons of the motor neurons extend out of the CNS directly to their targets. Voluntary motor axons are found in all spinal nerves, but are found in only 9 of the 12 cranial nerves (nerves 3 to 7, 9 to 12).

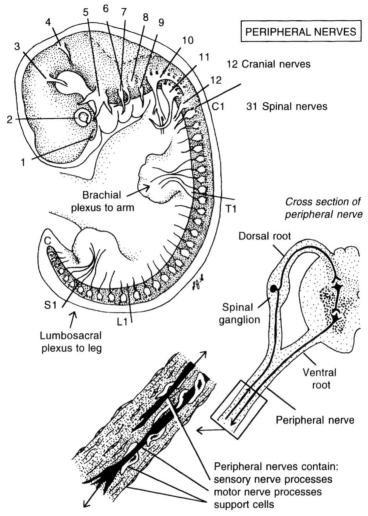

Figure 9-25
Peripheral nerves.

• **Differences in the composition of spinal and cranial peripheral nerves.**

All spinal nerves contain both sensory and voluntary motor fibers.

The major variation in the spinal nerves is whether they contain sympathetic or parasympathetic involuntary fibers. Most spinal nerves contain sympathetic autonomic fibers, while only a few at the caudal end contain parasympathetic fibers.

Cranial nerves are much more heterogeneous in the functional types of fibers they contain than are the spinal nerves.

Each cranial nerve contains a different combination of components, which do not follow any particular sequence. Cranial nerves can contain fibers of voluntary motor and involuntary parasympathetic motor nerves, whose cell bodies reside in nuclei in the brainstem. They can also contain sensory nerve fibers that synapse with sensory association nuclei in the brainstem. The nuclei are located at roughly the same level at which the cranial nerves enter or leave the brainstem. *There are no sympathetic motor fibers in cranial nerves.* Sympathetic innervation of the head comes from motor neurons located in the spinal cord which send axons to the head via cervical chain ganglia.

Many of the sensory and motor fibers in the cranial nerves belong to the "usual suspects" found at spinal cord levels (GSA, GVA, GSE, and GVE). Others belong to the special categories found only in the brain, which were introduced earlier in this chapter. Special visceral efferents supply voluntary motor innervation to "special" skeletal muscles formed in the pharyngeal arches (which were once considered to be derived from "visceral" mesoderm). Two special sensory nerve categories are formed in the brain: SVA and SSA, which innervate special senses in the head (SVA to smell and taste, SSA to sight and hearing).

• **A breakdown of the components of the 12 cranial nerves.**   The following detail is included for those who need it. Cranial nerve 1 (olfactory) is an entirely sensory nerve; its sensory fibers grow into the olfactory tract of the telencephalon. Cranial nerve 2 (optic) is also an entirely sensory nerve, but it originates from the diencephalon as an outgrowth called the *optic cup.* All subsequent cranial nerves originate from midbrain (3) or hindbrain (4 to 12) regions. Cranial nerves 3 and 4 (oculomotor and trochlear) and 6 (abducens) contain voluntary motor nerves that innervate specific extraocular skeletal muscles (to move the eyeball). Nerve 3 also contains parasympathetic nerves to smooth muscles associated with the eye. Nuclei for cranial nerves 4 to 12 originate in the hindbrain. A few migrate to the midbrain (sensory nucleus of cranial nerve 5 and the motor nucleus of nerve 4). Cranial nerve 8 (auditory) is an entirely sensory nerve that receives input from the inner ear. Cranial nerves 5 (trigeminal), 7 (facial), 9 (glossopharyngeal), 10 (vagus), 11 (spinal accessory), and 12 (hypoglossal) innervate structures of the head and neck, with mixtures of nerve types as delineated in the following list. Nerves 5, 7, 9, and 10 innervate structures formed in the pharyngeal arches. This is covered in more detail in Chap. 10 on the head and neck.

1. Nine cranial nerves contain voluntary motor fibers: 3 to 7, and 9 to 12; 4 contain *only* voluntary motor fibers: 4, 6, 11, and 12.
2. Four cranial nerves contain parasympathetic involuntary motor fibers: 3, 7, 9, and 10.
3. Seven cranial nerves contain sensory fibers: 1, 2, 5, 7, and 8 to 10; 3 contain *only* sensory fibers: 1, 2, and 8.
4. Five cranial nerves contain mixed fiber types: 3, 5, 7, 9, and 10.
   a. One contains voluntary and parasympathetic motor fibers: 3.
   b. One contains voluntary motor and sensory fibers: 5.
   c. Three contain all 3 fiber types: 7, 9, and 10.

FORMATION OF HEAD AND NECK

·

·   ·   ·   ·   ·   ·   ·   ·   ·   ·   ·   ·   ·

This chapter ties together the development of the tissues and the organ system components contained in the head and describes the development of features unique to the head and neck. These include the face, the internal features of the mouth (palate and tongue), nose, pharynx, and a number of special organs that develop in the neck (tonsils, thyroid, parathyroid, and thymus). Also covered are the development of the eyes and ears. This chapter builds on the development of component tissues presented in previous chapters—(primarily Chaps. 6, 7, and 8).

COMPONENTS OF THE HEAD

The head can be divided into two regions, the neurocranium and the viscerocranium, based on the major bones of the skull formed in each region (see Fig. 10-1). The neurocranium encases the brain and forms supporting structures for the eyes and ears. The viscerocranium forms the external structures of the face and the internal structures of the mouth, nose, and ears. The bony components of the ears and nose are formed from bones of both regions. The viscerocranial structures are largely derived from tissues of the pharyngeal arches, which develop around the ventral or inner curvature of the head. The structures of the neurocranium, however, are largely derived from components cranial to the arches. Both regions make extensive use of neural crest cells to form connective tissues which, in the rest of the body, would be formed by mesoderm.

Neurocranial components

The neurocranial portion of the head contains the brain, the portions of the skull that encase it, and the skeletal muscles that cover and move those bony supports. Many of the structures of the eyes, ears, and nose also form in this region. The development of their neural innervation are described in this chapter. The development of the brain is described in detail in Chap. 9.

   The neurocranial bones form in two groups by two methods. The base of the skull underlying the brain, or *chondrocranium*, is formed by endochondral ossification of cartilage models derived from both neural crest and mesoderm (the sclerotomes of occipital somites and cranial somitomeres). The bones of the base of the skull are the *sphenoid*, *ethmoid*, *temporal* and *occipital* bones. These bones also form capsules surrounding and protecting the sensory organs of the eyes, inner ears, and nasal cavities. The flat bones of the vault of the skull which surround the outer surface of the brain (*calvaria*) include the *frontal* and *parietal* bones, and the interparietal portion of the occipital bone. They are formed directly by membranous ossification from neural crest and are thus referred to as the *membranous neurocranium*.

   Most of the skeletal muscles of this portion of the head are developed from somitic myotome cells which first migrate into the pharyngeal arches, so their origins are discussed with the development of the viscerocranium. The development of the structures of the organs of special senses (eyes, ears, and nose) are described later in this chapter, since their complex structures also incorporate many elements derived from the arches. The details of bone and muscle development in the head are covered in Chaps. 7 and 8, respectively.

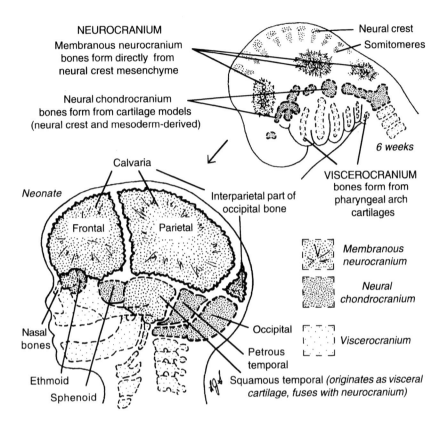

NEUROCRANIUM

Membranous neurocranium bones form directly from neural crest mesenchyme

Neural chondrocranium bones form from cartilage models (neural crest and mesoderm-derived)

Neural crest

Somitomeres

6 weeks

Calvaria

Neonate

Interparietal part of occipital bone

VISCEROCRANIUM bones form from pharyngeal arch cartilages

Frontal

Parietal

Membranous neurocranium

Neural chondrocranium

Nasal bones

Occipital

Viscerocranium

Petrous temporal

Ethmoid

Sphenoid

Squamous temporal *(originates as visceral cartilage, fuses with neurocranium)*

Figure 10-1
Neurocranial and viscerocranial regions of the head.

Viscerocranial components

The viscerocranial portion of the head includes the structures of the face and neck, the mouth and pharynx, the nasal cavities, and portions of the ears. These structures are largely formed from the tissues of the bilateral pharyngeal (or branchial) arches beginning in weeks 4 and 5 (see Fig. 10-2). Their development was first covered in Chaps. 6 to 8. The left and right components of each arch together form a semicircle which underlies the endoderm tube ventrally and surrounds it laterally on each side. Each arch begins as a condensation of lateral plate mesoderm around the most cranial portion of the forming endoderm tube, the pharyngeal endoderm. This region of the endoderm extends from the site of the future mouth, or *stomodeum*, to the site at which the respiratory diverticulum will form.

• **Pharyngeal arches are defined by clefts and pouches which partially separate them internally and externally.**   The arches become separated from each other on the exterior surface by deep pharyngeal clefts, or grooves, which form as ectoderm invaginates below the surface. Arches become separated internally by deep pharyngeal pouches which form by outpocketings of the pharyngeal endoderm at the same locations. Thus, each arch is a mesenchymal core with an ectoderm covering and an endoderm lining. The epithelia forming the cleft and pouch linings will form important derivatives.

• **Five pairs of arches form in sequence.**   A total of five pairs of arches are eventually formed, numbered 1, 2, 3, 4, and 6. Arch 5, if it ever exists, is a transitory structure with no derivatives. By the end of the embryonic period (8 weeks), the derivatives of the pharyngeal arches have been rearranged into their mature configuration.

• **Arch tissue derivatives include general connective tissues, cartilage and bone, and skeletal muscle.**   The connective tissue and cartilage components form first. Cartilages form in *all* arches, but bones will form only in the first three arches. Forming skeletal muscles attach to the incipient cartilages. Blood vessels and cranial nerves invade each arch. The cranial nerves synapse with the skeletal muscles as they form. As the cartilages and bones grow, in many cases they expand over ventral regions of the face. The muscles that are attached to them grow and, in many cases, migrate even further over the head. As a result, the original relationships between arch derivatives are often obliterated.

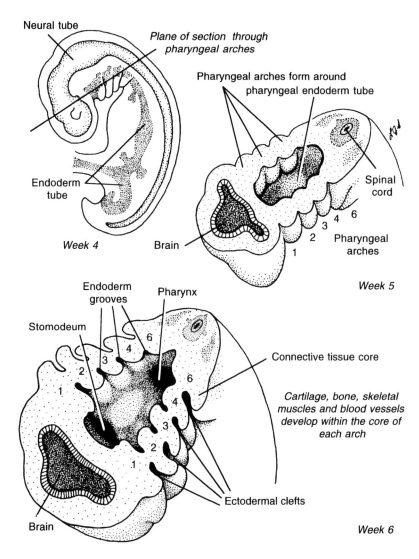

Figure 10-2
Formation of pharyngeal arch components.

Formation of pharyngeal arch tissues

• **Many connective tissue derivatives of the pharyngeal arches have atypical germ layer origins from the neural crest (see Fig. 10-3).**   Neural crest cells migrate into the mesodermal core of each pharyngeal arch as it forms. They give rise to general connective tissues in *all* arches. Neural crest also forms specialized connective tissue components, cartilage and bone, in some arches. Cartilage and most bones are formed by the neural crest in arches 1 to 3, while cartilages are formed from lateral plate mesoderm in arches 4 to 6, as they are in the rest of the body. These complicated origins are spelled out in the chapter on skeletal derivatives (Chap. 7).

> It is important to know that the neural crest is a source of tissue components in the head because congenital defects have been shown to result from inadequate migration and/or proliferation of neural crest cells into the arches (see congenital defects section later in this chapter). These defects include not only defects in bones or cartilages formed by the crest, but defects in arch blood vessels which are only indirectly affected by the smaller contribution of crest cells to their connective tissue components.

• **Each pharyngeal arch is supplied by a separate aortic arch artery.**   A separate artery grows into the ventral end of each arch in sequence from the outflow tract of the developing heart during week 4. These aortic arch arteries are formed from the local mesoderm and neural crest at the core of each arch. The arteries grow to the dorsal end of each arch, where they connect with a dorsal aorta forming on each side of the head. The bilateral dorsal aortae grow caudally into the body, where they merge into a single midline vessel, the descending aorta in the body cavity. Each arch's vessel supplies the tissues of that arch as they develop. With development, some of these aortic arch arteries and the section of the dorsal aorta connecting them merge or become obliterated entirely. The most important arch arteries that persist in the head are the third arch arteries, which give rise to the major vessels that supply the head and neck, the *common carotid arteries* and the start of the *internal carotid arteries*. The first and second arch arteries become small branches of the carotid arteries. The fourth and sixth arch arteries have different fates on the left and right. Together, they form the arch of the aorta, and the first portion of major vessels supplying the upper extremities, including the *right brachiocephalic* and *right subclavian arteries* and the vessels supplying the lungs, the *pulmonary arteries*. (The arch artery derivatives are fully described in Chap. 11.)

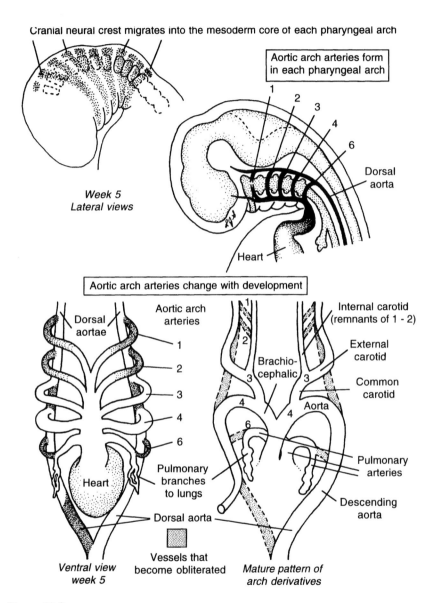

Cranial neural crest migrates into the mesoderm core of each pharyngeal arch

Aortic arch arteries form in each pharyngeal arch

Week 5
Lateral views

Dorsal aorta

Heart

Aortic arch arteries change with development

Dorsal aortae

Aortic arch arteries

1
2
3
4
6

Heart

Pulmonary branches to lungs

Dorsal aorta

Vessels that become obliterated

Ventral view
week 5

Internal carotid (remnants of 1 - 2)

External carotid

Brachio-cephalic

Common carotid

Aorta

Pulmonary arteries

Descending aorta

Mature pattern of arch derivatives

Figure 10-3
Origins of pharyngeal arch arteries.

• **Skeletal muscles form in the arches from invading myotome cells (see Fig. 10-4).**   Skeletal muscles formed in pharyngeal arches are derived from paraxial mesoderm that invades the arch mesoderm core, much as occurs in the limbs. This mesoderm originates from cranial somitomeres (arches 1 to 3), and myotomes of occipital somites (arches 4 to 6). (Remember that, although cranial somitomeres never proceed to the somite stage of organization, they give rise to the same types of derivatives as do somites.) Muscles that form in the pharyngeal arches include most of the muscles of the head and neck. These include the muscles of facial expression and mastication, as well as the internal pharyngeal and laryngeal skeletal muscles. Many of the developing muscles then migrate out of the arches over the face and head, obscuring the original boundaries of the arches.

The developmental origins of muscles can be determined from the nerves that innervate them.

Nerves grow into the arches and establish contact with skeletal muscles as they form and then remain connected to muscles as they migrate. Each arch is innervated by one cranial nerve. This applies not only to *motor* innervation of muscles, but also to all types of *sensory* innervation of arch derivatives (special senses, visceral senses, and general somatic senses).

The cranial nerves innervating each arch are the following:

Arch 1:   Trigeminal nerve, mandibular branch (cranial nerve 5)
Arch 2:   Facial nerve (cranial nerve 7)
Arch 3:   Glossopharyngeal nerve (cranial nerve 9)
Arches 4 and 6:   Vagus nerve branches (cranial nerve 10)

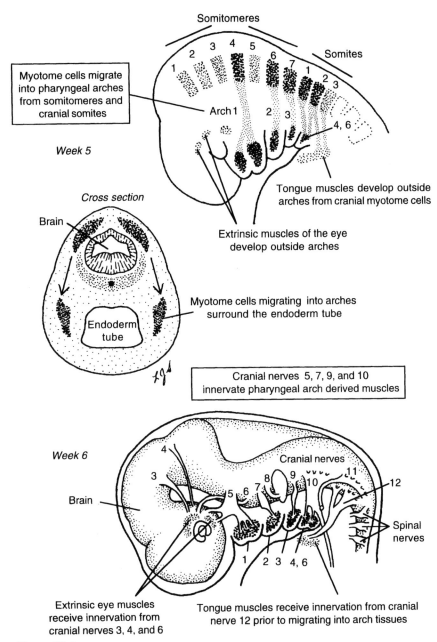

Figure 10-4

Formation of muscles in pharyngeal arches and their innervation patterns.

Specific tissue derivatives of each arch and their innervation

Arches 1 and 2 form the major viscerocranial structures: structures of the face, including the jaws, palate, and nasal septum; and many structures of the ear.

• **ARCH 1 DERIVATIVES: THE MANDIBULAR ARCH** The first and second arches are the only arches that have been given names. The names are based on their major derivatives. The mandibular arch makes the major contribution to the formation of the face, or *viscerocranium* (see Fig. 10-5). As it forms, two swellings termed the *maxillary* and *mandibular prominences* form within the arch. These prominences surround the cranial end of the endoderm tube. The mouth opening forms between the two parts of arch 1 when the endoderm and ectoderm meet and fuse to form the *buccopharyngeal membrane*. This membrane quickly breaks down to form the mouth opening, or *stomodeum*.

The mandibular prominences on each side form the lower jaw and many of its muscles, while the maxillary prominences on each side form the upper jaw and many of its muscles. Each prominence initially gives rise to a named cartilage formed by the neural crest: *palatopterygoquadrate* in the maxillary prominence and *Meckel's cartilage* in the mandibular prominence. Formation of these cartilages is essential for creating sufficient initial mass and correct relationship of arch prominences to each other. However, these cartilages largely regress and are replaced by bones formed around them by intramembranous ossification from separate arch cells. The *maxilla, palatine, zygomatic arch,* and *squamous temporal* bones form in the maxillary prominence, while the *mandible* forms in the mandibular prominence. The current evidence is that these bones are formed from neural crest, although there is some controversy on this point. The maxillary and palatine bones form the upper jaw, while the zygomatic arch links the maxilla to the squamous temporal bone. This part of the temporal bone originates in the arch and then fuses with the neurocranial portion of the temporal bone.

Both mandibular arch prominences form the skeletal muscles of mastication, along with several other muscles. Muscles of mastication close the jaw during chewing. Several other arch-derived muscles open the jaw via attachment to the hyoid bone (*mylohyoid* and *anterior digastric*). The arch also forms one soft palate muscle (*tensor palatini*) and one of the muscles that move the middle ear bones (*tensor tympani*; see next section on arch 2). All these muscles attach to cartilages or bones formed from arch 1. They are all innervated by *cranial nerve 5* (trigeminal).

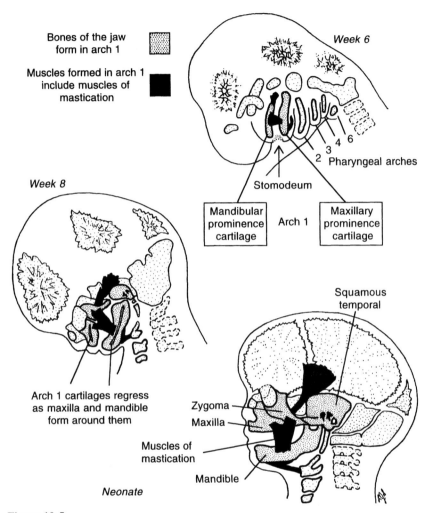

Figure 10-5
Derivatives of arch 1.

• **ARCH 2 DERIVATIVES: THE HYOID ARCH**   Arch 2 derives its name from its major bone derivative, the *hyoid bone* of the neck (see Fig. 10-6). Arch 2 cartilages and bones are derived from an original cartilage named *Reichert's cartilage* (which is derived from neural crest). The few bones derived from this arch are all formed by endochondral ossification from this cartilage model. The second arch develops in a line from the site of the developing ear dorsally to the surface of the future neck ventrally. The arch cartilage leaves derivatives behind at all these positions. It gives rise to the *styloid* process of the temporal bone dorsally, the *stylohyoid ligament* which extends ventrally from it to the hyoid bone, and to portions of the hyoid bone ventrally (the lesser horn and upper body). The hyoid bone is an essential brace that supports opening of the jaw during chewing, swallowing, and vocalization. It is positioned so that muscles use it as a fulcrum against which to contract from their origins on the mandible and tongue cranially, the styloid process of the temporal bone dorsally, and the laryngeal cartilages caudally.

While the first arch forms most of the bones and muscles which move the jaw, the second arch is a major player in formation of the face because it forms all muscles of facial expression.

These muscles move the surface features of the face by inserting into the connective tissues of the deeper layers of the skin. They surround all the openings on the head: the eyes, ears, nasal cavities, and mouth. The second arch also forms some jaw-opening muscles (*posterior digastric* and *stylohyoid*) and one muscle of the middle ear bones (*stapedius*). The facial muscles migrate up onto the head and face after formation. All these muscles are innervated by *cranial nerve 7* (facial nerve).

• **Arch 1 and 2 derivatives combine to form most structures of the ear and the anterior portion of the tongue.**   When these arches form, their dorsal ends mark the site of formation of the external ear. This helps to explain how they could also give rise to all three middle ear bones by endochondral ossification of remnants of the original arch cartilages. The dorsal end of the first arch cartilage gives rise to the *incus* and *malleus*. (These are the only bones that develop from cartilage precursors by endochondral ossification in arch 1.) The remaining bone of the middle ear (*stapes*) is formed by the dorsal tip of the second arch cartilage. The muscles that move these bones are derived from the same arches.

The tongue is formed by contributions from the ventral portions of the first four arches, but arches 1 and 2 together form the tissues of the anterior two-thirds of the tongue. (See p. 222 for details.)

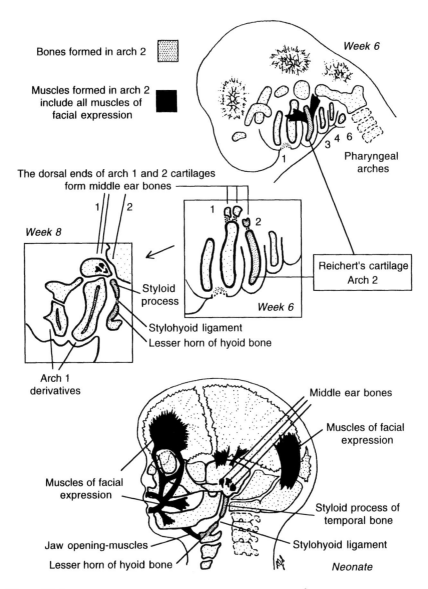

Figure 10-6
Derivatives of arch 2, and derivatives formed from arches 1 and 2 together.

> Arches 3, 4, and 6 form neck structures; some palate structures; and muscles of the neck, pharynx, and larynx (see Fig. 10-7).

• **ARCH 3 DERIVATIVES**   Arch 3 derivatives give rise to the remaining portions of the hyoid bone (greater horn and lower body). Arch 3 also gives rise to one muscle, the *stylopharyngeus*, which attaches to and raises the pharynx during swallowing and vocalization. It is innervated by *cranial nerve 9*, the glossopharyngeal nerve.

• **ARCH 4 AND 6 DERIVATIVES**   Arches 4 and 6 are never as large as the first three arches, and they merge during development. As a result, some of the specific arch origins of their derivatives are indistinguishable. These arches form the *laryngeal cartilages* (including the *thyroid* and *cricoid*) which surround the opening of the respiratory diverticulum. They are all derived from lateral plate mesoderm. These arches also form all but one of the *soft palate muscles*, all the *pharyngeal constrictor muscles*, and all *laryngeal muscles*. Both arches 4 and 6 are innervated by *cranial nerve 10*, the vagus nerve.

The movement of the laryngeal cartilages by the laryngeal muscles is important for controlling entry of air into the respiratory system, regulating movement of the vocal cords, and preventing entry of particles intended for the esophagus. The soft palate and pharyngeal constrictor muscles are involved in controlling the shape and size of the mouth and pharynx during chewing, swallowing, and vocalization.

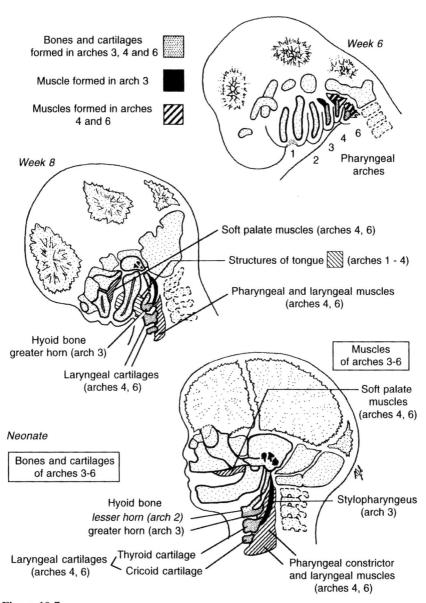

Figure 10-7
Derivatives of arches 3, 4, and 6.

DEVELOPMENT OF THE FACE

Formation of face primordia

The face begins to take shape when five face primordia develop late in week 4 and fuse during weeks 6 to 8 (see Fig. 10-8). Four of these primordia have already been described as the bilateral maxillary and mandibular swellings, or prominences, of the first pharyngeal arches. They are all filled with proliferating mesoderm and neural crest. The fifth prominence is a single midline *frontonasal (frontal) prominence*, which forms from the most cranial extension of the neurocranial region of the head. These five prominences encircle the stomodeum, or primitive mouth opening. The mandibular prominences fuse into a single structure as they form.

The frontonasal prominence develops two sets of bilateral swellings or placodes, called *nasal placodes*. They develop close to the stomodeum opening. They are the future site of the nasal cavities. *Lens placodes* develop more laterally at the future site of formation of the lens of each eye. As already seen, the dorsal end of the first pharyngeal cleft between the first two arches marks the spot of formation of the external ear. Thus, the stage is set for the formation of each sensory organ within the face primordia by week 5.

The nasal placodes of the frontonasal prominence then develop *medial* and *lateral nasal prominences* or swellings, which encircle the nasal pits as they form by invagination. The structure of all the facial prominences changes dramatically during weeks 6 to 8. The story of these changes continues on the next page.

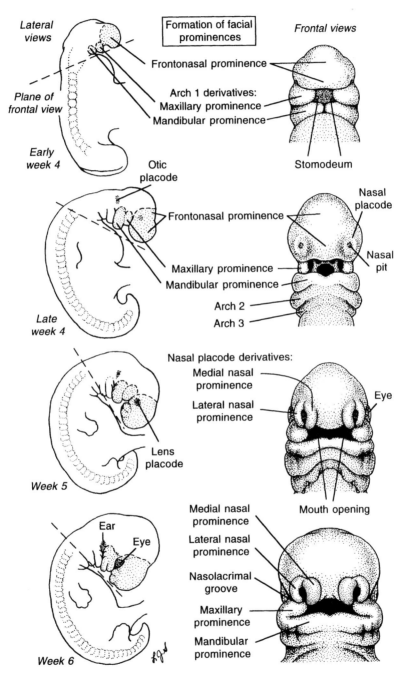

Figure 10-8
Development of the face from facial prominences.

Maturation of face primordia into mature facial structures

Differential growth of portions of the facial prominences, combined with fusion between several of them, creates the mature facial structures. First, the medial nasal prominences grow toward each other and fuse in the midline, forming the *intermaxillary segment*. This segment then elongates into the stomodeum opening between the maxillary prominences of arch 1. The intermaxillary segment then fuses with the maxillary prominences to each side of it. The nasolacrimal groove marks this line of fusion on each side.

Externally, the facial prominences form the structures of the forehead, nose, and all of the lower face surrounding the lips and extending down to the chin (see Fig. 10-9). The frontonasal prominence forms the forehead, as well as components of the nose. The nasal swellings of the prominence form the dorsum and apex of the nose, while the nasal pits deepen to form openings to the nasal cavities. The structures of the lip are formed by contributions from all the facial prominences. The medial intermaxillary segment forms the narrow medial portion of the upper lip, called the *philtrum*. The maxillary prominences form the lateral parts of the upper lip, while the mandibular prominences form the lower lip, and the face from the lips to the chin, and laterally along the jaw to the ears. The ears form at the dorsal end of the junction between the first two arches from the ectoderm, endoderm, and intervening mesoderm. The non-neural components of the eyes form from surface ectoderm and underlying mesoderm of the frontonasal prominence.

The final form of the face results from differential growth of several facial bones, which changes the proportions of the overlying structures. Air spaces, or paranasal sinuses, form within the maxilla and the bones of the frontonasal prominence (ethmoid, sphenoid, and nasal bones) causing extensive growth of these bones. Extensive growth of the mandible and maxillae also occur in part to accommodate the development of teeth within the jaw.

Failure of the face prominences to fuse with each other results in congenital defects of the face.

The most common defect is failure of the medial nasal swellings of the intermaxillary segment to fuse with the maxillary prominence in week 7, resulting in *cleft lip* (see Fig. 10-9). When this occurs on just one side, it results in unilateral cleft lip. When it occurs on both sides, it results in bilateral cleft lip. Cleft lip can vary in severity from a notch in the lip to complete division of the lip and the underlying maxilla, forming a combined cleft lip and palate in the roof of the mouth. These two defects are usually induced independent of each other.

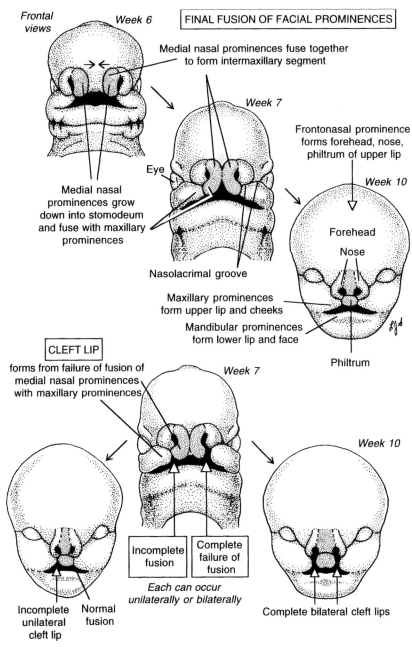

Figure 10-9
Development of the mature face and formation of cleft lip defects.

DEVELOPMENT OF INTERNAL VISCEROCRANIAL STRUCTURES

Formation of the mouth and nose

• **Structures of the mouth include the palate, tongue, and teeth (see Fig. 10-10).** The mouth or oral cavity is formed from the cranial end of the pharyngeal endoderm. The structures surrounding the mouth opening are formed by the maxillary and mandibular prominences of the first arch and the intermaxillary segment of the frontonasal prominence. The palate forms the roof separating the mouth from the nasal cavities, while the tongue forms its floor. Teeth are formed in connection with the maxilla and mandible.

• **The palate develops from the maxillary and intermaxillary prominences during weeks 5 to 10.** Development of the palate involves the formation and fusion of a primary palate and a secondary palate. Many abnormalities can occur in this process. The primary palate is a small midline structure which is formed from an internal swelling of the intermaxillary segment during week 5. It remains a small midline component of the mature palate. The four upper incisor teeth will arise from it. The bulk of the palate is formed by the secondary palate. This forms from two lateral palatine shelves which develop as internal projections of the maxillary prominences beginning in week 6. They grow toward the midline, where they fuse with each other, the primary palate, and the developing nasal septum in weeks 7 through 9. Fusion starts anteriorly. Bone develops in all but the most posterior portion of the palate by intramembranous ossification of precursor cells derived from the maxillary prominence, transforming these regions into the *hard palate*. The *premaxillary bone* forms within the small primary palate. *Palatine bones* form separately in the palatine shelves. The most posterior portion of the secondary palate forms the *soft palate*, which contains no bony or cartilaginous elements. Instead, it becomes invaded by skeletal muscles which will move the palate during breathing, chewing, and vocalizing. Most of the soft palate muscles are derived from myotome cells which first invade pharyngeal arch 4, and then migrate to the palate, carrying their innervation from the vagus nerve (*cranial nerve 10*). One muscle (*tensor veli palatini*) is derived from myotome cells which first invade arch 1, and is innervated by the trigeminal nerve (*cranial nerve 5*).

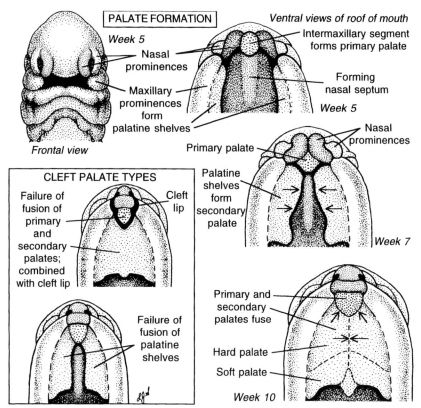

Figure 10-10
Normal formation of the mouth and palate, and defects in palate formation.

Cleft palate occurs when the palatine shelves fail to fuse during weeks 8 to 10.

Cleft palate can take several forms (see Fig. 10-10). A cleft in the anterior portion of the palate is caused by failure of fusion between the midline primary palate and one (or both) of the lateral palatine processes of the secondary palate. It is often continuous with a cleft lip on the same side. A long midline cleft can occur from failure of fusion of the lateral palatine processes with each other. These clefts can occur together. Cleft palate defects are multifactorial in causation, meaning genetic and teratogenic environmental factors interact.

• **Formation of nasal cavities and nasal septum is linked to formation of the palate.** The tissues lining the internal nasal cavities and making up the septum are formed by combinations of the first arch prominences and the frontonasal prominence. The first step in formation of the nasal cavities is the inward growth of the surface nasal placode epithelium covering the nasal pits (see Fig. 10-11). It grows through the mesoderm of the frontonasal prominence, remaining separate from the oral cavity by the primary palate forming in the intermaxillary segment. Continued growth causes the nasal cavities to break through to the oral cavity at the primitive choana. The nasal septum forms from another internal midline swelling of the frontonasal prominence, which grows down into the nasal cavity toward the tongue, where it encounters the primary palate and the developing secondary palate. The fusion of the palate and nasal septum separates the nasal cavities from each other, as well as from the mouth. Paranasal sinuses later form in the bones forming the lateral walls of the nasal cavities (maxilla, ethmoid, frontal, and sphenoid). Finally, some of the nasal placode cells, which line the nasal cavities, differentiate into primary sensory nerves. They meet and synapse with secondary neurons growing out in olfactory bulbs from each side of the forebrain to form cranial nerve 2.

• **Teeth are formed by neural crest and ectoderm derivatives.** Teeth begin to form in week 6 after the basic components of the mouth have been established. The surface ectoderm along the ridge covering the maxilla and mandible forms a thickened line called the *dental lamina*. Each lamina gives rise to ten *dental buds*, which grow into the underlying first arch mesenchyme during week 7. Each epithelial bud cups around a core of mesenchyme formed by neural crest, which condenses to form *dental papillae*. These two components mutually induce each other's differentiation. Beginning in week 10, cells of the papillae differentiate into *odontoblasts*, which produce *dentin*, a thick extracellular matrix at the core of the teeth. The core of the papilla is invaded by blood vessels and sensory nerve processes of the trigeminal nerve (the nerve of arch 1). While these developments are occurring, the outer epithelial cells of the dental cap differentiate into *ameloblasts* which form the *enamel* coating of teeth. The developing tooth is anchored to the jaw bone by *cementum*, a thin layer of specialized bone matrix produced by yet again another cell type of the dental papilla, the *cementoblast*. Outside this layer, other connective tissue mesenchyme forms *periodontal ligaments* which further anchor the teeth. With elongation of the roots of the teeth, they are pushed through the overlying soft tissues into the oral cavity. This occurs within the first two years after birth. Buds for permanent teeth are formed during fetal development in the jaw above the first teeth, but the teeth do not begin to develop until the sixth year of life. When they mature, they push the first teeth out of the jaw.

A. NASAL DEVELOPMENT

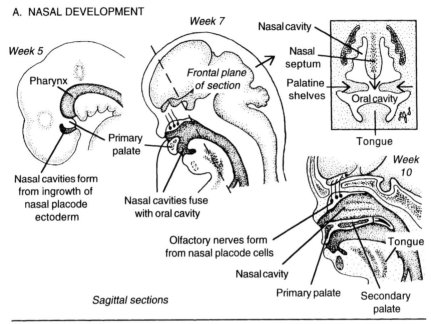

B. TOOTH DEVELOPMENT

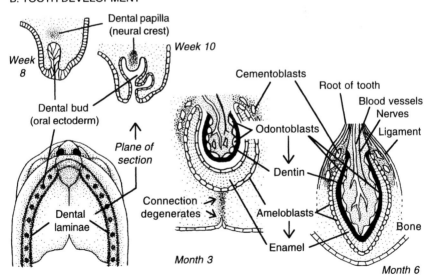

Figure 10-11
Formation of (A) the nasal cavities and (B) the teeth.

• **The tongue is formed by pharyngeal arch endoderm and arch tissues from the first four arches.** The floor of the mouth is formed by the tongue, which develops from the merger of a series of swellings of endoderm and underlying arch mesenchyme of the first four pharyngeal arches (see Fig. 10-12). The endodermal epithelium forms the surface of the tongue, as it does in most of the rest of the mouth. Arch lateral plate mesoderm and neural crest form its connective tissue core, while skeletal muscle cells invade from somites to form the bulk of the tissue mass of the tongue.

Arch 1 forms the anterior two-thirds of the tongue. It begins as a midline (median) swelling in the floor of the endoderm of arch 1. Lateral lingual swellings then form in arch 1 and overgrow the median swelling. Sensory innervation of the endodermal covering of this part of the tongue comes from cranial nerve 5, the nerve of arch 1.

Arches 2, 3, and part of 4 form the posterior one-third or root of the tongue. A median swelling (*copula*, or *hypobranchial eminence*) forms from these arches. Arch 3 overgrows most of the other two arches. Most sensory innervation is thus supplied by *cranial nerve 9*—the nerve of arch 3—and the remainder by *cranial nerve 10*—the nerve of arch 4. The boundary between the two parts of the tongue is marked by the *foramen cecum*, a depression that remains at the site of origin of the thyroid gland epithelium from the endodermal epithelium. The epiglottis and larynx develop at the caudal boundary of the tongue.

Intrinsic muscles of the tongue are derived from the first three somitic myotomes (occipital somites). The myotomes first receive innervation from *cranial nerve 12* (hypoglossal) and then migrate into the tongue, carrying their motor innervation with them. Thus, they are not originally arch structures.

As described earlier, general sensory innervation of the surface of the tongue is supplied by the cranial nerves of arches 1, 3, and 4, whose endoderm covers specific portions of the tongue. The endoderm also forms specialized epithelial structures called *taste buds* into which special sensory nerve endings penetrate. This innervation is supplied by branches of the facial nerve, the nerve of arch 2.

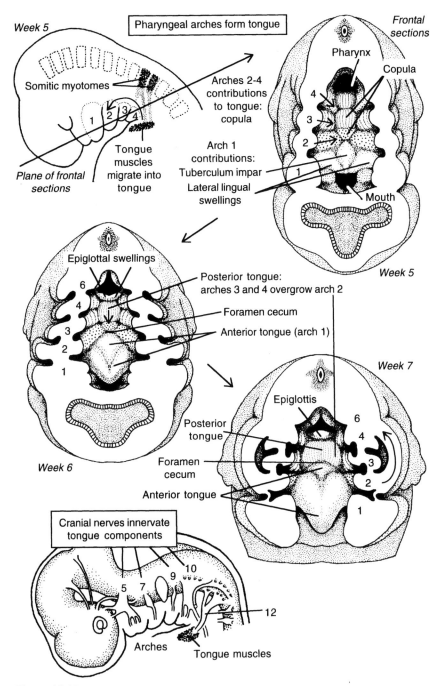

Figure 10-12
Development of the tongue.

EPITHELIAL DERIVATIVES OF PHARYNGEAL POUCHES AND CLEFTS

The epithelium that lines the pharyngeal pouches and clefts differentiates into a number of important structures, including components of several important lymphoid organs and endocrine glands. Descriptions of these derivatives are often incorrectly taken to mean that the *entire* organ is derived from pouch or cleft linings. That is not correct. The derivatives form epithelial components of organs. The mesoderm and neural crest within the arches surrounds these epithelial buds and forms the other tissues within these organs, although neural crest may form some specific epithelial components within some organs.

• **Numbering system of pouches and clefts.**   Pouches and clefts are *caudal* to the arch of the same number. Thus, pouch and cleft 1 are caudal to arch 1, or between arch 1 and arch 2. There are only four pairs of pouches and clefts, since there is no pouch or cleft caudal to arch 6.

• **Summary of pharyngeal pouch and cleft derivatives.**   This list of derivatives illustrates the complexity of the structures formed from pharyngeal arches. The formation of each of these derivatives is covered in the following pages.

Pouch and cleft 1:	Epithelial lining of middle and outer ear canals and tympanic membrane
Pouch 2:	Epithelial lining of palatine tonsils
Pouch and cleft 3:	
Ventral Portion:	Epithelial components of thymus gland
Pouch 3: Dorsal Portion:	Epithelial cells of inferior parathyroid gland
Pouch 4: Ventral Portion:	Epithelial parafollicular cells (incorporate into thyroid gland)
Dorsal Portion:	Epithelial cells of superior parathyroid gland
Clefts 2 and 4:	No derivatives

Specific derivatives of clefts and pouches

• **Derivatives of cleft and pouch 1 form ear structures.**   The first pharyngeal pouch and cleft elongate until they come together between arches 1 and 2. Together with the tissues of these two arches, they form many structures of the ear (see Fig. 10-13). The endodermal pouch forms the lining of the middle ear canal, or *auditory tube*. The ectodermal cleft forms the epithelial covering of the outer ear canal, or *external auditory meatus*. (Development of the ear is more fully covered at the end of this chapter.)

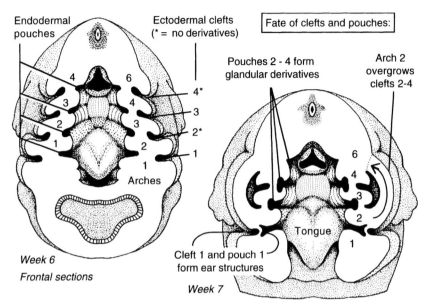

Figure 10-13
Derivatives of pharyngeal cleft and pouch 1 and clefts 2 to 4.

• **Ectoderm of clefts 2 and 4 does not form mature derivatives.**   Arch 2 obliterates clefts 2 to 4 by growing caudally over them. Initially this overgrowth leaves an ectoderm-lined cervical sinus, which is normally obliterated (see Fig. 10-13). Ectoderm of cleft 3 combines with pouch 3 to form thymus derivatives.

> Congenital defects can arise if cleft 2 or the cervical sinus are not obliterated.

Small blind cavities can persist, forming *cervical cysts*, or *sinuses* if the cavity is large. A channel can persist connecting to the surface, forming a *fistula*. These defects usually do not present serious complications unless they become infected.

• Endoderm of pouches 2 to 4 forms epithelial components of several lymphoid organs and endocrine glands (see Fig. 10-14). The endoderm at the base of each pouch forms an epithelial outgrowth that grows through the arch mesenchyme to its final location in the neck or upper thorax. Some of these outgrowths remain attached to the originating endoderm lining the mouth or pharynx, and others do not. When these migrations occur, they obscure the original source. These outgrowths form epithelial coverings of organs, epithelial networks within organs, and secretory cells within glands. The supporting connective tissues and smooth muscle components, as well as blood vessels of these organs, are formed by arch mesoderm or neural crest.

• Lymphoid organs receive endoderm contributions from pouches 2 and 3.

> Epithelia covering the palatine tonsils are formed from pouch 2.

Tonsils are lymphoid nodules that form in the walls of the pharynx just below the surface epithelium. The B lymphocytes housed here secrete antibodies that defend the body against foreign organisms. All tonsils are covered by the endoderm lining the mouth and pharynx; the palatine tonsils are specifically covered by the endoderm that forms pouch 2. The epithelial coverings also form deep crypts or invaginations which penetrate the underlying arch mesoderm, partially subdividing the tonsils. The connective tissue framework of the tonsils is formed by arch mesoderm and neural crest. The lymphocytes, which perform the work of these organs, invade the tonsils after their framework is established.

> Epithelial networks are formed within the thymus by ventral portions of pouch 3 endoderm and cleft 3 ectoderm which meet and fuse in the midline.

The thymus is another lymphoid organ. It is located in the neck inferior to the thyroid gland, where it extends under the sternum in the chest. The thymus houses T lymphocytes, which must mature within its framework during fetal life. As with the tonsils, the lymphocytes invade after the organ framework is established. Unlike all other lymphoid organs, the thymic framework is largely formed by an epithelial meshwork, or reticulum, which is formed in different parts of the thymus by endodermal cells of pouch 3, ectodermal cells of cleft 3, and arch 3 neural crest cells, all of which migrate caudally and to the midline.

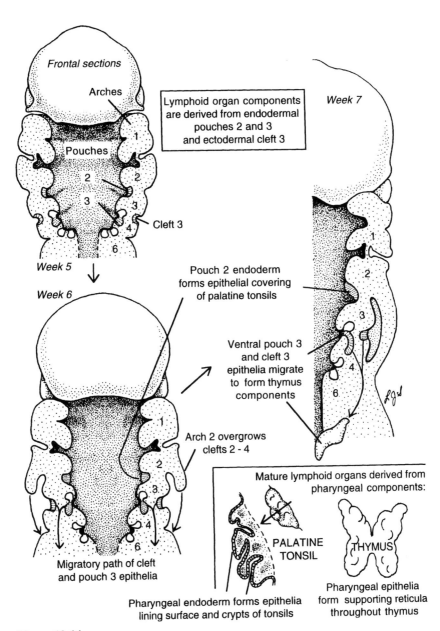

Frontal sections

Arches

Lymphoid organ components
are derived from endodermal
pouches 2 and 3
and ectodermal cleft 3

Week 7

Pouches

1

2   2

3   3

4   Cleft 3

6

Week 5

Week 6

Pouch 2 endoderm
forms epithelial covering
of palatine tonsils

Ventral pouch 3
and cleft 3
epithelia migrate
to form thymus
components

Arch 2 overgrows
clefts 2 - 4

Migratory path of cleft
and pouch 3 epithelia

Mature lymphoid organs derived from
pharyngeal components:

PALATINE
TONSIL

THYMUS

Pharyngeal endoderm forms epithelia
lining surface and crypts of tonsils

Pharyngeal epithelia
form supporting reticula
throughout thymus

Figure 10-14
Lymphoid organ derivatives of pouches 2 and 3 and cleft 3.

• **Glandular derivatives are formed by derivatives of pouches 3 and 4 (see Fig. 10-15).**

> Glandular secretory cells of the parathyroid gland are formed from the dorsal portions of endoderm pouches 3 and 4.

As their name suggests, these four small endocrine glands are located next to (para) the dorsal surface of the thyroid gland, within its connective tissue capsule. The endoderm outgrowths from the more cranial pouch 3 migrate a greater distance than those of the caudal pouch 4, so that pouch 3 cells contribute to the inferior parathyroid and pouch 4 to the superior parathyroid (see Fig. 10-15). These epithelial cells differentiate into glandular epithelial cells, called *chief cells*, which secrete parathyroid hormone into the blood vessels. The remaining tissues of the organs are formed by arch mesoderm and neural crest.

> Glandular parafollicular cells are formed from the ventral portions of pouch 4 endoderm and migrate into the thyroid gland.

The endoderm cells that originate from the ventral portions of pouch 4 migrate into the neck, where they penetrate the substance of the thyroid gland forming in the ventral midline of the neck. Here they differentiate into nests of glandular epithelial cells surrounding the forming thyroid glandular follicles, giving rise to the name *parafollicular* cells. The parafollicular cells, or *C cells*, secrete calcitonin into the blood stream. This endocrine hormone has the reverse effect of parathyroid hormone released by parathyroid glandular cells. Together, these two hormones regulate blood calcium levels by enhancing (parathyroid hormone) or inhibiting (calcitonin) calcium resorption from bone.

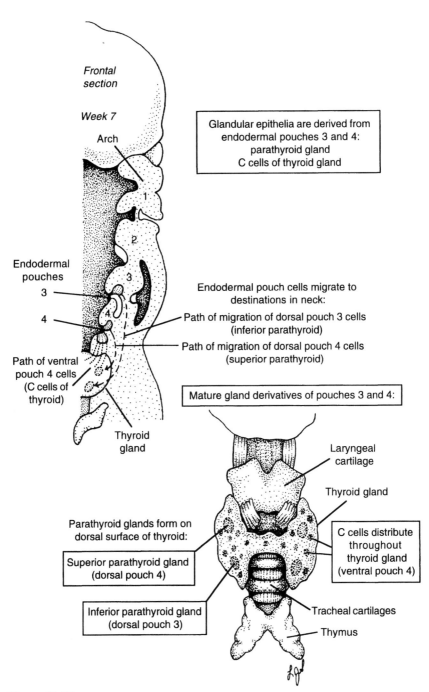

Frontal
section

Week 7

Arch

Endodermal
pouches
3
4

Path of ventral
pouch 4 cells
(C cells of
thyroid)

Thyroid
gland

Glandular epithelia are derived from
endodermal pouches 3 and 4:
parathyroid gland
C cells of thyroid gland

Endodermal pouch cells migrate to
destinations in neck:
Path of migration of dorsal pouch 3 cells
(inferior parathyroid)
Path of migration of dorsal pouch 4 cells
(superior parathyroid)

Mature gland derivatives of pouches 3 and 4:

Laryngeal
cartilage

Thyroid gland

Parathyroid glands form on
dorsal surface of thyroid:

Superior parathyroid gland
(dorsal pouch 4)

Inferior parathyroid gland
(dorsal pouch 3)

C cells distribute
throughout
thyroid gland
(ventral pouch 4)

Tracheal cartilages

Thymus

Figure 10-15
Glandular derivatives of pharyngeal pouches 3 and 4.

Other glandular derivatives of pharyngeal epithelia

• **THYROID GLAND**   The thyroid is an endocrine gland whose glandular epithelia forms from a midline outgrowth of the endoderm in the floor of the future pharynx between arches 1 and 2 (see Fig. 10-16). This endoderm outgrowth, or thyroid *diverticulum*, descends through the developing tongue, retaining its connection to the pharynx temporarily via a *thyroglossal duct*. Its point of origin marks the *foramen cecum* of the future tongue. The thyroid diverticulum forms the epithelial components of the thyroid gland, which become the glandular cells that manufacture and secrete *thyroid hormone*. The connective tissue framework and blood vessels around the thyroid follicles are formed by lateral plate mesoderm.

Congenital defects can arise from persistence of the thyroglossal duct.

If any portion of the thyroglossal duct persists, a *thyroglossal cyst* (small blind cavity), *sinus* (large cavity), or *fistula* (open channel) can form from these remnants anywhere along the path within the tongue, containing nests of thyroid gland tissue. In addition, if the thyroid outgrowth fails to descend out of the forming tongue tissue altogether, this results in an ectopically located *lingual thyroid* gland embedded within the tongue.

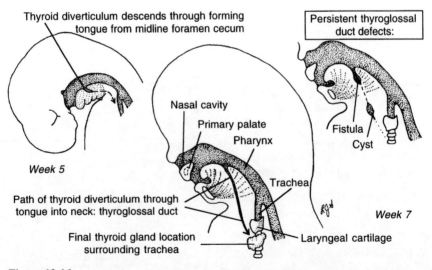

Figure 10-16
Formation of the thyroid gland.

• **PITUITARY GLAND**   The pituitary gland (*hypophysis*) is composed of two portions: the *anterior* and the *posterior pituitary* (see Fig. 10-17). These two portions reflect the dual embryonic origin of this gland. The endocrine glandular portion, or the anterior pituitary, originates from an upgrowth of pharyngeal epithelium lining the roof of the primitive mouth (oral) cavity. This upgrowth is called *Rathke's pouch*. Its connection with the oral cavity is obliterated by week 8. These cells secrete a number of important hormones, which are described in Chap. 16.

This upgrowth is derived from ectoderm, not endoderm. Why is there ectoderm on the inside of the mouth? Initially the ectoderm and endoderm meet at the cranial and caudal ends of the gut tube. The two layers initially fuse to form membranes that break down to form the mouth opening (stomodeum) and anal opening (cloaca). However, the original boundary of this meeting point is actually carried a short way into the interior of the body at both openings.

The posterior pituitary is formed by a downgrowth of neuroectoderm from the developing brain called the *infundibulum*. This downgrowth connects with Rathke's pouch to form one organ. (More specifics of pituitary formation are covered in Chaps. 9 and 16.)

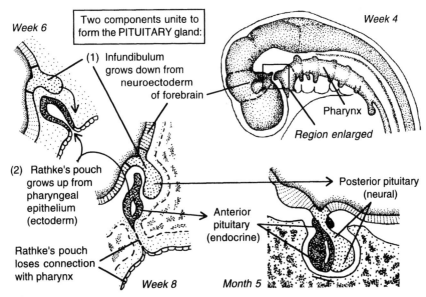

Figure 10-17
Pituitary development.

DEVELOPMENT OF THE EYE AND OPTIC NERVE

Mature structures of the eye (see Fig. 10-18)

The important structures of the eye include the *eyeball* itself, which consists of the transparent *cornea* and opaque *sclera*; the *lens*; the *eye chamber* in front of the lens and *vitreous body* behind it; the *retina* and the *optic nerve*, which receive and transmit visual signals to the brain. The important structures of the eye also include the surrounding muscular structures which permit the eye to function. These include the *ciliary body*, whose muscles focus the lens; the *iris* muscles, which regulate pupil diameter; and the *extraocular* muscles, which move the eyeball. Finally, the *conjunctiva* lining the interior surface of the eyelids are important to the maintenance of the structures of the eye.

Formation of the eye

The structures of the eye are formed by three different germ layer contributions: neuroectoderm, surface ectoderm, and mesoderm. Each forms specific structures.

• **NEUROECTODERM CONTRIBUTIONS.** Neuroectoderm of the forebrain gives rise to the retina and optic nerve and the structures of the iris and ciliary body (see Fig. 10-18).

• **The retina and optic nerve form from optic vesicles.** The neuroectoderm of the forebrain region evaginates on each side of the developing forebrain during week 4 to form *optic vesicles*, which grow toward the surface ectoderm. The distal ends of the vesicles enlarge to form *optic cups*, while their connections with the forebrain narrow to become *optic stalks*. Each of these gives rise to different structures of the eye.

• **The optic cup differentiates into the retina, while the optic stalk becomes the optic nerve.** The optic cup is composed of two layers with an intervening space. The inner layer forms the light-sensing neural layer of the retina as its cells differentiate into light sensitive rods and cones bordering the intraretinal space. These nerve cells send out axonal processes through the optic stalk into the developing forebrain, turning the optic stalk into the optic nerve. The outer layer of the optic cup forms the pigmented layer of the retina. The optic stalk develops a deep invagination called the *choroid fissure* along its length, into which the hyaloid artery grows to supply the optic cup derivatives. It later becomes the central artery of the retina. The mesenchyme that forms this artery also fills the space between the developing lens and retina, forming a gelatinous substance called the *vitreous body*.

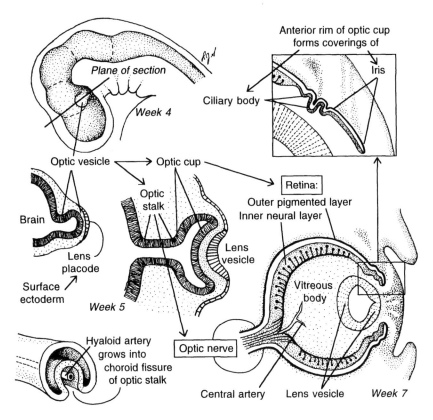

Figure 10-18
Mature structures of the eye and development of neuroectoderm contributions.

• **The optic cup also forms the iris and ciliary body.**   The anterior rim of the optic cup differentiates into the epithelial covering of the ciliary body and the epithelial covering of the iris, which controls the size of the pupil. Both structures contain muscles that connect to them (see next section).

• **NON-NEURAL (SURFACE) ECTODERM CONTRIBUTIONS TO THE EYE.**   Surface ectoderm of the frontonasal prominence just above the maxillary prominences is induced to form optic structures after contact with the underlying optic vesicles (see Fig. 10-19). These structures include the lens and cornea, as well as the epithelial coverings of the lacrimal glands, and eyelids (conjunctiva).

• **The lens is formed from the lens vesicles.**   Thickenings of the surface ectoderm called *lens placodes* are induced to form by the optic vesicles. The placodes invaginate below the surface ectoderm and separate from it to form lens vesicles. These vesicles then differentiate into the lenses, which focus the incoming light rays by changing their curvature.

• **The cornea is formed by surface ectoderm and mesoderm.**   The cornea overlying the anterior surface of the lens is subsequently formed from mesenchyme formed from both surface ectoderm and mesoderm. Corneal precursor cells separate from the surface ectoderm and become mesenchymal, surrounding themselves with substantial extracellular matrix. These cells and matrix components mature into the anterior portion of the cornea. Inner portions of the cornea are derived from mesoderm that also forms the walls of the anterior chamber. The anterior chamber of the eye then develops between the cornea and lens.

• **The epithelial coverings of the lacrimal glands, eyelids, and conjunctiva are all formed by surface ectoderm.**   *Conjunctiva* is the name given to the covering of the inner surface of the eyelids that face the eyeball. Lacrimal glands form by invagination of ectoderm at the lateral angles of the conjunctiva. They mature after birth to secrete tear fluids into the conjunctival space.

• **MESODERM CONTRIBUTIONS TO THE EYE.**
• **All connective tissues and vascular structures are formed by surrounding lateral plate mesoderm (see Fig. 10-19).**   Connective tissues around the eye form an inner vascular choroid layer and an outer connective tissue sclera layer. The sclera becomes continuous with the dura mater surrounding the optic stalk, and the choroid becomes continuous with the pia-arachnoid.

• **Muscles of the eyes are formed from mesoderm and neuroectoderm.**   The ciliary muscle (smooth muscle that focuses the lens) is formed by lateral plate mesoderm, which invades the ciliary body. The pupillary muscles of the iris, which control pupil diameter, are probably derived from neural crest. They are myoepithelia: nonstriated muscle similar to smooth muscle in organization. Both ciliary muscle and iris muscle cells invade these structures as they form. Extrinsic skeletal eye muscles, which move the eyeball, are formed by the first three somitomeres. They are innervated by three *cranial nerves* (*3*, *4*, and *6*).

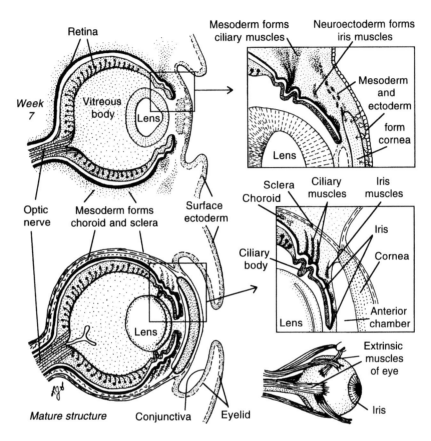

Figure 10-19
Surface ectoderm and mesoderm contributions to the eye.

DEVELOPMENT OF THE EAR
Mature components of the ear

The ear is composed of inner, middle, and outer ear portions (see Fig. 10-20). They are derivatives of all three germ layers. Development of the middle and outer ear were introduced earlier in this chapter. The outer ear, or *auricle*, is a collection device to channel sounds to the tympanic membrane which forms the boundary between the outer and middle ears. The middle ear transmits sound vibrations to the inner ear. It contains three bones, the *malleus*, *incus*, and *stapes*, whose movements transmit sounds across the tympanic cavity. The middle ear also contains the auditory tube, which connects the tympanic cavity to the pharynx. Inner ear structures are designed to amplify sound waves and convert them into nerve signals (cochlear duct), as well as to sense the position of the body (vestibular apparatus). The structures of the inner ear are referred to collectively as the *membranous labyrinth*. These structures are housed within the bony labyrinth of the petrous part of the temporal bone. The labyrinth is divided into two structural and functional regions. The *saccule* region forms the *cochlear duct*, whose epithelial lining (the *spiral organ of Corti*) is composed of sensory "hair" cells which transmit signals to the acoustic portion of the auditory nerve (cranial nerve 8). The *utricle* region forms the vestibular apparatus, which consists of the *semicircular canals* and *endolymphatic ducts*. Their sensory epithelial cells are involved in sensing and maintaining equilibrium.

Formation of the ear

The first pharyngeal pouch and cleft elongate until they come together. Together with the surrounding tissues of arches 1 and 2, they form the structures of the middle and outer ear. The structures of the inner ear are formed by the *otic placodes*, thickenings of the surface ectoderm which develop at the dorsal tip of the first pharyngeal cleft and invaginate below the surface to form *otic vesicles*.

• **Outer ear development involves formation of the external acoustic meatus and auricles (see Fig. 10-20).**   The outer ear canal, or external acoustic meatus, is formed by the invagination of pharyngeal cleft 1. The cleft ectoderm then forms the epithelial lining of the canal. The auricles of the outer ear are formed by six auricular swellings, which form from tissues of arches 1 and 2. These tissues surround the first pharyngeal cleft. The swellings fuse together and their cores become filled with arch mesoderm, which forms connective tissue components of the auricles, including cartilaginous supports. Initially, these swellings fuse in the lower neck region, but ascend to the level of the eyes primarily due to the growth of the mandible.

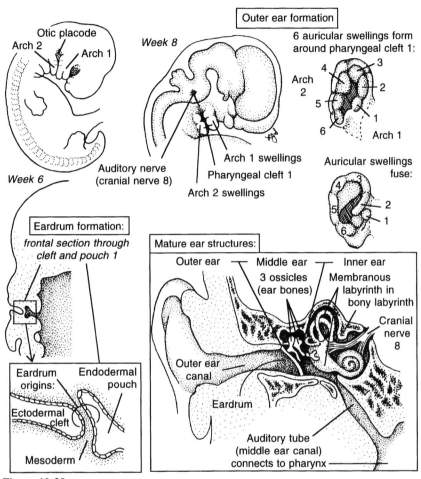

Figure 10-20
Structures of the mature ear and development of the outer ear.

• **The eardrum is formed by tissues from all three germ layers.**   The ecto-dermal invagination from cleft 1 meets the endoderm evagination from pouch 1, with a narrow layer of mesoderm sandwiched between them. These three layers fuse to form the eardrum, or *tympanic membrane*, which separates the outer ear from the middle ear.

• **Middle ear components are formed from derivatives of pharyngeal arches 1 and 2 and the pouch and cleft between them.**   These derivatives form bones, skeletal muscles, and epithelial linings which compose the middle ear (see Fig. 10-21). The first pharyngeal pouch expands to form a long tube, which widens at its distal end to become the tympanic cavity, while its proximal end remains narrow and forms the *auditory*, or *eustachian, tube* connecting the middle ear cavity with the pharynx. Endoderm of pharyngeal pouch 1 forms the epithelial lining of these cavities. The tympanic lining forms around the middle ear bones, or ossicles, as they develop by endochondral ossification from the dorsal tips of the cartilages of arches 1 and 2. The malleus and incus are derived from the cartilage of arch 1, and the stapes from the cartilage of arch 2. Initially these bones are surrounded by mesenchyme. It dissolves, leaving the bones attached to the wall of the tympanic cavity by the endodermal epithelium, which is subsequently transformed into ligaments by invading arch mesenchyme. Skeletal muscles move the malleus (tensor tympani) and stapes (stapedius). They are derived from mesoderm of somitomeres, which migrates into arches 1 and 2, respectively. During postnatal development, the epithelium lining the tympanic cavity invades the mastoid process of the temporal bone to form epithelial-lined *mastoid air sacs*. These connections provide the basis for infections of the middle ear, which begin in the pharynx and spread into the auditory tube, tympanic cavity, and mastoid air sacs.

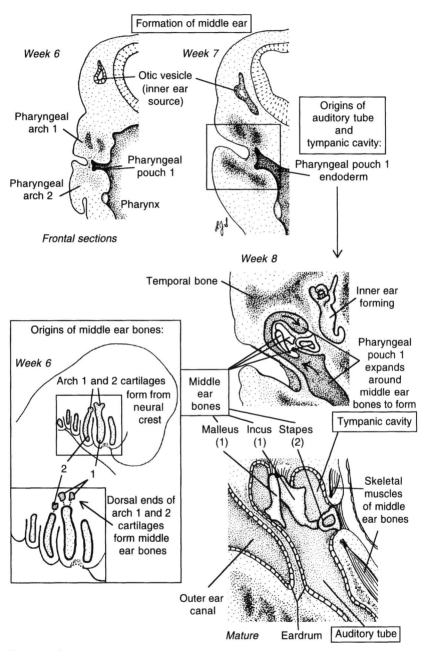

Figure 10-21
Development of the middle ear.

• **The inner ear is derived from surface ectoderm of the otic placode.**   The inner ear forms from the otic placode, a thickening of surface ectoderm which forms in week 4 at the dorsal tip of the first pharyngeal cleft (see Fig. 10-22). It invaginates below the surface and separates from it to form the otic vesicle. It moves inward to become surrounded by the mesenchyme, which will form the petrous portion of the temporal bone. Here the vesicle differentiates into all structures of the inner ear, which are collectively referred to as the *membranous labyrinth*. During weeks 6 to 8, it expands into dorsal and ventral portions, which each give rise to separate components of the membranous labyrinth. The ventral component, the *saccule*, forms the structures involved in transmitting sound: the cochlea and organ of Corti within it. It initially forms an elongated outgrowth, the cochlear duct, which spirals to form the cochlea. Part of its epithelial lining differentiates into sensory hair cells (the spiral organ of Corti), which transform sound wave vibrations into impulses which can be transmitted by the auditory nerve fibers of cranial nerve 8 which contact them. The dorsal portion of the otic vesicle, the *utricle*, forms the vestibular apparatus, which is involved in maintaining equilibrium. It begins as a broad extension, whose walls become flattened against each other centrally, leaving three semicircular canals connected to the utricle at both ends. Each of these semicircular canals is oriented in a different plane. Cells lining these canals, as well as the utricle and portions of the saccule, become sensory hair cells which detect changes in position. These changes are transmitted to the vestibular fibers of cranial nerve 8, which invade the canal walls. The utricle also forms a long extension, the *endolymphatic duct*, which removes excess endolymphatic fluid from the interior of the membranous labyrinth space into blood vessels surrounding its saccular ending. The vestibulocochlear nerve, or cranial nerve 8, is formed by cells from both the otic vesicle and neural crest. Together, they form sensory ganglion cells that form separate cochlear and vestibular branches which receive auditory and vestibular impulses. Beginning in week 9, the mesenchyme surrounding the membranous labyrinth forms a cartilaginous otic capsule, which will ossify to form the petrous part of the temporal bone. The bony spaces surrounding the elements of the membranous labyrinth are called the *bony labyrinth*. The space between the two becomes filled with perilymphatic fluid.

CONGENITAL DEFECTS OF THE HEAD AND NECK

Congenital defects of the head and neck are both genetically and teratogenically induced. Most originate from defects in formation of the pharyngeal structures, either from abnormal persistence of arch structures that normally disappear or underdevelopment of structures. Most of these malformations are uncommon. Many defects that occur in localized structures in the head have already been covered in this chapter. In addition, defects that affect multiple structures can occur. The most common of these are described on page 242.

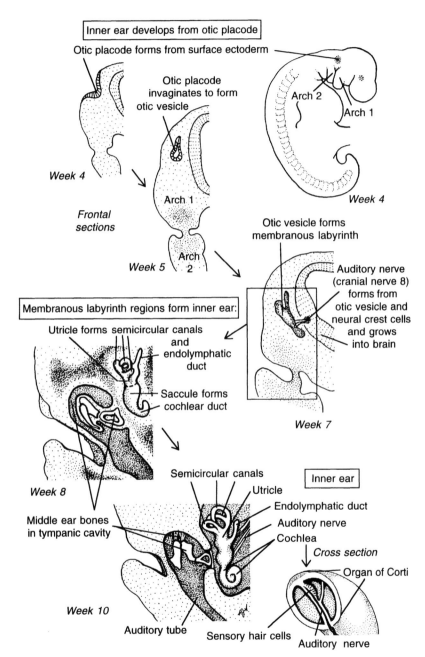

Figure 10-22
Development of the inner ear.

• **Defects in formation of the neurocranium and brain are tied together.**
Anencephaly refers to the absence of the brain and failure of the vault formation
of the skull, whereas *microencephaly* refers to the severe underdevelopment of
the skull and cerebral hemispheres. The primary cause is usually failure of the
neural tube to close in the head region, which interferes with proper formation of
the skull. These defects have already been discussed in Chaps. 7 and 9.

• **Defects in formation of many arch structures can result in facial anomalies.**   A host of defects in development of facial structures can result from failure of the neural crest to migrate into appropriate arches in adequate numbers or
from failure to proliferate once there. The same complexes of defects often occur
together, and so are classified as syndromes. Syndromes can be caused by either
genetic factors or teratogenic insults. It is beyond the scope of this book to go into
the range of syndromes or their precise causes. It is important to recognize that
defects that appear disconnected can be tied together by the involvement of
neural crest cells. It has been demonstrated that neural crest cells are more susceptible to teratogens and susceptible to different teratogens than is mesoderm.
In the head, where crest cells form a host of connective tissues, this distinction is
critical. Depending on the timing of the insult, different syndromes will result.
First arch syndrome refers to a spectrum of defects primarily involving development of first arch structures. Defects occur primarily in bony structures of the
eyes, ears, jaw, and palate (craniofacial dysostosis). Defects can also occur in
external epidermal features of the eyes and ears. *DiGeorge syndrome* refers to a
spectrum of defects primarily involving development of structures derived from
the third and fourth arches and their pharyngeal pouch derivatives. These include
hypoplasia (underdevelopment) or absence of the thymus, since crest cells form
some of its reticular framework. They also include hypoplasia or absence of the
parathyroid glands, and defects in the blood vessels leading out of the heart (see
also Chap. 11). The latter defects are caused by failure of adequate neural crest
migration into these arches, even though crest cells do not form major structural
components of either. However, crest cells do form the associated connective tissues. Any loss of appropriate connective tissue mass can affect the mass of structures that must develop within the arch.

• **Defects in formation of the eye and ear.**   Defects in formation of structures
of the eyes and ears can occur independently of larger defects in pharyngeal arch
derivatives. Maternal rubella infection can cause defects in both, depending on
when the infection occurs. Infection in weeks 4 to 6 can lead to congenital
cataract, or opacity, of the lens of the eye. Infection during weeks 7 to 8 can cause
congenital deafness due to defective formation of the sensory cells of the organ
of Corti. Other causes of congenital deafness can result in maldevelopment of
membranous or bony labyrinths, ossicles, or tympanic membranes.

TABLE 10-1
PHARYNGEAL ARCH DERIVATIVES

ARCH	CRANIAL NERVE	CARTILAGES[a] AND BONES	SKELETAL MUSCLES
1: Mandibular arch Maxillary prominence		Palatopterygoid[a, b] maxilla, palatine, zygoma, squamous temporal, incus	All muscles of mastication: masseter, temporalis, pterygoids
	Trigeminal (5)		
Mandibular prominence		Meckel's[a, b], mandible, malleus	Mylohyoid, anterior digastric, tensor veli palatini, tensor tympani
2: Hyoid arch	Facial (7)	Reichert[a], styloid, hyoid (part), stapes, stylohyoid ligament	All muscles of facial expression[c] Posterior digastric, stylohyoid, stapedius
3	Glosso-pharyngeal (9)	Hyoid (part)	Stylopharyngeus
4	Vagus (10): Superior, laryngeal branch Pharyngeal branch	All laryngeal cartilages[a]: thyroid, cricoid, arytenoid, corniculate, cuneiform, epiglottis (Arches 4 and 6)	Pharyngeal constrictors All soft palate muscles *except* tensor veli palatini (1) All intrinsic laryngeal muscles (arches 4 and 6)
6	Recurrent laryngeal branch		

[a]Cartilage.
[b]Temporary structures in arches.
[c]Muscles of facial expression: scalp (frontalis, occipitalis), ears (auricular), eyes (orbicularis oculi, corrugator), nose (procerus, dilator nares, depressor septi, nasalis), mouth (buccinator, orbicularis oris, platysma; depressor labii and anguli, mentalis, levator anguli and labii, zygomaticus, risorius).

CARDIOVASCULAR SYSTEM

·

· · · · · · · · · · · ·

The cardiovascular system consists of one central organ, the heart, and a complex system of blood vessels and lymphatic vessels that distribute and collect the blood and tissue fluids to every organ system in the body. This chapter covers the development of the heart and the major blood and lymphatic vessels. While all the tissue components of these structures are derived from one part of the mesoderm germ layer, the splanchnic lateral plate mesoderm, the events involved in the formation of the heart and vasculature are complex ones. A knowledge of cardiac embryology provides the basis for understanding the many ways in which the development of the heart can go awry. Congenital defects in heart formation are among the most common types of congenital defects.

COMPONENTS OF THE MATURE
CARDIOVASCULAR SYSTEM

The cardiovascular system consists of the heart and the vasculature, which distributes blood to the body (*arteries*) and returns it to the heart (*veins*) (see Fig. 11-1). It also consists of a separate *lymphatic* vascular system, which retrieves blood fluids that regularly seep into body spaces and returns them to the venous system.

The mature heart has four chambers: left and right *atria* and *ventricles*. Venous blood enters both atria. Deoxygenated blood returns to the right atrium from the body via the *vena cavae*. *Pulmonary veins* return oxygenated blood from the lungs to the left atrium. *Mitral* and *tricuspid* [*atrioventricular* (AV)] valves regulate flow from the atria into the ventricles. Blood flows from there into the main arteries past *semilunar valves*. Oxygenated blood flows from the left ventricle to the body via the *aorta*. Deoxygenated blood flows from the right ventricle to the lungs via the *pulmonary arteries*.

• **TISSUE COMPONENTS**   The heart walls consist of cardiac muscle (or *myocardium*) criss-crossed by coronary vessels and supporting connective tissue. The chambers are lined by an epithelial layer, the *endocardium*. Cardiac valves consist of connective tissue cores covered by endocardium. Blood vessel walls consist of smooth muscle and connective tissue, and are lined by an epithelial layer, the *endothelium*. The outer surface of the heart is covered by *epicardium*. This layer consists of an epithelial covering, and an underlying layer of fat through which coronary arteries penetrate the myocardium.

The myocardium of both atrial and ventricular chambers is trabeculated on its inner layers. *Trabeculae* are networks or chords of myocardium, which facilitate complete chamber emptying. The ventricular walls are thicker and more heavily trabeculated than the atrial walls, reflecting their function as the main pumping chambers of the heart. Extensions of ventricular myocardium, called *papillary muscles*, control the opening and closing of the AV valves by their connection to *chordae tendineae* ("tendinous cords"), which insert along the edges of the valves.

Cardiac contraction is initiated by pacemaker, or conduction, cells, which are specialized myocardial cells, many of which are grouped into nodes. The stimulus goes from the *sinoatrial node* to the *AV node*, then along the *bundle of His* to a network of *Purkinje* pacemaker cells. Autonomic innervation helps to regulate the rate of cardiac contraction, but is not required for contraction itself.

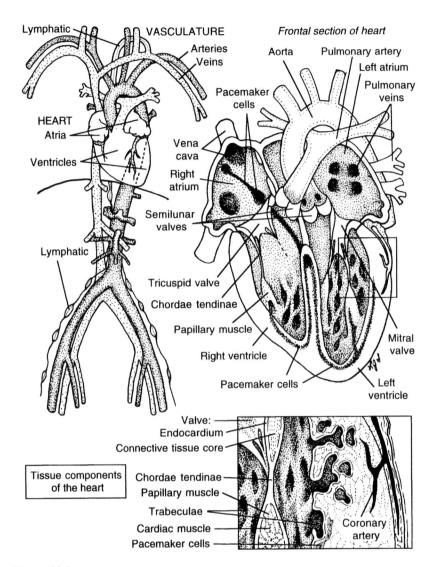

Figure 11-1
Mature cardiovascular system and its tissue components.

GERM LAYER ORIGINS

• **Tissues that compose the cardiovascular system are formed by splanchnic lateral plate mesoderm (see Fig. 11-2).** Mesoderm is the expected source for connective tissues and all muscle. However, this is one of two systems in which the epithelial components are also formed by mesoderm (the urogenital system is the other). In addition, the ubiquitous neural crest cell contributes to the outflow vessels of the heart.

HEART FORMATION

Formation and fusion of bilateral heart tubes

• **Bilateral endocardial and myocardial tubes form from splanchnic lateral plate mesoderm in week 3.** The splanchnic mesoderm, which will form the heart, is a horseshoe-shaped region that extends around the cranial end of the neural plate and to each side of the forming endoderm tube. Endocardial tubes form on each side by mesoderm coalescing into epithelial tubes. Premyocardial tubes then form from the splanchnic mesoderm surrounding the endocardial tubes. Together they form heart tubes to either side of the endoderm tube (see Fig. 11-2). The thin epicardial covering of the heart is believed to form later from mesodermal cells that grow over the surface of the heart tube.

• **The heart tubes are brought together by embryonic folding.** The lateral body folds bring the heart tubes to the midline ventral to the endoderm tube. The cranial head fold pushes the heart tubes caudal to the developing brain.

• **Fusion creates a single heart tube with an endocardial lining inside a myocardial wall.** Fusion begins at the cranial end during week 3 (see Fig. 11-2). The endocardial tubes fuse into one tube first. Then the myocardial sheaths fuse around the endocardial tube. A thick extracellular matrix layer forms between them, called the *cardiac jelly.*

• **A pericardial cavity is formed around the fusing heart tubes.** The pericardial cavity is formed by the cranial portion of the intraembryonic coelom into which the developing heart tubes protrude. The lateral plate mesoderm, which lines this cavity, forms the pericardial membrane. The pericardial cavity is limited caudally by a shelf of somatic lateral plate mesoderm, called the *septum transversum*, which grows across the body cavity at the caudal end of the heart tube. This important structure will help form venous connections to the heart, as part of its formation of tissues of the liver and diaphragm (see vasculature development later in this chapter and in Chap. 12).

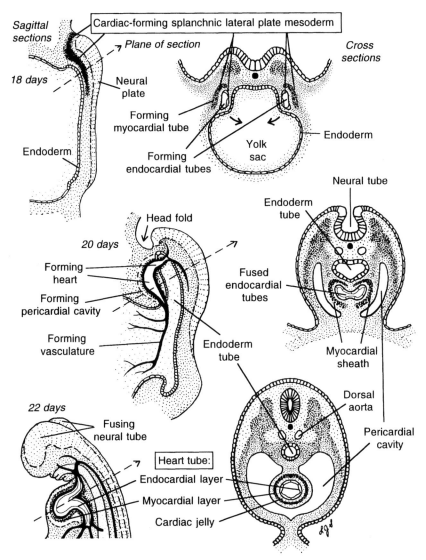

Figure 11-2
Formation and fusion of bilateral heart tubes.

Formation of regions of the heart tube

• **The origins of each region of the heart are determined as the bilateral heart tubes fuse (see Fig. 11-3).**   You can get a preview of how the single heart tube forms all the structures of the heart by following the path of blood flow through the heart tube. From entry at the caudal end, blood flows through regions that become externally recognizable as *sinus venosus, primitive atrium, AV canal, primitive ventricle, bulbus cordis,* and *truncus arteriosus,* emerging at the cranial end.

• **Specific derivatives of each region of the heart tube.**

1.   The sinus venosus forms the veins entering the right atrium and is partially incorporated into the right atrium.
2.   The primitive atrium forms the remainder of the right atrium and all of the left atrium.
3.   The AV canal between the primitive atrium and ventricle forms the valves between the chambers.
4.   The primitive ventricle forms the left ventricle.
5.   The bulbus cordis forms the right ventricle and the muscular outflow channels from both ventricles.
6.   The truncus arteriosus forms the arterial outflow, or "great vessels": the pulmonary arteries and aorta.

Heart tube looping

The midsection of the heart tube loops ventrally, caudally, and to the right during week 4. Looping begins as the heart tubes complete their fusion. This brings the primitive ventricle and bulbus cordis ventral to the primitive atrium and sinus venosus. The rightward looping also moves the bulbus cordis to the right of the ventricle, while the truncus arteriosus remains anchored in the midline. The result is a heart tube in which the components assume positions that come close to the mature relationship of their derivatives: the ventricles are mostly ventral and caudal to the atria, while the outflow vessels originate from the ventricles in the midline.

> Looping is the first sign of left-right *sidedness*, or *situs*, in the heart. Situs is under genetic regulation. In the syndrome known as *situs inversus*, the sidedness of many organs is reversed; the heart may loop to the left. Since situs is rarely perfectly reversed, it is usually accompanied by a range of defects, including congenital heart defects.

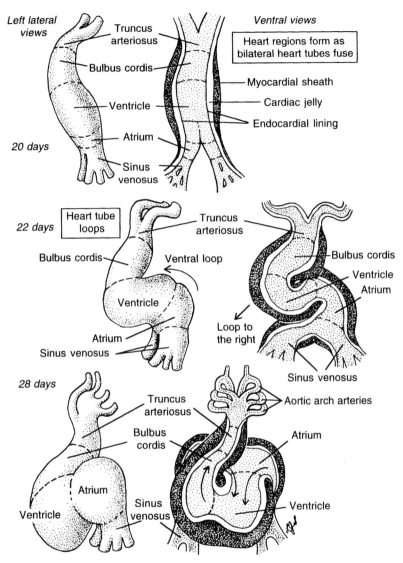

Figure 11-3
Heart tube looping and development of regions.

• **CARDIAC FUNCTIONING BEGINS DURING LOOPING.** Cardiac muscle begins to differentiate in the myocardial layer while the heart tube is still looping, and the heart then begins to beat (see Fig. 11-4). Circulation begins early in week 4, when connections are established with the blood vessels to the developing placenta.

> Circulation must replace diffusion for the embryo to develop beyond the germ layer stage. Thus, the cardiovascular system is the first to develop, the only system that fully functions in the embryo and whose function is essential to the development of other organs.

Unlike skeletal muscle, cardiac myocytes continue to divide after differentiating. This proliferation accounts for most growth in myocardial mass during fetal life. Continued increases in mass after birth are due to *hypertrophy* (or growth in size) of individual cardiac myocytes. This is one of the few tissues in which cellular hypertrophy is a significant factor in development. As looping proceeds, the myocardium becomes several cell layers thick. As septation begins, the ventricular myocardium becomes much thicker than that of the atria, and its inner layers become extensively *trabeculated*. Specialized conduction cells form from myocytes in each heart region as it forms. These cells pace the rate of contraction of the remaining myocardium. Autonomic nerves first contact the heart during septation, but functional innervation occurs much later.

• **SEPTA BEGIN TO DIVIDE THE HEART TUBE INTO LEFT AND RIGHT SIDES DURING CARDIAC LOOPING.** Keep in mind that septation happens simultaneously in each region of the heart tube. During weeks 5 and 6, septa create two atria and ventricles and divide the AV canal and ventricular outflow tract into two channels. Valves then form in those channels from dilations called *endocardial cushions*. Division of the distal outflow tract forms the great vessels leaving the heart.

> Knowledge of the embryology of the cardiovascular system is essential to understanding the many congenital heart defects.

One fifth of all congenital defects occur in this system. Their causation is not well understood, but the vast majority are of multifactorial origin, meaning

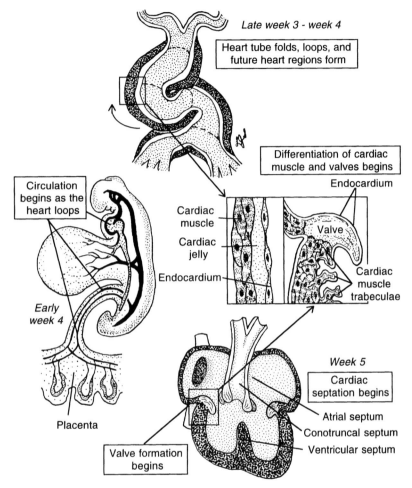

Late week 3 - week 4

Heart tube folds, loops, and
future heart regions form

Differentiation of cardiac
muscle and valves begins

Endocardium

Circulation
begins as the
heart loops

Cardiac
muscle

Valve

Cardiac
jelly

Endocardium

Cardiac
muscle
trabeculae

Early
week 4

Week 5

Cardiac
septation begins

Atrial septum

Conotruncal septum

Placenta

Ventricular septum

Valve formation
begins

Figure 11-4
Overview of cardiac development.

that environmental factors (teratogens) interact with genetic "predisposition."
Because of the differences between fetal and postnatal circulatory patterns, most
of these defects create no problems until birth, at which time many would prove
rapidly fatal without surgical intervention. One important determinant of postnatal status is whether or not defects cause *cyanosis*: deficient oxygenation of blood.

Atrial development

• **ATRIAL SEPTATION**   The primitive atrium is divided into left and right atria by formation of two parallel septa during weeks 4 and 5 (see Fig. 11-5). The *septum primum* is a crescent-shaped ridge that grows from the dorsal roof of the primitive atrium down toward the AV canal. Its advancing edge leaves an opening called the *ostium primum*, which is closed by endocardial cushion tissue from the atrioventricular canal.

While the ostium primum is closing, a second opening, called the *ostium secundum*, forms in the septum primum by the coalescing of many small perforations. A thick *septum secundum* then forms to the right of the septum primum. It grows from the ventral roof of the atrium, completely covering the ostium secundum. It then stops, leaving a crescent-shaped opening called the *foramen ovale*. These two septa do not fuse together, and a channel between them remains patent during fetal life. Thus, blood can (and does) cross the atrial septum throughout fetal life. This shunt is essential for delivery of oxygenated placental blood to the left side of the heart, from which it enters the forming aorta to the fetal body.

Defects in atrial septation are common.

Most atrial septal defects permit blood to continue to flow across the septum after birth (see Fig. 11-5). The higher blood pressures on the left side of the heart after birth cause left-to-right flow, which can eventually overburden the right side of the heart and lead to cardiac failure.

1. An *ostium primum atrial septum defect* forms if this opening isn't closed by fusion of the septum primum with the endocardial cushions.
2. An *ostium secundum atrial septal defect* is formed either by excessive resorption of the septum primum or incomplete development of the septum secundum.
3. If the foramen ovale doesn't seal physically after birth, blood can be shunted across it through the *patent foramen ovale*.
4. *Premature closure of the foramen ovale* during fetal life causes *left heart hypoplasia* (or underdevelopment), due to lack of flow on the left side of the heart. This is incompatible with postnatal life, since there is inadequate blood flow to the body from the aorta.

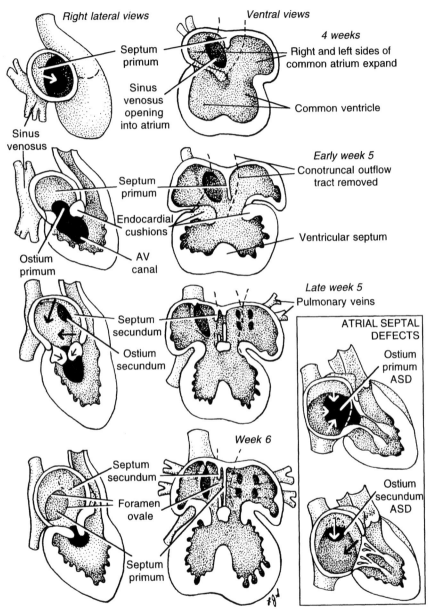

Figure 11-5
Atrial septation and defects in atrial septal formation.

• VENOUS RETURN TO THE ATRIA

• Venous return from the body comes to the right atrium via the sinus venosus. The sinus venosus becomes the "antechamber," or entrance, to the heart, since all venous drainage from the body returns to it (see Fig. 11-6). Venous return to the sinus venosus is initially from vessels called *cardinal veins*, which will become the ends of the vena cavae leading into the sinus venosus on both sides. During week 5, the right horn of the sinus venosus expands to receive all venous drainage from the body and opens into the right atrium. The left horn of the sinus venosus forms a narrow venous return channel to the right atrium. It sinks into the crevice between the left atrium and ventricle on the back (dorsal) side of the heart. It becomes the *coronary sinus*, which receives venous drainage from the myocardial walls.

• The right horn of the sinus venosus becomes largely incorporated into the right atrium. It forms the dorsal, smooth-walled part of the atrium, while the primitive atrium forms the trabeculated walls of the right atrial appendages. The primitive atrium also forms the entire left atrium, including the left atrial appendage. The atrial appendages expand ventrally to cup, like fingers of an appendage, around the truncus arteriosus.

Defects in formation of venous return from the body can alter the configuration of either the left or right horn of the sinus venosus, and the atria, into which they drain. (This is covered later in this chapter in the section on formation of the venous system.)

• Pulmonary venous drainage from the lungs returns to the left atrium. Pulmonary veins form as outgrowths from the dorsal wall of the left atrium beginning in week 4. Two veins grow out into each developing lung. During fetal life only enough blood enters and leaves the lungs to nourish their development. After birth, the lungs expand and flow increases into and out of the lungs. The pulmonary veins then receive large volumes of oxygenated blood for the left atrium.

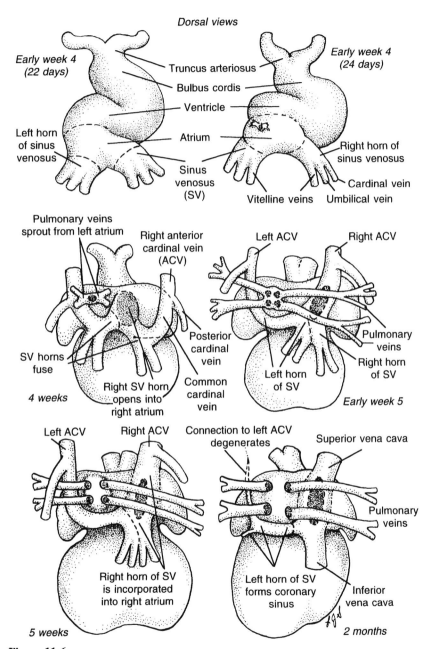

Figure 11-6

Formation of venous drainage to the right atrium via the sinus venosus and formation of pulmonary veins draining to the left atrium.

Partitioning of the atrioventricular canal

• **Endocardial cushions divide the AV canal and form the AV valves.**   During atrial and ventricular septation, endocardial cushions form and begin to grow across the AV canal (see Fig. 11-7). Initially, in week 4 the canal is positioned so that it connects the left side of the common atrium with the left side of the common ventricle. With expansion of the right sides of both cardiac chambers in week 5, the AV canal widens to the right. As it does, the endocardial cushions grow across the canal from its dorsal and ventral surfaces until they meet and fuse with each other, creating left and right AV canals. These cushions, in conjunction with cushions that form along the lateral walls of each canal, will grow and differentiate to form the AV valves (mitral and tricuspid valves) separating the atria from the ventricles. In the interim, they function like valves in helping to prevent backflow of blood during contraction of the heart tube.

• **Mechanisms of formation of the endocardial cushions.**   The endocardial cushions develop as specializations of the endocardium and its underlying "cardiac jelly" during month 2. The myocardium in the valve regions (and *only* these regions) induces cushion formation. First, it generates an extracellular matrix called cardiac jelly that expands to form thick "cushions." Myocardial signals then induce the endocardial cells to disattach and migrate into the cushions. The endocardial cells differentiate into the connective tissue core of the valves. The final formation of valves involves remodeling and hollowing out of the ventricular side of the cushions and myocardial walls to which they are attached. This remodeling results in connection of valve leaflets to papillary muscles extending from the ventricular walls via connective tissue strands called *chordae tendineae.*

• **Endocardial cushions also participate in the final closure of atrial and ventricular septa.**   Portions of the dorsal and ventral endocardial cushions must fuse with both atrial and ventricular septa and contribute tissue for their septa to be complete. The cushion contribution forms the final portion of the atrial septum primum and the final portion of the ventricular septum, which is a membranous septum.

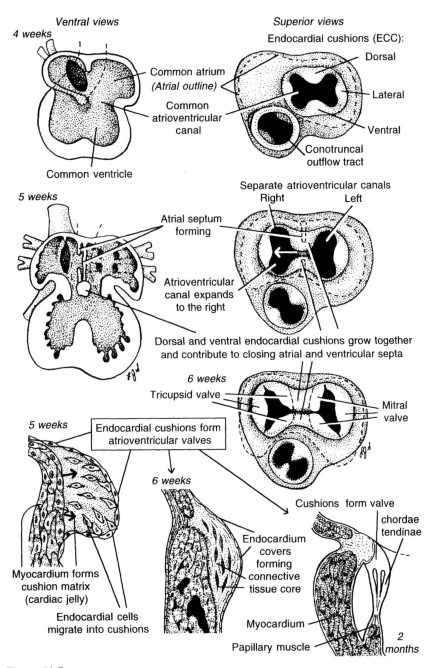

Figure 11-7
Partitioning of the atrioventricular canal by endocardial cushions.

> Defects in formation or fusion of the atrioventricular endocardial cushions can produce a spectrum of congenital defects.

Defects can occur not only in valve formation, but also in formation of atrial and/or ventricular septa (see Fig. 11-8). These defects will all result in left-to-right shunts after birth, which will eventually, if left untreated, overload the right heart and lead to heart failure.

1. At the mildest end of the spectrum, abnormal mitral or tricuspid valve cusps may be formed, which may permit backflow on ventricular contraction, resulting in incomplete emptying.
2. Inadequate development of the cushions can cause failure of final closure of either the atrial septum (*ostium primum atrial septal defect*) or ventricular septum (*membranous ventricular septal defect*). Medial leaflets of the AV valve cusps are often also abnormal, as they cannot form normally when a hole persists in the very area they should be crossing.
3. At the most severe end of the spectrum, both atrial and ventricular septa and the medial AV valve leaflets are incomplete, leaving a *persistent AV canal defect*. This is the most common defect in trisomy 21 (Down syndrome). It leaves a large hole and produces signficiant left-to-right shunting. It is difficult to fix surgically because of all the structures involved.
4. *Mitral* or *tricuspid atresia* can occur if the AV valve leaflets fuse during development. Since this leaves no opening for flow into the affected ventricle, it results in *hypoplasia*, or underdevelopment, of the affected ventricle and hypertrophy of all other chambers. Severe stenosis of the valves can produce the same result.

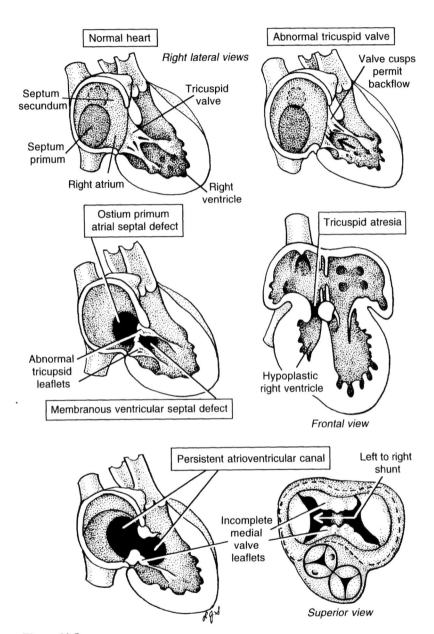

Figure 11-8
Defects in atrioventricular canal septation.

Ventricular development

• **Formation of a septum between the primitive ventricle and bulbus cordis forms two ventricles.**   Ventricular septation begins at the end of week 4, at the same time as atrial septation (see Fig. 11-9). A thick muscular septum forms at the junction of the primitive ventricle and bulbus cordis. It forms by a combination of infolding of their walls and growth of the advancing edge of the septum. The primitive ventricle forms the left ventricular chamber, while the proximal bulbus cordis forms the right ventricular chamber. Final closure of the remaining interventricular foramen is achieved by week 7 by fusion of the muscular septum with two separate structures: endocardial cushion tissue of the AV canal and a separate muscular septum, which forms in the distal bulbus cordis.

• **Septation of the distal bulbus cordis, or conus cordis, forms muscular ventricular outflow tracts and helps close the ventricular septum.**   The conus cordis forms the outflow regions of both ventricles. During month 2, it becomes septated (along with the distal truncus arteriosus) by ridges that form in a spiral along opposite sides of the conus, much like a spiral staircase. This spiral lines up one outflow tract with each ventricle. The ventral (or anterior) outflow tract remains connected to the right ventricular chamber, forming a long muscular outflow tract called the *infundibulum*. The dorsal (or posterior) outflow tract forms a short connection with the left ventricle. The fusion of the muscular conal septal ridges with the ventricular septum helps to close the ventricular septum ventrally.

• **The interventricular foramen is finally closed by the membranous ventricular septum.**   A membranous septum is formed from the ventral endocardial cushion tissue in the AV canal. It grows across the foramen to close the septum by the end of month 2.

Ventricular septal defects are the most commonly occurring congenital heart defects.

These defects usually result in left-to-right shunts of blood after birth, which overload the right side of the heart and can lead to heart failure if left untreated (see Fig. 11-9).

1. *Membranous ventricular septal defect* (VSD) is the most common congenital heart defect. Membranous VSD is formed when the muscular and mem-

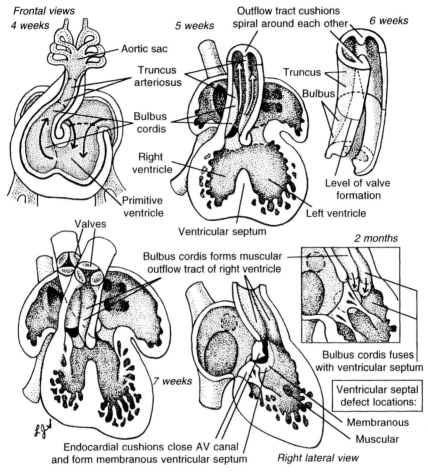

Figure 11-9
Ventricular development and defects in septation.

branous septal portions fail to fuse with each other. It can be caused by underdevelopment of the muscular septum, misalignment of the conal and ventricular muscular septa, or underdevelopment of the endocardial tissue.

2. *Muscular VSDs* occasionally occur in the trabeculated regions of the lower muscular ventricular septum. They are usually small when they occur as isolated defects. They often close spontaneously.

Partioning of great vessel outflow trunks

• **Two spiral ridges form in the truncus arteriosus which fuse to form the aorticopulmonary septum.**   When the truncal ridges fuse with each other, they create two separate "great vessels" which spiral around each other (see Fig. 11-10). The truncal ridges become continuous with the ridges forming in the conus cordis at the same time. The point of junction of the truncus arteriosus and the conus cordis is the point at which the *semilunar valves* of the aorta and pulmonary artery form. The spiraling conotruncal septum positions the aorta in the left ventricle, and the pulmonary artery in the right ventricle.

• **Neural crest participates in formation of the great vessel walls.**   That neural crest migrates into the pharyngeal arches should not be a surprise if you have read Chap. 6 or 10. The relevance to cardiovascular development is that crest cells become incorporated into the walls of the blood vessels that grow into the arches as outgrowths from the truncus. The crest cells then migrate caudally along the endothelium of these aortic arch vessels into the truncus arteriosus. They participate in formation of the aortic arch vessels, in formation and septation of the truncus outflow tract, and possibly in formation of the semilunar valves. Crest cells form connective tissues and perhaps smooth muscle within the walls of the vessels. Whether crest cells migrate further into the heart to contribute to formation of the pacemaker cells of the heart or the AV valves, as some evidence suggests, is not yet clear.

> Congenital defects in formation of the great vessels or their aortic arch outgrowths occur as a result of inadequate migration of neural crest into one or more pharyngeal arches. Vessel defects are frequently associated with defects in formation of other structures derived from neural crest in the pharyngeal arches. Together, the combined defects comprise the *DiGeorge syndrome*.

This syndrome includes a spectrum of defects in facial structures (formed from the first two arches), absence of thymus or parathyroid components (formed by third and fourth arch derivatives), as well as vessel defects (formed from all arches). The specific defects and severity probably reflect differences in timing of teratogenic insults. Alcohol has been shown to have a teratogenic effect on development of this neural crest population.

• **Formation of aortic and pulmonary semilunar valves and coronary arteries.**   The great vessel valves are called *semilunar valves*, because their cusps form in the shape of half-moons. The valves are formed by endocardial

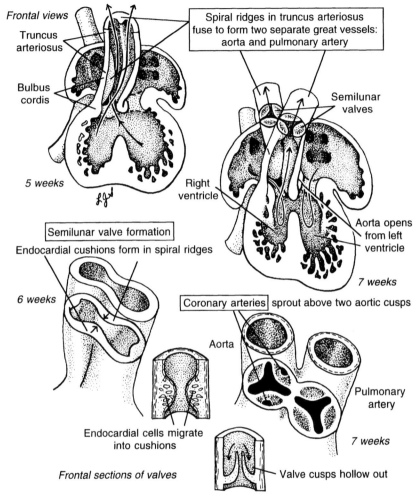

Figure 11-10
Partitioning of the great vessels and formation of their valves.

cushions, which form at the junction of the conal and truncal ridges by the same process that forms the AV valves. Coronary arteries form by sprouting as buds above two of the aortic valve cusps. The mechanisms directing their outgrowth into the ventricular and atrial walls are not well understood.

> Defects in aorticopulmonary septation.

Defects in septation of the outflow vessels are often accompanied by defects in the heart, because anything that alters hemodynamics (or blood flow) in one affects the other by altering either the path or volume of flow (see Fig. 11-11). In particular, defects in aorticopulmonary septation often result in ventricular septal defects underlying one or both great vessels.

1. *Persistent truncus arteriosus* occurs when the aorticopulmonary septal ridges fail to form. Since the conal ridges also fail to form normally, the persistent truncus overrides a ventricular septal defect. Oxygenated and deoxygenated blood mix in the outflow tract, resulting in a cyanotic defect. This defect is difficult to fix surgically.

2. Abnormal location of the truncal and conal septa are the most common causes of aorticopulmonary septal defects. These defects are, collectively and individually, among the most common and most serious congenital defects of the cardiovascular system:

   a. *Tetralogy of Fallot* is the most common conotruncal defect and the most common cyanotic defect. It results from unequal division of the truncus and conus. The aorticopulmonary septum is displaced anteriorly, resulting in a complex of 4 defects: narrow right ventricular outflow tract (pulmonary stenosis), large VSD, overriding aorta, and hypertrophy of the right ventricular wall due to the higher pressures on the right side of the heart.

   b. *Transposition of the great vessels* occurs when the septum grows almost straight down the truncus. The aorta is transposed to the right ventricle, and the pulmonary artery to the left. There is usually an atrial or ventricular septal defect or a patent ductus arteriosus, which provides some mixing of blood. Even so, this severely cyanotic defect can be fatal if not treated quickly, because most of the blood entering the aorta for distribution to the body is deoxygenated blood that just returned to the right heart from the body.

   c. In *double outlet right ventricle*, the abnormal truncal septation causes the aorta to override both ventricles via a membranous ventricular septal defect. This sends deoxygenated right ventricular blood into the aorta, causing another cyanotic defect.

3. *Semilunar valvular atresia* or *stenosis* can affect either the aortic or pulmonary valves. Atresia results from complete fusion of valve material early in development. The left side of the heart is underdeveloped or hypoplastic because of lack of flow through it.

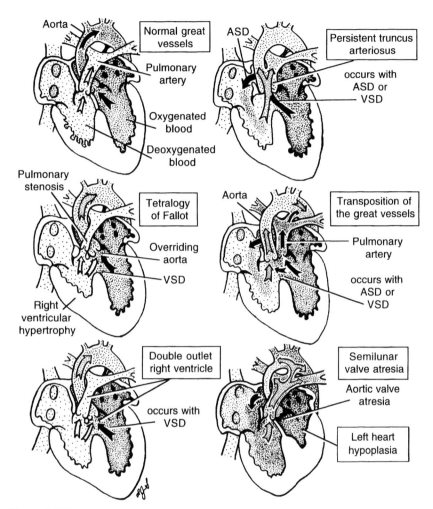

Figure 11-11
Defects in great vessel septation.

FORMATION OF THE VASCULATURE

Blood vessels form throughout the embryo as the heart is forming. The main arteries form as outgrowths from the aorta and pulmonary arteries, while the main veins from the body lead into the sinus venosus. Both arterial and venous systems initially consist of three sets of paired vessels (see Fig. 11-12). The arterial vessels include the *aortic arches* and *dorsal aortae*, which form as extensions of the truncus arteriosus, and the *vitelline* and *umbilical arteries*, which then form as outgrowths from the dorsal aorta. The three major pairs of veins that form are the *cardinal veins*, *vitelline veins*, and *umbilical veins*, which all initially enter the sinus venosus.

• **EARLY BLOOD VESSEL FORMATION**   Blood vessels begin to form in the embryo and yolk sac in week 3. The initial circuitry between placenta and embryo is established by week 4. The early vessels cannot be distinguished as arteries or veins except by location and connections. Almost all are formed by splanchnic mesoderm which coalesces in many locations. Many small cavities form within this coalesced mesoderm. The cells that line the cavities, called *angioblasts*, become the endothelial lining of vessels. The separate endothelial cavities fuse together to form extensive networks. This process is called *vasculogenesis*. In many places, *angiogenesis* then takes over: the endothelium of existing vessels buds and grows into organs under the direction of angiogenesis factors secreted by those target organs. In all cases, the local mesoderm will later form any connective tissue and smooth muscle walls.

• **The formation of blood vessels is intimately associated with the initial formation of blood cells, or hematopoiesis.**   It is believed that the first blood cells differentiate from cells at the center of the cavities, or blood islands, formed in the yolk sac. These cells (and possibly cells formed in as yet undetermined locations in the embryo) migrate into the embryo within the forming vessels and seed several organs as they form: the liver, spleen, thymus, lymph nodes, and finally the bone marrow. These organs then become sites of hematopoiesis. (This is explored in more depth in Chap. 17.)

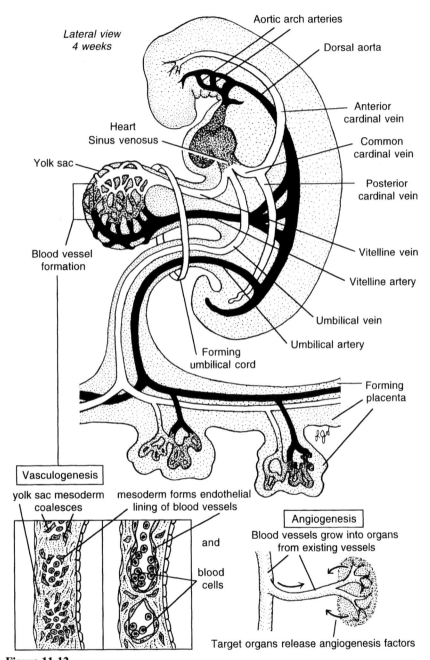

Figure 11-12
Overview of the formation of the earliest arteries and veins.

Formation of the arterial system

The formation of each of the three sets of paired vessels that form the arterial system is examined in sequence (see Fig. 11-13). The aortic arch arteries and *dorsal aortae* form as extensions of the truncus arteriosus. The *vitelline* and *umbilical* arteries then form as outgrowths from the caudal end of the dorsal aorta.

• AORTIC ARCHES AND DORSAL AORTAE
• The aortic arch arteries and the dorsal aorta form the aorta and its main branches, as well as the main pulmonary artery.   Aortic arch arteries form bilaterally during week 4 as extensions of the distal end of the truncus arteriosus. They grow into the pharyngeal arches as they form around the cranial end of the endoderm tube. Arteries form in cranial-caudal sequence in each of the five pharyngeal arches. They are numbered 1 to 4, and 6, since no arch 5 forms in higher vertebrates. The vessels grow through the arches to their dorsal limits, where they unite with the dorsal aortae forming on each side of the body. Each dorsal aorta grows caudally into the body cavity, where they fuse together to form a single dorsal aorta.

> The septation of the truncus arteriosus in week 5 places the first four pairs of aortic arch arteries into the aortic trunk, while the aortic arch arteries of arch 6 arises from the pulmonary trunk.

The originally symmetrical aortic arches transform into an asymmetric adult branching pattern. The arteries of the first two arches regress on each side, except for branches to the head whose origins migrate onto the third arch arteries. The third arch arteries form the *common carotid arteries* to the head. The fourth arch arteries have a different fate on each side. The left fourth arch artery forms the *arch* of the definitive aorta. It remains connected to the left dorsal aorta, which forms the *descending aorta*. The right fourth arch artery and adjoining part of the right dorsal aorta form the *right subclavian artery*. The rest of the right dorsal aorta degenerates. A *brachiocephalic* trunk is created on the right when the origin of the right common carotid artery moves onto the right subclavian artery. The descending aorta gives rise to a series of *intersegmental arteries* which supply the thoracic and abdominal body walls. Those at the level of the limbs form the main arteries to the limbs by hooking up with axial arteries that develop there.

The definitive pulmonary arteries to the lungs form as outgrowths from the arch 6 arteries. The sixth arch arteries themselves have different fates distal to

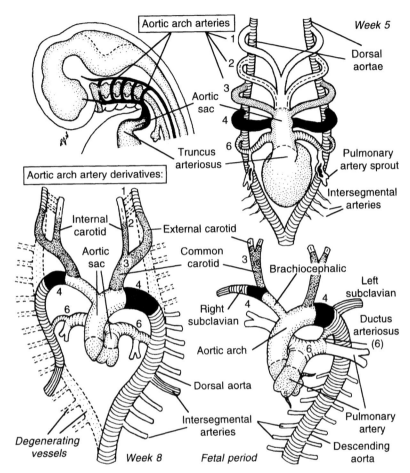

Figure 11-13
Formation of aortic arch derivatives.

these pulmonary artery outgrowths. The distal right arch artery degenerates, while the left arch artery persists throughout fetal life as the *ductus arteriosus*.

The ductus arteriosus shunts most of the blood from the right side of the heart past the fetal lungs to the descending aorta. In the fetus, this is largely oxygenated blood from the placenta.

Defests in formation of aortic arch artery derivatives (see Fig. 11-14).

1. *Patent ductus arteriosus*: The ductus arteriosus normally closes after birth to form the *ligamentum arteriosum*. When it does not close, patent ductus arteriosus can create problems because blood will be shunted from the aorta to the lungs, eventually causing irreversible pulmonary hypertension. Sometimes, however, when the ductus is associated with other congenital heart defects, a patent ductus provides just the life-saving shunt needed to buy time. For the same reason, the ductus is sometimes kept open medically to provide this shunt.

2. *Coarctation of the aorta*: The aorta can become severely constricted or even obliterated at a single point on one side or the other of the ductus arteriosus. In *preductal coarctation*, the ductus persists, providing a shunt around the obstruction during fetal, as well as postnatal, life. However, after birth, the flow to the descending aorta comes entirely from deoxygenated blood from the right side of the heart and subsequently requires surgical correction. In the more common *postductal coarctation*, however, an alternative route must develop to get flow to the descending aorta even during fetal life. Usually, intersegmental arteries enlarge to form "collateral vessels" around the coarctation.

3. Abnormal persistence or obliteration of fourth aortic arch segments, or the dorsal aorta distal to them, can occur in several forms:

    a. *Interrupted aortic arch* results when the artery of the fourth arch, or a segment of the dorsal aorta distal to it, is abnormally obliterated on the left side (as well as on the right). The ductus arteriosus again provides the necessary flow to the descending aorta during fetal development. It must be kept open after birth to maintain this flow.

    b. *Right aortic arch* results when the right fourth arch artery and dorsal aorta persist, while the left arch and aorta regress. Without other defects, this can result in normal circulation.

    c. *Double aortic arch* results when both the left and right arteries of the fourth arch and dorsal aorta persist. The problem here is that the bilateral aortic arches form a ring around the esophagus as they form from the ventral truncus arteriosus to the dorsal aortae; if they persist on both sides, they form a constricting vascular ring around the trachea and esophagus.

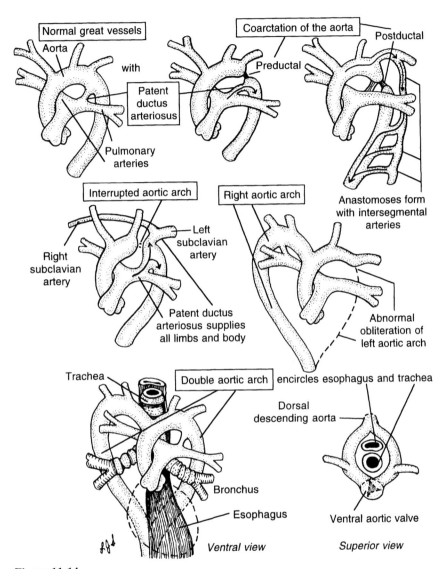

Figure 11-14
Defects in arterial vessel formation.

• **VITELLINE ARTERIES FORM MESENTERIC ARTERIES** The vitelline arteries form as paired vessels from the abdominal portion of the dorsal aorta (or future descending aorta) (see Fig. 11-15). They grow along the wall of the yolk sac, which retains a narrow connection with the midgut section of the endoderm tube. The long-term importance of the vitelline arteries lies in their formation of the arteries supplying the gastrointestinal tract, digestive organs, and their mesenteries—*celiac, superior,* and *inferior mesenteric arteries.*

The vitelline arteries serve a significant function during fetal life: blood cells form within their lumens as the vessel walls are forming and are then transported to the body in these arteries, where they seed the hematopoietic organs (see Chap. 17 for more details).

• **UMBILICAL ARTERIES FORM IMPORTANT LINKS TO THE PLACENTA** This third major pair of vessels develops from the caudal end of the dorsal aorta (see Fig. 11-15). The umbilical arteries (and veins) use the wall of the allantois to grow into the mesodermal core of the umbilical stalk, just as the vitelline vessels use the yolk sac wall. The allantois is described more fully in Chaps. 14 and 18. It is one of those obscure embryonic structures that we inherited from our nonplacental evolutionary ancestors. For now, just realize that it is a diverticulum of the hindgut endoderm which grows out into the mesoderm core of the forming umbilical stalk. After birth, the proximal portions of the umbilical arteries within the body persist as the internal iliac and superior vesical arteries, while their distal extents are transformed into the medial umbilical ligaments.

Umbilical vessels do the reverse of what all other veins and arteries do: the veins carry *oxygenated* blood to the fetus, while the arteries carry *deoxygenated* blood from the fetus to the placenta.

• **Arteries branch ventrally, laterally, and dorsally from the descending aorta.** Vitelline and umbilical arteries develop as ventral branches from the descending aorta. Thus, the arteries that eventually supply the gastrointestinal tract are ventral branches of the aorta. Lateral branches of the aorta develop to supply visceral organs derived from the intermediate mesoderm, including the urinary and genital systems. Finally, the intersegmental arteries that supply the body walls and limbs develop as dorsal branches of the aorta.

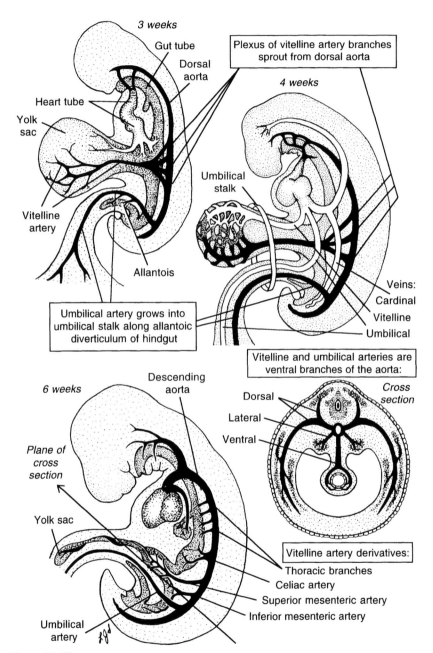

Figure 11-15
Derivatives of vitelline and umbilical arteries.

Formation of the venous system

All venous return from the embryo connects initially to the sinus venosus. (Venous return from the lungs via the pulmonary veins to the left atrium was already covered in the section on venous return to the atria.) Just as with the arterial system, three major pairs of vessels form: *cardinal veins*, *vitelline veins*, and *umbilical veins* (see Fig. 11-16). However, venous development is more varied. Multiple connections, or anastomoses, form between the left and right veins in each pair. Most of the left-sided veins then regress, leaving their anastomoses to drain the left body into the right-sided veins.

• **CARDINAL VEINS**
• **The cardinal veins form the initial venous drainage of the embryo to the heart via the sinus venosus.**   Anterior cardinal veins drain the head and arms, while posterior cardinal veins drain the body and legs. These veins converge to form short left and right common cardinal veins which enter their respective sinus venosus horns. The right common cardinal vein and right sinus horn enlarge, shifting the left common cardinal vein to open into the right common cardinal vein. All cardinal vein flow then enters the right atrium via the right common cardinal vein.

• **The superior vena cava and its branches that drain the head and arms are derived from the right anterior cardinal vein.**   The left anterior cardinal vein drains the left head and arms into the right-sided superior vena cava via the development of an anastomosis, which becomes the left brachiocephalic vein. The connection of the left anterior cardinal vein to the sinus venosus then degenerates. The most proximal segment of the left sinus venosus persists as the coronary sinus, which drains the myocardial walls to the right atrium.

• **The inferior vena cava is formed in several segments, mostly derived from outgrowths of the right posterior cardinal vein.**   The posterior cardinal veins are transient structures, from which a series of other "cardinal" veins develop as outgrowths on both sides. Collectively, these veins will form the mature drainage of the body and legs and several segments of the inferior vena cava. *Supracardinal veins* form most cranially and drain the thoracic body walls and contents via their formation of right-sided *azygos* and left-sided *hemiazygos* veins. *Subcardinal veins* form first at the abdominal level and drain the dorsal abdominal body wall and dorsal organs (the kidneys and gonads). Caudal *sacrocardinal veins* drain the lower limbs. In each pair, the left-sided veins regress after forming anastomoses to shunt their blood to the right-sided veins.

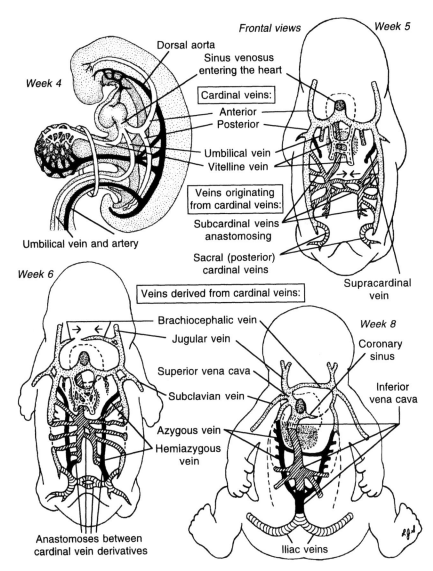

Figure 11-16
Cardinal venous drainage.

• VITELLINE VEINS

• **The vitelline veins form the venous drainage of the digestive organs and the terminal portion of the inferior vena cava.**   The vitelline veins arise in the yolk sac. They initially grow into the abdominal region to connect with the sinus venosus on both sides (see Fig. 11-17). However, this soon transforms into another right-sided connection with left-right anastomoses. The vitelline veins form anastomoses around the foregut and midgut sections of the endoderm tube, and the left vein regresses beyond that point. The anastomoses sprout *celiac*, *mesenteric*, and *splenic veins*, which drain the future gastrointestinal tract, its mesenteries, and associated digestive organs. These veins enter the right vitelline vein as a single *portal vein*. Where the vitelline veins pass through the forming liver cords, they sprout another venous plexus, which forms the *hepatic sinusoidal veins*. A direct channel through the liver then forms from coalescing vitelline sinusoids. It opens into the terminal portion of the right vitelline vein, which enlarges to form the hepatic portion of the inferior vena cava.

> The definitive inferior vena cava is constructed from portions of four separate veins: the right vitelline vein (terminal or hepatic segment), right subcardinal vein (renal segment), right supracardinal vein (abdominal segment), and sacral cardinal veins (sacral segment).

• UMBILICAL VEINS

• **Umbilical veins bring oxygenated blood to the fetus from the placenta.** The umbilical veins grow through the umbilical stalk into the abdomen and then through the forming liver area to connect independently with the left and right horns of the sinus venosus. However, these independent connections degenerate and are replaced by anastomoses with the hepatic sinusoidal veins. The right umbilical vein then degenerates completely (providing the only shift to the left in all these venous changes). The left umbilical vein forms a direct channel through the liver, called the *ductus venosus*, which shunts blood directly into the portion of the right vitelline vein that becomes the inferior vena cava. The ductus venosus will shut down after birth.

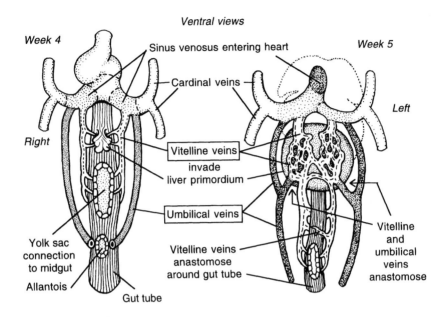

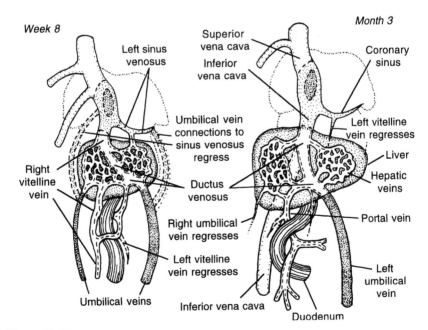

Figure 11-17
Vitelline and umbilical venous contributions.

Congenital defects in vein formation (see Fig. 11-18).

1. *Persistent left superior vena cava* (or *double superior vena cava*) occurs when the *left anterior cardinal vein* persists, draining into the right atrium by way of its abnormal persisting connection to the coronary sinus.
2. *Double inferior vena cava* occurs when the left sacrocardinal vein persists; it eventually drains to the renal segment of the inferior vena cava (formed by the subcardinal vein).
3. *Absent inferior vena cava* occurs when the right subcardinal vein fails to connect to the liver vessels and, instead, continues to shunt its blood directly into the right supracardinal vein (future azygos vein).
4. *Anomalous pulmonary venous return* occurs when the pulmonary veins are pulled away from their left atrial origins to open into the right atrium or other systemic veins, either partially or entirely. This results in the mixing of blood on both sides of the heart.

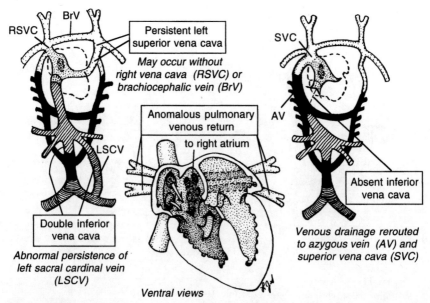

Figure 11-18
Defects in vein formation.

LYMPHATIC VASCULATURE

For lymphatic vessels to retrieve fluids lost to the tissue spaces from capillaries and small veins, they must develop parallel to them. Lymphatic channels form from lateral plate mesoderm throughout the body, much as the venous system forms (see Fig. 11-19). They begin forming late in week 5. Structurally, lymphatics resemble small veins in that they consist of an epithelial lining, with a small amount of surrounding connective tissue. Initially a series of *lymphatic sacs* form bilaterally (*jugular, cysterna chyli, retroperitoneal,* and *iliac*), which serve as drainage sites for proliferating lymph vessels. These sacs become connected to each other by channels during month 2. The channels coalesce into right and left *thoracic ducts.* They empty into the venous system at the junction of the forming subclavian and internal jugular veins on each side. The ducts are then reshaped by anastomoses. Ultimately, the definitive thoracic duct forms from the left duct proximally and, via anastomoses, the right duct distally. A smaller right lymphatic duct usually persists from just the proximal part of the embryonic right duct. Lymph nodes develop along the path of lymphatic vessels. They filter the lymph components on their way back to the venous circulation (see Chap. 17).

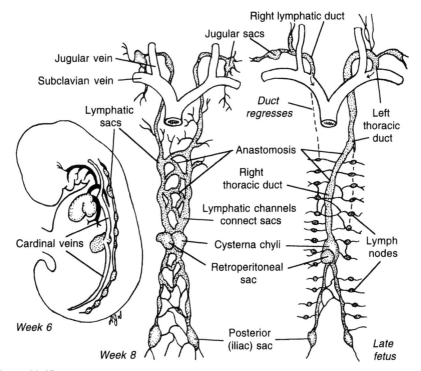

Figure 11-19
Development of lymphatic system.

CIRCULATION PATTERNS BEFORE AND AFTER BIRTH

The heart tube begins contracting during the cardiac looping stage. Circulation begins as the bilateral heart tubes are still fusing, and blood vessels connect to either end of the heart (see Fig. 11-20). Fetal circulation shunts oxygenated blood from the placenta past the liver into the inferior vena cava via the *ductus venosus*. The oxygenated blood bypasses most of the right side of the heart into the left side of the heart via the *foramen ovale* and bypasses the lungs to enter the aorta via the *ductus arteriosus*. The result of these shunts is that the majority of oxygenated blood bypasses the liver and right side of the heart for the left side of the heart, from which it travels out the aorta to the body. The blood in the right side of the heart is mixed: some of the placental oxygenated blood is mixed with the deoxygenated blood returning from the head and upper limbs and propelled through the right ventricle and out the pulmonary artery. This mixture is still sufficient to nourish the lungs; when some of it enters the descending aorta at the ductus arteriosus, the reduction in total oxygenation is still sufficient to supply the more caudal portions of the body. What this circuit ensures is that the head and upper limbs, as well as the heart via the coronary arteries, receive the most highly oxygenated blood.

• **After birth, all these shunts shut down.**   Oxygenated blood ceases to enter the newborn via the umbilical veins and begins to enter the circulation from the pulmonary veins to the left atrium. These changes in flow cause differences in pressure, which reroute flow and help to close these shunts. The uninflated fetal lungs present high resistance to flow. When the newborn lungs expand with the first breath, they then present low resistance to flow, just as they need that flow to oxygenate blood. The new volume of blood to the lungs returns to the left atrium, increasing volume and pressure in the left side of the heart. The higher left atrial pressure closes the foramen ovale, stopping the shunt of blood across the atrial septum. The ductus arteriosus is signaled to shut down by changes in oxygen content and hormones released into the circulation from the lungs during initial inflation. The ductus arteriosus degenerates into the ligamentum arteriosum. The ductus venosus through the liver from the umbilical vein is also signaled to shut down at birth, forming the *ligamentum venosum*.

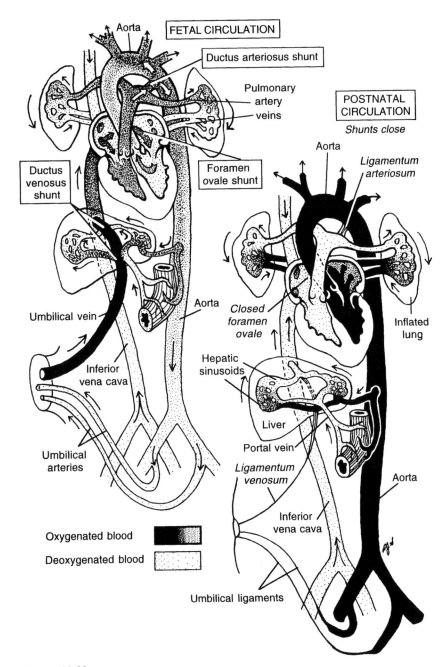

Figure 11-20
Fetal and neonatal circulation patterns.

GASTROINTESTINAL SYSTEM

·

·   ·   ·   ·   ·   ·   ·   ·   ·   ·   ·   ·

The gastrointestinal, or digestive, system consists of the gastrointestinal (GI) tract and associated digestive organs. The GI tract takes in food, mechanically and enzymatically digests it so that it can be absorbed into the circulation, and eliminates the solid wastes of that digestion. Associated digestive organs assist the digestion process. They include the *salivary glands, liver, gallbladder*, and *pancreas*. The mature structure and development of the gastrointestinal system are intimately connected with the membranes and structures that line the body cavity and separate internal organs from each other. These structures are the *peritoneum, mesenteries, ligaments*, and *diaphragm*. Their development was first described in Chap. 6. Developments of particular relevance to the digestive system are described in more detail in this chapter.

COMPONENTS OF THE GASTROINTESTINAL SYSTEM
The gastrointestinal tract

The GI tract begins at the mouth (see Fig. 12-1) . Formation of most structures of the mouth (teeth, tongue, and muscles of mastication and of the palate) were covered in Chap. 10. The first accessory digestive organs, the salivary glands, secrete the first digestive enzymes here. From the mouth, ingested food enters the pharynx. Swallowing is initiated as a voluntary action in the pharynx and is continued through the esophagus, from which food enters the stomach. The dilated lumen of the stomach curves to the right to enter the small intestines, which contain three regions, the *duodenum, jejunum,* and *ileum.* The first serious enzymatic digestion takes place in the stomach, while the majority of enzymatic digestion, and virtually all nutrient absorption, takes place in the small intestines. The ileum leads into the shorter, wider *large intestines* or *colon,* which also has three regions: *ascending, transverse,* and *descending* limbs. The descending limb merges into the *rectum* and *anus* that opens to the outside at the anal sphincter. The major function of the large intestines is concentration of waste by reabsorption of water and controlled elimination of wastes.

Associated digestive organs: pancreas, liver, and gallbladder

These organs are located together in the abdominal cavity. The pancreas is a combined endocrine and exocrine gland. Its exocrine secretions are largely digestive enzymes that are emptied into the duodenum by a duct. Its endocrine secretions are hormones, principally insulin and glucagon, which are secreted into the bloodstream. The liver is a large organ that performs many functions essential to metabolism. It is in direct contact with the diaphragm cranial to it and wraps ventrally around the junction of the stomach and small intestines. The gallbladder is tucked under its ventral rim. A knowledge of the blood supply of the liver is critical to understanding its functioning. The portal vein delivers nutrients to it that were just absorbed from the small intestines, and the hepatic artery supplies oxygenated blood from the aorta. After this blood is filtered through liver lobules, it leaves the liver via the *hepatic vein* to return to the vena cava. One of the products of liver hepatocytes is *bile,* which is carried via channels called *bile canaliculi* from the liver to the hepatic duct. This then drains into the gallbladder via the cystic duct. Bile is stored in the gallbladder until needed for digestion of fats, when it is released into the *bile duct,* which has a common opening into the duodenum with the main pancreatic duct.

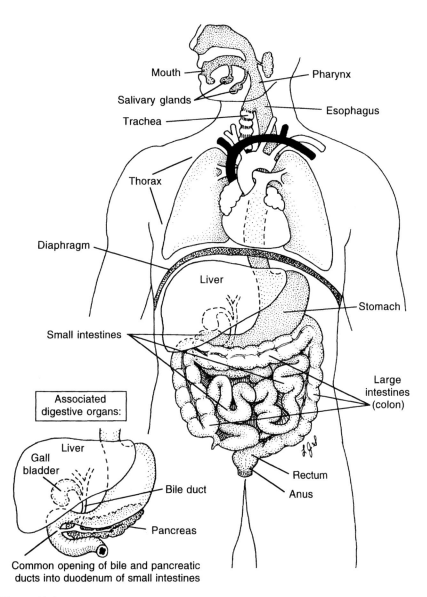

Figure 12-1
Components of the gastrointestinal (GI) system.

• RELATIONSHIP OF GASTROINTESTINAL ORGANS TO THE BODY CAVITIES AND LININGS

• **The diaphragm is a skeletal muscle septum dividing the body cavity into thoracic and abdominal cavities.**   The GI system extends through the thoracic and abdominal cavities (see Fig. 12-2). The esophagus extends the length of the thoracic cavity, passing through an opening in the diaphragm and into the abdominal cavity just prior to its junction with the stomach. There are separate openings for major blood vessels in the diaphragm. The remainder of the GI system is contained in the abdominal cavity.

• **The epithelium lining the thoracic cavity extends into the cavity to divide it into two cavities.**   A central pericardial cavity contains the heart, while two dorsolateral pleural cavities contain the lungs. They are separated by epithelial septa of the same names. The dorsomedial part of the cavity, or *mediastinum*, contains the esophagus, trachea, and descending aorta. Connective tissue surrounds these vessels, and reflections of the pleural epithelium cover their surfaces.

• **The epithelium lining the abdominal part of the body cavity is called the** *peritoneum*.   Portions of the gastrointestinal tract and associated organs are *retroperitoneal*, or fixed in place to the dorsal body wall behind the peritoneum. These include the duodenum, the pancreas, and terminal parts of the system (ascending and descending colon, rectum, and anus). The remaining portions of the system are *intraperitoneal*, that is, within the body cavity. These portions are attached to the dorsal body wall by mesenteries and peritoneal ligaments. Mesenteries are double layers of peritoneum that surround and enclose an organ and connect it to the body wall. They provide pathways for vessels, nerves, and lymphatics to reach these visceral organs. They also suspend portions of the GI tract within the peritoneal cavity. Mesenteries are usually broad sheets. In places they form narrow dense cords that are called *peritoneal ligaments*. They pass between specific organs, or between organs and the body wall.

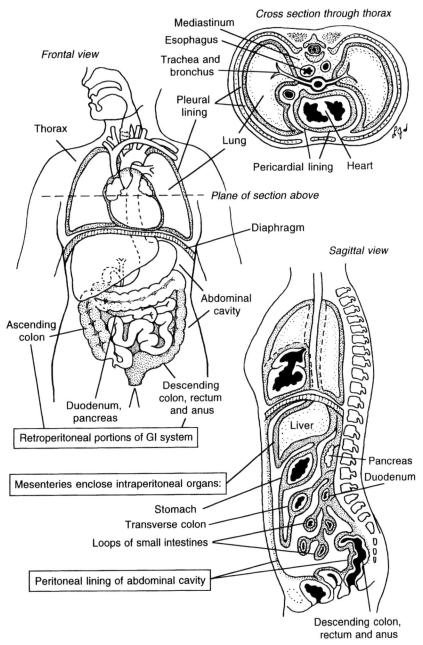

Figure 12-2
Relationship of the GI system to the peritoneum, mesenteries, and diaphragm.

• HISTOLOGIC STRUCTURE OF THE GASTROINTESTINAL SYSTEM

The GI tract is composed of a series of layers (see Fig. 12-3). Its lumen is lined by an epithelium, which is supported by underlying connective tissue richly supplied with blood vessels and lymphatics. Lymphoid follicles are embedded in the connective tissue in many places. These layers are surrounded by two or three layers of smooth muscle that cause *peristalsis*, a coordinated wave of contraction that carries contents along the tract. Small autonomic nerve ganglia that innervate the smooth muscle are sandwiched between the muscle layers. At both ends of the tract, skeletal muscle replaces smooth muscle, permitting voluntary control of the initial steps of swallowing and defecation.

• The histologic structure of the GI tract differs along its length, reflecting differences in function.   The tract differs in the width of its lumen; the thickness of its walls; and the presence of folds, or rugae, glands, and fingerlike projections called *villi*. Each region also differs in the specific types of absorptive, secretory, and protective cells in its epithelial lining. It is necessary to know about these regionally specific characteristics to fully appreciate the complexities of embryonic development of this system.

In most places along the GI tract, the epithelium forms glands that are contained within the wall of the tract. Glands are epithelial tubes that extend down into the connective tissue layers. They differ in length, complexity, and epithelial cell types. In the small intestines, villi are formed that extend into the lumen to increase surface area for absorption of nutrients. They are formed by epithelia covering interior cores filled with loose connective tissue, blood vessels, and lymphatics.

• The histologic structure of the associated digestive glands have certain features in common.   The functional cells of each organ are epithelial cells, surrounded by small amounts of connective tissue. Of the three, only the gallbladder contains a morphology similar to the GI tract, with an epithelial lining thrown into folds, surrounded by thin connective tissue and smooth muscle layers. The liver is organized into a series of lobules, each formed by a series of epithelial channels, or cords, of *hepatocytes* between which blood is filtered. The pancreas contains both *exocrine* secretory cells, which release their digestive enzymes through epithelial ducts into the lumen of the small intestines, and separate epithelial clumps called *islets of Langerhans*, which form *endocrine* cells that secrete hormones into the bloodstream.

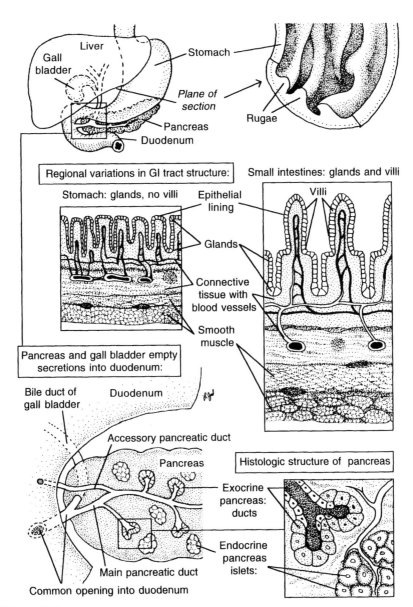

Figure 12-3
Histologic organization of the GI tract and regional variations.

GERM-LAYER ORIGINS OF THE GASTROINTESTINAL SYSTEM

• **The endoderm tube forms the epithelial lining of the entire GI tract and the epithelial components of its associated digestive organs (see Fig. 12-4).** The endoderm tube is created during weeks 3 and 4 when embryonic folding causes the flat endoderm sheet to fold ventrally into a tube that runs the length of the embryo, as first covered in Chap. 4. The epithelial components derived from the endoderm are the "business" cells of each organ. That is, the epithelial cells perform the secretory, absorptive, metabolic, and protective functions that characterize the function of each region of the organ system.

• **Splanchnic lateral plate mesoderm forms the connective tissue and smooth muscle components of the GI system.**

The formation of all components of the GI system requires that the mesoderm and endoderm components mutually induce each other's development. The development of specific regional characteristics along the GI tract is also directed by these inductive interactions. It is known that the mesoderm carries the region-specific instructions. However, it is not understood how it receives those instructions.

Mesoderm induces the endoderm to form specific types of epithelial cells, such as cells secreting acid in the stomach and digestive enzymes in the small intestines. It also directs the specific location of formation of villi and glands and their specific configuration. The endoderm induces the mesoderm to form appropriate arrangements and types of connective tissue and smooth muscle components, and blood vessel patterns.

• **Skeletal muscle that forms at both ends of the GI tract is derived from mesoderm of the somitic myotomes.** These cells migrate into the lateral plate mesoderm, where they begin their differentiation.

• **Diverticula of the endoderm tube foreshadow the formation of the liver, gallbladder, and pancreas.** The associated digestive organs form as diverticula that bud out from the endoderm tube into the surrounding splanchnic mesoderm beginning in week 4. These diverticula form close together. The ventral diverticulum gives rise to the *hepatic diverticulum* and the *ventral pancreatic bud*, while the *dorsal pancreatic bud* forms separately. Together, these diverticula give rise to the epithelial components of the liver, gallbladder, and pancreas.

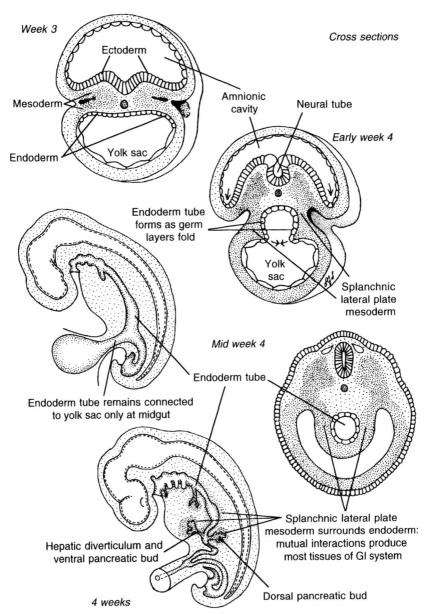

Figure 12-4
Germ-layer origins of the GI tract.

FORMATION OF THE GASTROINTESTINAL TRACT

• **Different regions of the GI tract become clear within the endoderm tube as it forms.**   The endoderm tube forms three separate regions as it folds (see Fig. 12-5). The *foregut* and *hindgut* regions are formed by the folding that occurs first at either end of the endoderm tube during week 3. The midsection of the tube remains a broad, open sheet longer than the rest. As it folds into a tube, the *midgut* is identifiable by the end of week 4. It remains in communication with the *yolk sac* via the *yolk stalk*, or *vitelline duct*. This connection becomes the core of the umbilical cord.

• **The foregut, midgut, and hindgut regions each give rise to specific portions of the GI lining.**

> The junctions between the regions of the endoderm tube are marked by specific landmarks. Further, each of these regions in the mature gut is supplied by different blood vessels.

• **Foregut derivatives extend from the mouth to the first part of the small intestines.**   The foregut can be subdivided into the *pharyngeal gut* and the *foregut proper*. The pharyngeal gut forms the lining of the mouth and pharynx. It ends at the point of origin of the respiratory diverticulum that forms the lining of the respiratory system. An added complexity in the development of the pharyngeal region is that the initial part of the mouth cavity actually becomes lined by ectoderm that is drawn into the interior of the body after the two germ layers meet and fuse. The foregut proper forms the lining of the esophagus, stomach, and first third of the duodenum. The point of foregut termination remains identifiable as the site of pancreatic and hepatic diverticula outgrowth.

• **Midgut derivatives extend from the small intestines through the first part of the large intestines.**   The midgut forms the lining of the remainder of the small intestines (the remaining duodenum, the jejunum, and ileum) and the proximal portion of the large intestines (the *ascending colon* and first two-thirds of the transverse colon). A diverticulum called the *cecal bud* arises at the end of the midgut region, which forms the lining of the dilated start of the large intestines, the cecum, and the appendix that extends from it.

• **Hindgut derivatives form the lining of the distal portion of the large intestines.**   This includes the distal one-third of the transverse colon, the descending colon, and the rectum and anal canal.

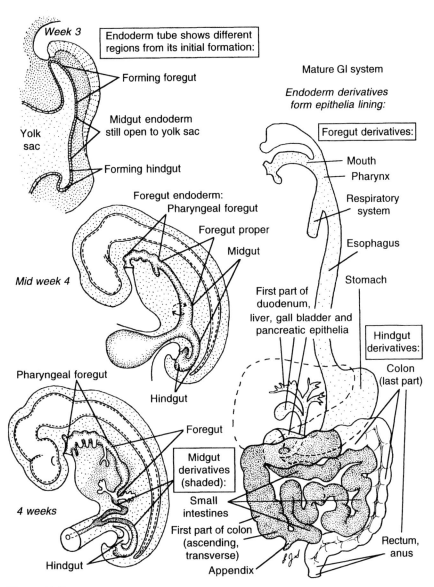

Figure 12-5
Regional derivatives of the endoderm tube.

• **The formation of the rectum and anal canal are complex.** The lining of these structures is formed from a portion of the terminal hindgut that first dilates to form the *cloaca* (see Fig. 12-6). The cloaca becomes partitioned into two compartments by a ridge of mesoderm (the *urorectal septum*). The more caudal compartment becomes the lining of the rectum and anal canal. (The more cranial compartment, the *urogenital sinus*, forms the epithelial lining of the terminal part of the urinary system; covered in Chap. 14.)

The terminal part of both canals is lined by ectoderm in the same way that the mouth cavity becomes partially lined by ectoderm. That is, the endoderm tube fuses with the ectoderm, creating a *cloacal membrane* that rapidly breaks down. The ectoderm-endoderm junction point is then drawn into the interior of the body in both canals.

Anorectal agenesis (failure to develop) can occur if the cloacal membrane does not break down overlying the anal canal. The rectum then ends in a blind pouch.

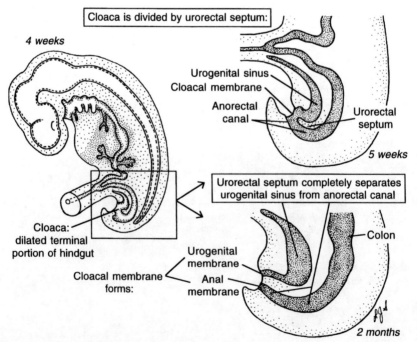

Figure 12-6
Development of the rectum and anal canal.

Arterial and venous supply of the gastrointestinal tract

Each part of the gut is supplied by a different main artery and drained by different groups of veins (see Fig. 12-7). The pharyngeal foregut is supplied by derivatives of the *aortic arch arteries* that form in the pharyngeal arches, and is drained by *anterior cardinal vein* derivatives. All parts of the GI tract from this point on are supplied by derivatives of the vitelline vessels, which originally develop as the vessels supplying the yolk sac. (Remember that the yolk sac is continuous with the midgut.) The foregut proper is supplied by the *celiac artery* and drained by *supracardinal vein* derivatives (azygous and hemiazygous veins) and *portal veins*. The midgut is supplied by the *superior mesenteric artery* and *vein*. The hindgut is supplied by the *inferior mesenteric artery* and vein.

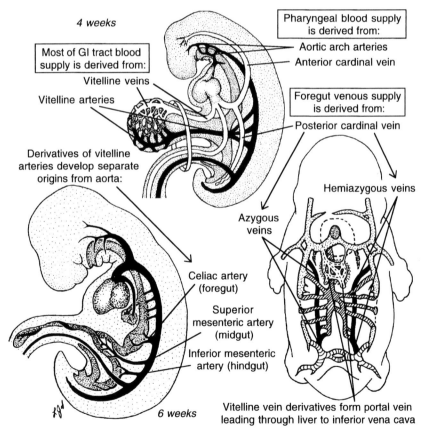

Figure 12-7
Blood supply of the GI tract.

Events in maturation of the gastrointestinal tract

• **HISTOLOGIC MATURATION OF THE GI TRACT (see Fig. 12-8)**

• **The GI tract becomes temporarily solid and then recanalized.** Many regions of the tract temporarily lose their patent lumens when the endodermal epithelium proliferates to form multiple layers in weeks 6 to 7. Recanalization reopens the lumen by weeks 8 to 10. This is essential not only to normal postnatal function, but also to maintaining normal amniotic fluid volume during fetal development. This is because amniotic fluid is continually created, and some must be continually removed. The fetus swallows the fluid, which is absorbed through the epithelial lining of the patent GI tract into blood vessels and returned to the maternal circulation through the placenta.

Stenosis (narrowing) or atresia (closed lumen) of portions of the GI tube can result from failure to recanalize. The most common sites are the esophagus and duodenum. Atresia leads to *polyhydramnios*, or excess amniotic fluid accumulation.

• **Villus and glandular morphology develop during weeks 8 to 10.** In the small intestines, mesoderm proliferates to form projections that push out the covering epithelium to form villi. Mesoderm also directs downgrowth of epithelial buds into mesoderm along most segments of the GI tract, forming simple tubular glands. Epithelial cells differentiate into specific secretory and absorptive cell types during the second trimester. However, only some cell types secrete their products prior to birth.

• **Autonomic innervation of the smooth muscle of the GI tract causes peristalsis to begin by week 10.** The autonomic or involuntary nervous system has both sympathetic and parasympathetic components (described more fully in Chap. 9). In most organ systems, these components form normally. However, formation of parasympathetic innervation of the terminal part of the descending colon and rectum can go awry. This segment is innervated by primary neurons derived from the sacral spinal cord levels and secondary neurons derived from the sacral neural crest. The secondary neurons form ganglia within the wall of the terminal part of the GI tract.

Aganglionic megacolon (or Hirschsprung's disease) results from defective parasympathetic innervation of the descending colon.

The GI tract lumen becomes solid and then recanalized while villi and glands form:

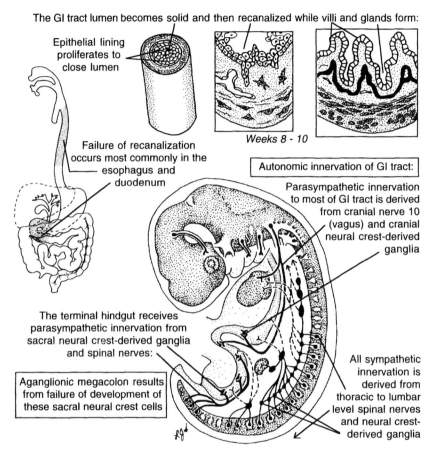

Epithelial lining proliferates to close lumen

Weeks 8 - 10

Failure of recanalization occurs most commonly in the esophagus and duodenum

Autonomic innervation of GI tract:

Parasympathetic innervation to most of GI tract is derived from cranial nerve 10 (vagus) and cranial neural crest-derived ganglia

The terminal hindgut receives parasympathetic innervation from sacral neural crest-derived ganglia and spinal nerves:

Aganglionic megacolon results from failure of development of these sacral neural crest cells

All sympathetic innervation is derived from thoracic to lumbar level spinal nerves and neural crest-derived ganglia

Figure 12-8
Histologic maturation of the GI tract.

The sacral neural crest cells fail to migrate into the walls of the developing colon, or they fail to penetrate the wall once there. This lack of innervation causes dilation and obstruction due to lack of peristalsis. These consequences can be fatal.

By contrast, development of parasympathetic innervation of the remainder of the GI system, as well as most other internal viscera, goes normally. This occurs even though the primary nerves must send their fibers all the way from the brain via the vagus nerve and the neural crest forming their ganglia must migrate all the way from their cranial level origins as well.

• ANATOMIC MATURATION OF THE GASTROINTESTINAL TRACT

• Esophageal-tracheal septation (see Fig. 12-9).   A respiratory diverticulum forms from the ventral surface of the endoderm tube at the end of the pharyngeal region. This diverticulum forms the epithelial lining of the entire respiratory system (as covered in Chap. 13). An *esophageal-tracheal septum* forms to narrow the communication between the two to a narrow *laryngeal orifice*. Surrounding mesoderm pushes endoderm ahead of it to create the septum.

> The esophageal-tracheal septation process can be abnormal. Too complete septation can result in esophageal *stenosis*, or narrowing. Septation can completely cover the common opening, resulting in esophageal *atresia*, or a blind lumen.

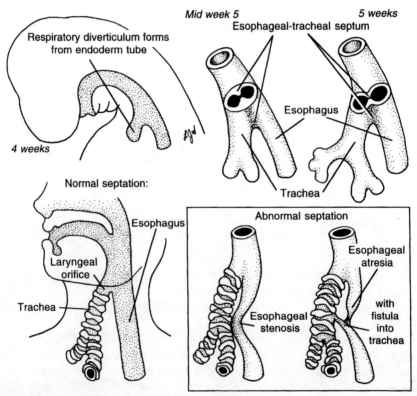

Figure 12-9
Esophageal-tracheal septation.

• **Stomach rotation (see Fig. 12-10).**   The stomach first appears as a dilated region of the midgut endoderm during week 4. As the result of differential rates of growth during weeks 5 to 6, it rotates around both its longitudinal and cranial-caudal axes. More rapid growth of the dorsal side causes it to expand to form the *greater curvature* and rotate to the left. The slower growing ventral side forms the *lesser curvature* and rotates to the right. This growth also causes the esophageal end of the stomach to move caudally and to the left, while the distal (or future pyloric end) moves cranially and to the right. These rotations also affect the formation of the attached mesenteries (see the final section of this chapter).

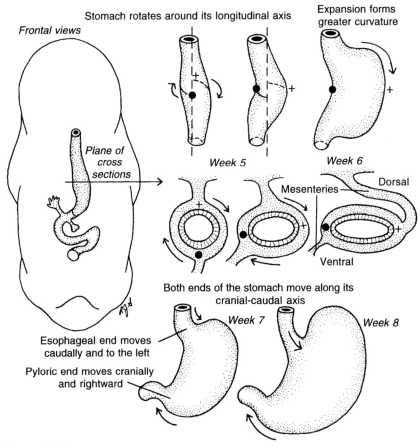

Figure 12-10
Rotation of the stomach.

• **Midgut elongation, herniation, retraction, and rotation (see Fig. 12-11).**
A rapid elongation of the midgut and its attached mesenteries begins during week
5, forming a loop. By weeks 6 and 7, this elongation causes the midgut to leave
the abdominal cavity, or herniate into, the yolk stalk, which is still broadly connected to the body. The first part of the large intestines is also drawn into this herniation. The apex of the herniated loop is the point at which the endoderm of the
midgut is still continuous with the yolk sac endoderm through a narrow vitelline
duct. This duct connects to the future ileum. Midgut rotation occurs around the
axis of the herniated loop, which is formed by the superior mesenteric artery
growing into the forming dorsal mesentery. A total rotation of 270° counter-
clockwise occurs. The initial rotation during herniation is 90°. By weeks 8 to 9,
the abdominal cavity is large enough to accommodate the elongated gut, and
retraction begins. During retraction, a final rotation of 180° occurs. Rotation
changes the relationships among the different portions of the intestines. The
colon now crosses in front of (or dorsal to) the small intestines and assumes an
inverted U-shaped configuration. The duodenum rotates to the right to form a C-
shaped loop.

Abnormal persistence of the vitelline duct from the ileum can occur. The
vitelline duct can persist as either a patent diverticulum of the ileum
(called *Meckel's diverticulum*) or as a ligament, sometimes with a cyst
within it. Intestinal loops can twist around these ligaments, becoming
obstructed. If the diverticulum is patent, fecal material can emerge.

Abnormalities of herniation and retraction of the intestines can occur. In
omphalocele, the gut remains partially herniated through the body wall,
covered only by amniotic membrane epithelium. An *umbilical hernia*
results from failure of normal closure of all layers of the ventral body wall
due to incomplete mesoderm proliferation in the region. The herniated
intestines are covered by both peritoneal lining and amnion.

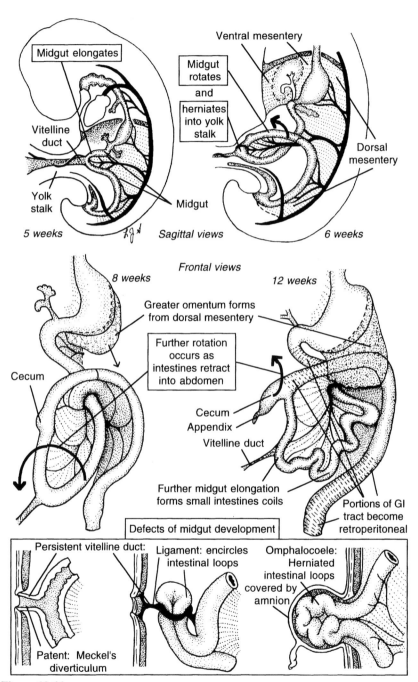

Figure 12-11
Midgut looping, herniation, and retraction, and defects in these processes.

FORMATION OF ASSOCIATED DIGESTIVE ORGANS: LIVER, GALLBLADDER, AND PANCREAS

These organs are all derived from endodermal diverticula that push out into the surrounding splanchnic mesoderm at the boundary of the foregut with the midgut (see Fig. 12-12). The endoderm tube forms the epithelial components of these organs. The mesoderm gives rise to the connective tissue, smooth muscle, and blood vessel components of these organs.

• **Dorsal and ventral endodermal diverticula form specific derivatives.**   The ventral diverticulum branches to form a *hepatic diverticulum* and a *ventral pancreatic bud*. The hepatic diverticulum branches repeatedly to form the epithelial components of the liver and gallbladder, while the dorsal and ventral pancreatic buds branch to form the epithelial components of the pancreas.

Formation of the liver

The hepatic diverticulum first grows into the surrounding splanchnic lateral plate mesoderm. Both tissues then push out into the *septum transversum*, a plate of dense somatic lateral plate mesoderm that grows out from the ventral body wall. It supplies a portion of the mesoderm that forms the liver connective tissue stroma, while most of it is formed by splanchnic lateral plate mesoderm.

The hepatic diverticulum branches repeatedly to form *liver cords*, which become disconnected from the diverticulum to form cords of *hepatocytes*. They group together to form *hepatic lobules*. The cords become invaded by mesodermal blood vessels through which nutrient-rich blood is filtered. Small channels called *bile canaliculi* also develop between hepatocytes. Bile formed by the hepatocytes will be secreted into these channels, which coalesce to enter *hepatic ducts* formed from the terminal ends of the branches of the hepatic diverticulum.

• **During embryonic life the only function of the liver is hematopoiesis, or formation of blood cells from mesoderm-derived stem cells.**   Blood cells are first formed from mesoderm surrounding the yolk sac in week 3. By week 5, hematopoiesis begins in the liver. During weeks 6 to 8, the liver entirely replaces the yolk sac, and maintains a hematopoietic role even after birth. By month 6, however, the bone marrow has taken over as the primary source of hematopoiesis (see Chap. 17 for details of this progression). Hepatocytes gradually begin to perform some other functions during fetal life, including conversion of glucose into its storage form, glycogen, and bile formation. It is not until after birth that hepatocytes begin to perform all of their functions.

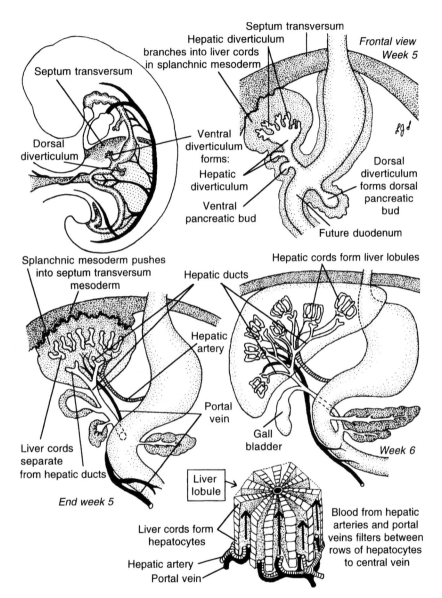

Septum transversum
Hepatic diverticulum
branches into liver cords
in splanchnic mesoderm

Frontal view
Week 5

Septum transversum

Dorsal
diverticulum

Ventral
diverticulum
forms:

Hepatic
diverticulum

Ventral
pancreatic bud

Dorsal
diverticulum
forms dorsal
pancreatic
bud

Future duodenum

Splanchnic mesoderm pushes
into septum transversum
mesoderm

Hepatic ducts

Hepatic cords form liver lobules

Hepatic
artery

Portal
vein

Liver cords
separate
from hepatic ducts

Gall
bladder

Week 6

End week 5

Liver
lobule

Liver cords form
hepatocytes

Hepatic artery
Portal vein

Blood from hepatic
arteries and portal
veins filters between
rows of hepatocytes
to central vein

Figure 12-12
Formation of the liver.

Formation of the gallbladder

• **The hepatic diverticulum gives rise to the epithelial components of the gallbladder, cystic duct, and bile duct (see Fig. 12-13).** The terminal end of the diverticulum forms hepatic ducts that coalesce to transport the bile salts to the gallbladder. The gallbladder itself forms as a separate dilation of the distal end of the hepatic diverticulum. Its connection with the hepatic diverticulum narrows to form the cystic duct. The most proximal portion of the hepatic diverticulum forms the common bile duct that drains into the duodenum with the pancreatic duct.

> Biliary atresia (interruption) or stenosis (narrowing) can occur at any level of the bile channels. *Intrahepatic* defects in bile canaliculi are rare. More commonly, *extrahepatic* defects occur in the cystic duct or the main bile duct.

Formation of the pancreas

• **Dorsal and ventral pancreatic diverticula form all the secretory cells and ducts of the pancreas (see Fig. 12-13).** As with liver formation, the pancreatic diverticula grow into the surrounding splanchnic mesoderm, which forms the connective tissue stroma and blood vessels of the pancreas. The proximal ends of the dorsal and ventral pancreatic diverticula form the pancreatic ducts leading into the small intestines. The ventral pancreatic bud is an outgrowth from the hepatic diverticulum. The entire hepatic diverticulum rotates dorsally and to the left to open on the left side of the duodenum just below and behind the opening of the dorsal pancreatic duct. With further development, the ventral bud forms the opening of the main pancreatic duct into the duodenum at the same point as the bile duct. The dorsal pancreatic bud then sends an offshoot to open into the main duct, forming one long duct. Its original connection to the duodenum usually regresses.

Secretory cells are formed from cells at the tips of the pancreatic buds. They form both exocrine cells that secrete digestive enzymes into the pancreatic ducts, as well as endocrine cells that secrete hormones into the bloodstream. The endocrine cells break away from the tips of the buds to form separate clumps of cells. Pancreatic secretory cells first differentiate in month 3, but few secrete products during fetal life. The exceptions are the endocrine cells that begin to secrete insulin in month 5.

> An *annular pancreas* completely encircles the duodenum and obstructs its lumen.

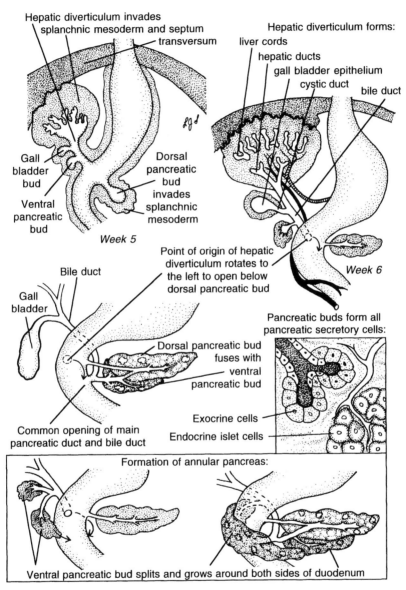

Figure 12-13
Formation of the gallbladder and pancreas.

This may result from an abnormal outgrowth of the ventral pancreatic bud that grows around the ventral side of the duodenum to meet the existing pancreas.

FORMATION OF PERITONEUM, MESENTERIES, LIGAMENTS, AND DIAPHRAGM

The abdominal body cavity is formed between the two layers of lateral plate mesoderm (see Fig. 12-14). The surface cells of both portions of lateral plate mesoderm form the peritoneal lining of the cavity. The splanchnic mesoderm then forms mesenteries and ligaments.

• **The dorsal mesentery is formed by splanchnic lateral plate mesoderm.**
All parts of the gut tube are initially in broad contact with the dorsal abdominal wall via the splanchnic mesoderm. During week 4, the splanchnic mesoderm forms a narrow stalk dorsal to the gut tube called the *dorsal mesentery*. Its surface cells become its peritoneal covering, while the interior cells form connective tissue stroma into which blood vessels and nerves penetrate. The dorsal mesentery thus becomes the only connection of the GI tube to the dorsal body wall.

• **Different regions of the embryonic dorsal mesentery are given names based on the part of the GI tract to which they are attached.** The *dorsal mesogastrium* connects the stomach to the dorsal body wall. Rotation of the stomach pulls the dorsal mesogastrium to the left, creating the *omental bursa* and *greater omentum*. The omental bursa is a blind pouch behind (dorsal to) the stomach. The dorsal mesogastrium expands as a double-layered sac over the small intestine and transverse colon like an apron. It fuses into a single layer called the *greater omentum*, which hangs from the greater curvature of the stomach.

A portion of the splanchnic mesoderm sandwiched between the layers of the dorsal mesogastrium proliferates to form the tissues of the *spleen*. Its development is covered in Chap. 17, since it is a major organ of the hematopoietic system. Ligaments then develop from the dorsal mesogastrium that attach the spleen to the stomach (gastrolienal) and to the dorsal body wall overlying the kidneys (*lienorenal*).

Progressing caudally, the *dorsal mesoduodenum* attaches the duodenum to the body wall. Most of the duodenum and pancreas press against the dorsal body wall during midgut rotation, becoming fixed in a retroperitoneal position. The *dorsal mesenteries* connecting the jejunum and ileum to the body wall persist as the mesentery "proper," while the mesentery attaching the large intestines or colon to the body wall forms the *dorsal mesocolon*.

• **The ventral mesentery forms along only the ventral surface of one portion of the GI tube.** It extends along the inner curvature of the stomach as far as the upper duodenum. Along with contributions from the septum transversum, the ventral mesentery forms the *falciform ligament* which attaches the liver to the

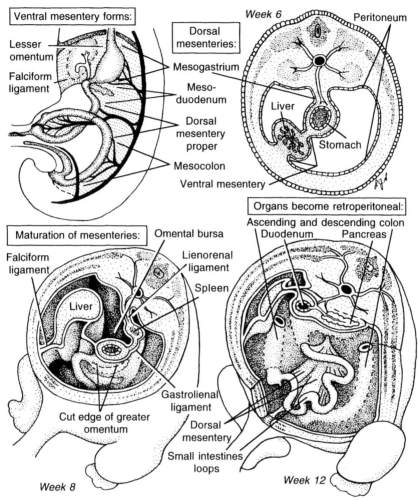

Figure 12-14
Formation of mesenteries and ligaments.

ventral body wall the *coronary* and *triangular ligaments* (which attach the cranial surface of the liver to the diaphragm) and the *lesser omentum* (which attaches the stomach and duodenum to the liver). *Hepatoduodenal* and *hepatogastric ligaments* form from parts of the lesser omentum.

• **Diaphragm formation (see Fig. 12-15).** The coelomic cavity becomes divided into the thoracic cavity and peritoneal (or abdominal) cavity by formation of transverse septa. These septa eventually unite to form the diaphragm. First, somatic lateral plate mesoderm projects from the ventral body wall to start this division. It forms the *septum transversum*. The septum transversum forms the central connective tissue core of the diaphragm. *Pleuroperitoneal membranes* form the dorsal and lateral parts of the diaphragm. They form as ingrowths from the more lateral and dorsal portions of the somatic lateral plate mesoderm. The muscular component of the diaphragm forms from skeletal muscle cells invading it from thoracic level somites (see Chap. 7).

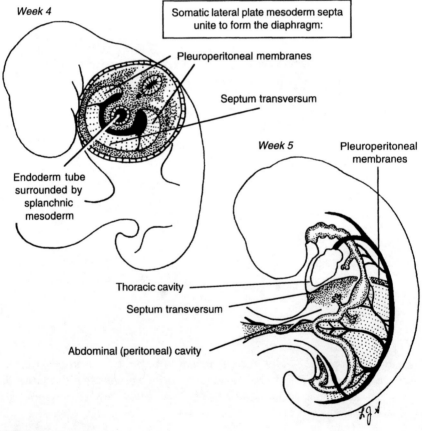

Figure 12-15
Diaphragm formation.

RESPIRATORY SYSTEM

·

•   •   •   •   •   •   •   •   •   •   •   •   •

The respiratory system consists of collecting portions and respiratory exchange portions. The collecting portions begin with the nasal cavities, and then share the pharynx with the gastrointestinal system, before proceeding into conducting airways in the chest cavity, the trachea and bronchi. These airways enter the lungs, where they branch into smaller conducting portions which finally give rise to respiratory exchange passages within the lungs. Here oxygen and carbon dioxide are exchanged between the airways of the lungs and the pulmonary blood vessels within the lungs. The germ layer origins, and subsequent development of, the respiratory system differs somewhat between the collecting portions in the head and the rest of the system contained within the chest cavity. What unites the development of these portions of the respiratory system is that most regions are lined by endoderm-derived epithelia, which interacts with surrounding mesoderm to form the other components of the system. An understanding of the basic development of the initial portion of the endoderm tube helps in understanding the development of the respiratory system.

ELEMENTS OF THE MATURE RESPIRATORY SYSTEM

The respiratory system can be divided into upper and lower respiratory tracts (see Fig. 13-1). The upper portion, the nasal cavities and pharynx, is entirely a collecting portion or a conduit for air, as well as an air filter. The lower portion contains the portions of the respiratory tract within the thoracic cavity: the end of the collecting portion, which begins at the larynx, and all of the functional portion, in which gaseous exchange between the vascular system and airways occurs. The lower portion of the respiratory system also can be considered to include the structures that support the breathing process. These include the muscular diaphragm and the intercostal muscles.

Upper respiratory system: collecting airways

The collecting portion starts at the *nasal cavities* and proceeds through the *pharynx* across the *larynx* into the *trachea*. From there, the trachea branches into two main *bronchi* which enter the substance of each lung medially at its hilus, along with the pulmonary blood vessels. Several levels of branching of the bronchi into *bronchioles* are still part of the collecting system. Portions of the collecting tract contain a number of cartilages which provide structural support and keep the structures of the airway from collapsing. The larynx, or voice box, marks the point of division between upper and lower respiratory systems. It contains nine cartilages joined by ligaments (the largest being the *thyroid cartilage*), as well as the *vocal cords*, which are actually epithelial folds to each side of the laryngeal opening, or *glottis*.

Lower respiratory system: collecting and respiratory exchange portions

The collecting portion of the lower respiratory system begins with the trachea. The tracheal wall contains 16 to 20 C-shaped cartilages distributed along its length. The main bronchi also contain partial cartilage rings distributed in somewhat more irregular fashion. Cartilage stops at the point where the bronchioles form. Considerable amounts of elastic and smooth muscle are present in the walls of the airways down through the bronchioles to help make them flexible and distensible and able to recoil after distension.

The functional exchange portion of the lungs begins with the *respiratory bronchioles* of the lungs, from which *alveolar ducts*, *sacs*, and, finally, individual *alveoli* arise. The simple squamous epithelial walls of alveoli permit gaseous exchange between them and the capillary epithelium of the pulmonary vessels against which they are directly opposed. Certain alveolar cells secrete a *surfac-*

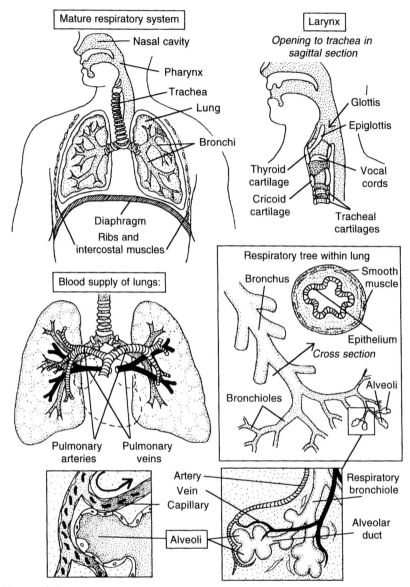

Figure 13-1
Mature respiratory system.

tant into the air spaces, a lipoprotein that decreases surface tension, thereby keeping the alveolar walls from collapsing on expiration. Deoxygenated blood enters the lungs via the pulmonary arteries from the right side of the heart and leaves via the pulmonary veins to return the newly oxygenated blood to the left atrium.

ORIGINS OF THE RESPIRATORY SYSTEM

The origins of the upper and lower portions of the respiratory system differ in several ways. The dividing point between the upper and lower respiratory systems is the larynx, which serves as the gate to the trachea. The upper respiratory tract is formed in the head, while the lower respiratory tract is formed in the body.

Origins of the upper respiratory tract: nasal cavities and pharynx

The entrance to the respiratory system is formed by the nasal cavities (see Fig. 13-2). These cavities form by invagination of surface ectoderm specializations called *nasal placodes*. The placodes form epithelial diverticula which dive into the mesodermal substance of the nasal swellings of the face, uniting temporarily to form a single cavity which eventually meets and opens into the pharygneal region of the endoderm tube. Thus, the start of the respiratory system is lined by ectoderm-derived epithelium.

The ectodermal placode cells form not only the epithelial linings of the nasal cavities, but also the primary olfactory sensory receptors (neurons).

These primary neurons then grow into the outgrowing first cranial nerve, where they connect with its olfactory association neurons. The surrounding head mesoderm forms the other components of the nasal walls and the palate separating the nasal cavities from the pharynx, as well as the nasal septum. These developments are covered more extensively in Chap. 9.

The portion of the pharyngeal cavity into which the nasal cavities open is lined by the epithelium of the endoderm tube, and the tissues of its wall are formed by surrounding mesoderm (mostly lateral plate mesoderm of the pharyngeal arches).

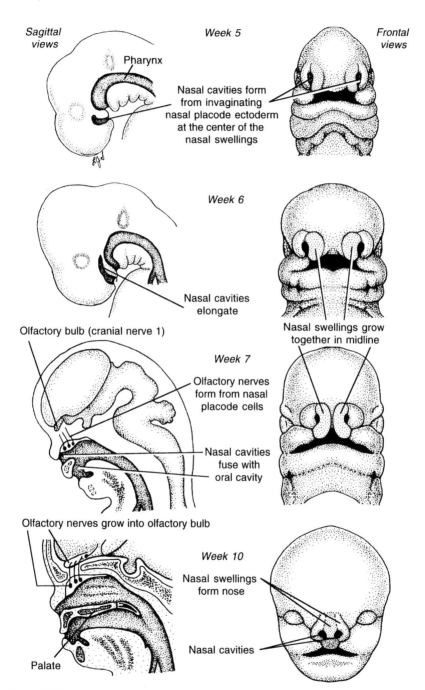

Figure 13-2
Formation of the upper respiratory tract.

Origins of the lower respiratory tract

• **The respiratory diverticulum is formed by an endoderm bud.**   The respiratory system begins in week 4 with the formation of a respiratory diverticulum or lung bud, from the ventral wall of the foregut endoderm just caudal to the pharyngeal arches (see Fig. 13-3).

> The endoderm of the respiratory diverticulum will form the epithelial lining of all the respiratory airway passages, starting with the laryngeal orifice to the trachea and extending all the way down to the terminal alveoli.

In the terminal alveoli, this epithelium will form the "business" cells of the respiratory system, which means the epithelial sacs that perform the gaseous exchange between the lungs and pulmonary blood vessels.

• **Respiratory diverticulum meets splanchnic lateral plate mesoderm.**   The respiratory diverticulum expands into the lateral plate mesoderm, which surrounds the endoderm tube from the point at which it enters the body cavity. The most cranial end of the endoderm tube is surrounded by the lateral plate mesoderm formed in the pharyngeal arches, while the lung bud extends into the forming body coelom where it is surrounded by the splanchnic lateral plate mesoderm, which surrounds all of the endoderm tube.

Splanchnic mesoderm forms the smooth muscle and connective tissues (including the cartilages) of the trachea, bronchi, and all airways in the lung. It also forms all the tissues of the pulmonary blood vessels.

> Mesoderm contains the primary instructions for epithelial budding and the patterning of its branches in all organs which form by such budding. (Other organs formed by such epithelial-mesenchymal inductive interactions include the liver, pancreas, and kidneys.) In the formation of the lungs, the mesoderm at the tips of the lung buds directs when and where the buds branch.

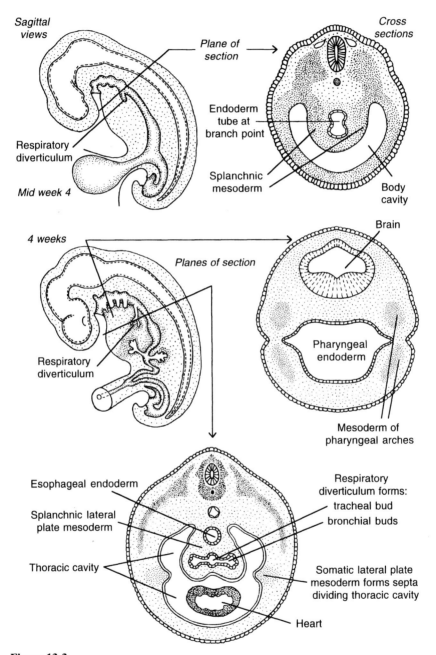

Figure 13-3
Formation of the endoderm diverticulum and its initial interaction with splanchnic lateral plate mesoderm.

• Formation of the laryngeal opening to the respiratory tract (see Fig. 13-4). Since the lung bud forms just caudal to the pharyngeal arches, it should not be surprising that some of the mesoderm derivatives formed in the walls of the first portions of the lung bud are derived from the lateral plate mesoderm of the pharyngeal arches. Specifically, these include the cartilages and muscles of the larynx. These are derived from arches 4 and 6 and are innervated by cranial nerve 10 (the vagus), the nerve of these arches. During month 2, proliferation of cartilagenous precursors around the lung bud opening changes the round shape of the orifice to a T-shaped opening. These cartilages then form the laryngeal cartilages. True and false vocal cords form from folds of epithelium around the laryngeal orifice.

• Formation of the trachea, main bronchi, and bronchial tree of the lungs. During month 2, the main stem of the lung bud forms the trachea and then branches into two bronchial buds, which form the main bronchi. The right bronchus forms three secondary bronchi, and the left bronchus forms two, setting up the pattern for three lobes to form in the right lung and two in the left. These secondary bronchi then divide repeatedly over an extended period of fetal development. The initial bronchial tree branches will all form portions of the collecting system. The final branches in this collecting component are called *"terminal" bronchioles*.

Splanchnic mesoderm forms all the "expected" mesoderm derivatives from the trachea on into the lungs. It forms all the smooth muscle and connective tissues, including elastic fibers and cartilages. The cartilage rings of the trachea and cartilages of the bronchi form from mesoderm cells which coalesce in the walls of the lung bud diverticula as they form.

During the same period, splanchnic mesoderm also forms all the tissues of the pulmonary blood vessels (which include smooth muscle and an epithelial lining). The pulmonary arteries form from branches of the arteries of the sixth aortic arches which arise from the outflow trunk of the heart. The pulmonary veins grow in from their origins in the dorsal wall of the left atrium of the heart.

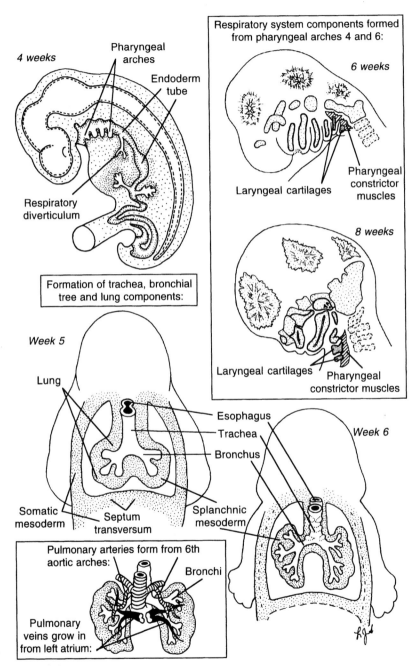

Figure 13-4
Formation of trachea, bronchi, and lungs.

• **Formation of respiratory bronchioles and alveoli.**   The lung buds undergo many levels of branching to form all the branches of the respiratory tree. By the end of month 6, roughly 17 generations of branches have been formed (see Fig. 13-5). As many as 6 additional divisions will be formed during postnatal life.

The first branches of the respiratory exchange portion of the respiratory tree are appropriately called *respiratory bronchioles*. They form as extensions of the terminal bronchioles beginning at month 4 and continue to form in large numbers through month 6. During this same period, the vascular tree also proliferates within the connective tissue stroma of the lungs between the respiratory branches.

Beginning in month 6, the respiratory bronchioles begin to bud to form *primitive alveolar ducts* and *alveoli. Capillaries* become closely associated with them as they form. Although fully mature alveoli do not develop until after birth, the maturation necessary for the switch to gaseous exchange begins in month 7. The epithelial cells lining the respiratory bronchioles and primitive alveoli change into flat squamous epithelial cells. The majority of them will differentiate into the definitive exchange cells of the lung alveoli, *type I pneumocytes*. The remaining lining cells form *type II pneumocytes*, which produce *surfactant*. The air passages of the lung become filled with fluid that contains surfactant during the last two fetal months; surfactant levels increase during the last two weeks before birth. When the alveoli become filled with air after birth, surfactant prevents their collapse during expiration. During month 7, a sufficient capillary network also develops to permit adequate gas exchange should birth occur prematurely.

Morphogenesis of lung tissue continues after birth. Postnatal growth of the lungs is due mostly to an increase in the number of respiratory bronchioles and alveoli, either by formation of new primitive alveoli or by septation of existing alveoli. In fact, 90 percent of alveoli are formed after birth.

Respiratory distress syndrome develops in premature infants due to inadequate levels of surfactant in the lung airways. (The syndrome is also known as *hyaline membrane disease* because of hyaline membrane debris released with the surfactant.) It can account for as many as 20 percent of all infant deaths in the neonatal period. Treatments have been developed to permit premature babies as young as 6.5 months of gestation to survive. These include the use of artificial surfactant and treatment of newborns with glucocorticoids to stimulate surfactant production.

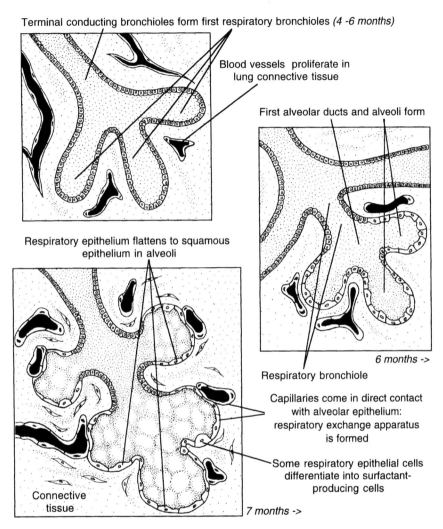

Terminal conducting bronchioles form first respiratory bronchioles *(4 -6 months)*

Blood vessels proliferate in lung connective tissue

First alveolar ducts and alveoli form

Respiratory epithelium flattens to squamous epithelium in alveoli

6 months ->

Respiratory bronchiole

Capillaries come in direct contact with alveolar epithelium: respiratory exchange apparatus is formed

Some respiratory epithelial cells differentiate into surfactant-producing cells

Connective tissue

7 months ->

Figure 13-5
Development of functional units in lungs.

Formation of the pleural cavities around the lungs

As the lung buds grow caudally into the splanchnic mesoderm, they push the mesoderm ahead of them into the intraembryonic body coelom (see Fig. 13-6). As this is happening in week 4, the single body cavity is also being divided. The forming lungs and heart are contained in the thoracic portion of the body cavity. The thoracic cavity is partially separated from the abdominal (or peritoneal) cavity by the ingrowth of the *septum transversum* from the ventral-lateral body wall. This important structure is intimately involved not only in the formation of the linings of the thoracic cavity, but also in the formation of the diaphragm and tissues of the liver. Since the body cavity is lined by both arms of lateral plate mesoderm, the linings of each of its derivative cavities will be formed by this mesoderm.

The lungs continue to expand caudally into the openings that still remain between the thoracic and peritoneal cavities on each side of the endoderm tube, called the *pleural canals*. The thoracic cavity then becomes divided into a ventral pericardial cavity, which houses the heart, and dorsolateral pleural cavities, which house the lungs. This division occurs when additional septa grow in from the body wall's lateral plate mesoderm. First, the thoracic cavity becomes separated from the abdominal (peritoneal) cavity by the fusion of the ventral septum transversum with *pleuroperitoneal folds*, which grow in from the dorsal body wall at the caudal limits of the forming lungs. Together, they form the diaphragm. The heart and lungs become separated from each other into their own cavities by the ingrowth of two *pleuropericardial folds* from the lateral body walls. These are more longitudinally oriented folds.

The lateral plate mesoderm, which covers the outside of the lung and lines the inside of the pleural cavity, then forms the *pleural membranes*.

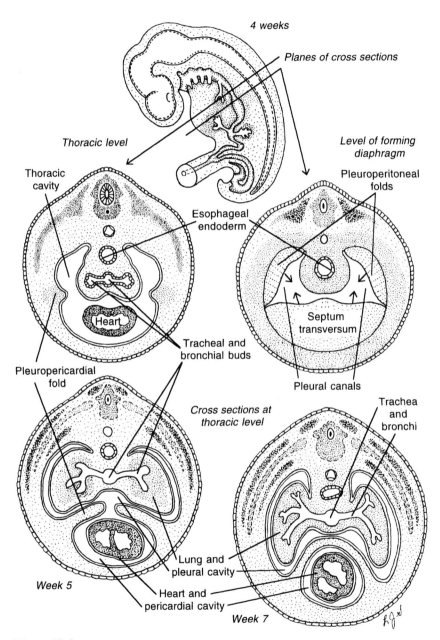

Figure 13-6
Formation of the pleural cavities around the lungs.

CONGENITAL DEFECTS OF THE RESPIRATORY SYSTEM

• **Abnormal partitioning of the esophagus and trachea leads to tracheoesophageal fistulas (see Fig. 13-7).** This spectrum of defects is rare, although it is the most common structural defect of the respiratory system. Almost all involve stenosis (narrowing) or atresia (obliteration) of a segment of the esophagus or, rarely, the trachea. The lung bud originally forms quite a long common opening with the foregut from which it originates. This opening is normally closed down to a round laryngeal opening by fusion of two longitudinal tracheoesophageal ridges which form along the opening. If these ridges do not fuse properly, a narrow patent connection called a *tracheoesophageal fistula* may be formed. Most commonly, abnormal septation causes the esophagus to become completely interrupted, with the upper (proximal) portion ending blindly and the lower (distal) portion forming a *fistula* with the trachea. Several rarer variations also occur, in which the esophagus is interrupted at both ends, or a fistula into the trachea forms with the proximal end of the esophagus. These abnormalities are often associated with other defects, particularly cardiac abnormalities. Many of these defects cause the fetus to develop *polyhydramnios*, or excess amniotic fluid. This is the result of the inability to pass swallowed fluid along through the gastrointestinal tract, from which most of it is normally absorbed into the fetal circulation and eliminated into the maternal circulation via the placenta.

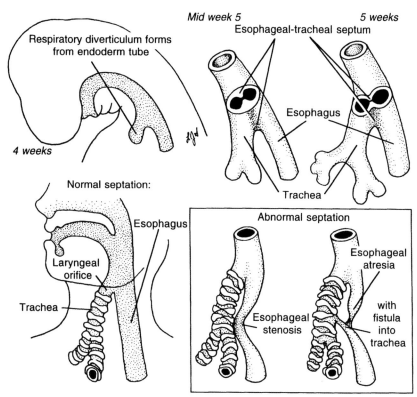

Figure 13-7
Tracheoesophageal fistulas.

· C H A P T E R · 14 ·

URINARY SYSTEM

·

•   •   •   •   •   •   •   •   •   •   •   •

The urinary system consists of bilateral kidneys, which filter wastes from blood to form urine, as well as the ureters which carry urine to the bladder, where it is stored until excreted via the urethra. This final structure of the urinary system, the urethra, is part of the reproductive ducts in the male as well, while in the female the two systems remain separate. However, the development of the urinary system is intertwined with that of the reproductive system to a very considerable degree in both sexes. Since the major structures of the urinary system develop first, it is covered first in this book. Both systems develop almost all of their components from the intermediate mesoderm, a region of mesoderm which you have not encountered in the development of organ systems described so far in this book. The urinary and genital systems are its major derivatives. Thus, the chapter begins by taking you back to the formation of the various subdivisions of the mesoderm germ layer.

COMMON ORIGINS OF URINARY AND GENITAL SYSTEMS

The urinary and genital systems develop in conjunction with each other from the same germ layer derivatives (see Fig. 14-1). They are formed almost entirely from intermediate mesoderm, with a dash of endoderm and splanchnic lateral plate mesoderm. It is easier to examine the development of the urinary system first. This is because the urinary system gets a head start on the genital system in development. In addition, some of the structures formed in the early urinary system are retained and transformed for their own uses by the reproductive systems.

• **Intermediate mesoderm forms all the typical mesoderm derivatives in the urogenital systems.** Intermediate mesoderm is named for its location in the mesoderm layer: between paraxial mesoderm (a.k.a. somites) and lateral plate mesoderm. As the embryonic body folds, the intermediate mesoderm remains confined to the dorsal body wall. Intermediate mesoderm forms all the derivatives in the urogenital systems you would expect to be derived from mesoderm: the connective tissues, smooth muscle, and blood vessels. However, that doesn't mean that this part of the story is a simple one, since the intermediate mesoderm subdivides into different regions before giving rise to these components.

• **Endoderm and intermediate mesoderm both form the epithelial linings of the urogenital systems.** Most of the epithelial linings of these systems are derived from intermediate mesoderm. Endoderm forms the epithelial linings of the terminal portions of the systems: that is, the structures closest to the openings to the outside of the body. How does the endoderm become recruited into the urogenital systems? After all, most of it lines the gastrointestinal tract. In this chapter, we will review the early dilation of the terminal portion of the endoderm tube to form the *cloaca*, its division to form the *urogenital sinus*, and how this sinus hooks up with the other urogenital system structures.

• **Splanchic lateral plate mesoderm forms the mesoderm derivatives in those urogenital organs lined by endoderm.** Since endoderm is surrounded by splanchnic mesoderm, it makes sense that this mesoderm should take over the job of making the smooth muscle and connective tissue walls of the endoderm-lined organs.

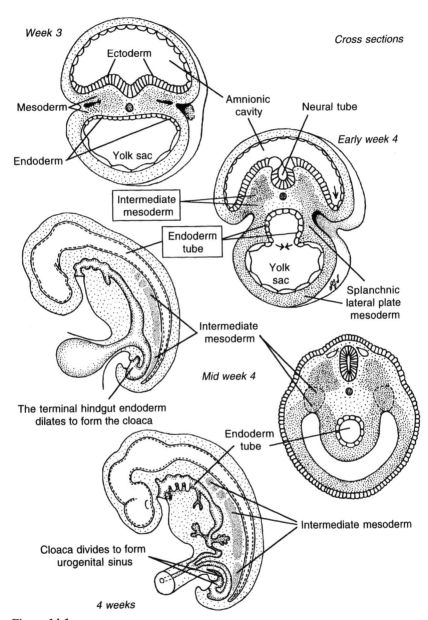

Figure 14-1
Common origins of urinary and genital systems.

ELEMENTS OF THE ADULT URINARY SYSTEM

To understand the formation of the urinary system, let's first outline the components of the adult system. The excretory components, which make urine, are contained within the *kidneys*. The collecting components, which collect, store, and transport the urine out of the body, begin in the kidneys (see Fig. 14-2). They continue into the *ureters*, which lead to a single *urinary bladder* and *urethra*. All the urinary structures are formed and remain retroperitoneal, meaning that they are covered by peritoneum on the surface facing the body cavity.

Kidneys

The two kidneys are compact organs, located in the upper abdominal cavity, whose shape inspired the name "kidney bean." The renal artery and vein, as well as the ureter, supply the kidney on its indented medial side (the hilus). The kidney contains both excretory and collecting elements in the form of epithelial tubes and cavities, which are separated and supported by connective tissue laced with blood vessels. Distinctions between excretory and collecting elements are important in development, because these elements originate from different regions of the intermediate mesoderm and must connect with each other for a functional system to form. If they don't, defects occur.

The excretory portion, the *nephron*, consists of the renal corpuscle and tubules. It filters out waste products and regulates water, electrolyte, and ion balance in the blood. The nephron starts in the outer cortex at the renal corpuscle. The corpuscle consists of *Bowman's capsule*, a double-layered squamous epithelial cup that cradles around a *glomerulus*, or tuft, of capillaries, which bring in the blood to be filtered. The excretory portion then continues through an elongated series of tubules lined by cuboidal epithelium: the *proximal convoluted tubule*, the *loop of Henle*, and the *distal convoluted tubule*. Excretory tubules begin in the cortex, extend down into the medulla, and then loop back to the cortex. This elongated, looping architecture maximizes the area for exchange between the excretory tubules and surrounding blood vessels.

The collecting components of the kidney drain the urine from the excretory tubules. They begin with the collecting tubules, which converge to form wedge-shaped pyramids in the medullary region. These empty into cavities called the *minor* and *major calyces*, which empty into the *renal pelvis*. The calyces and renal pelvis are lined by a type of epithelium which is unique to the urinary system: *transitional epithelium*. This is a thick (stratified) epithelium named for the transition its surface layers undergo from a rounded to a flattened profile as the structures become distended with urine.

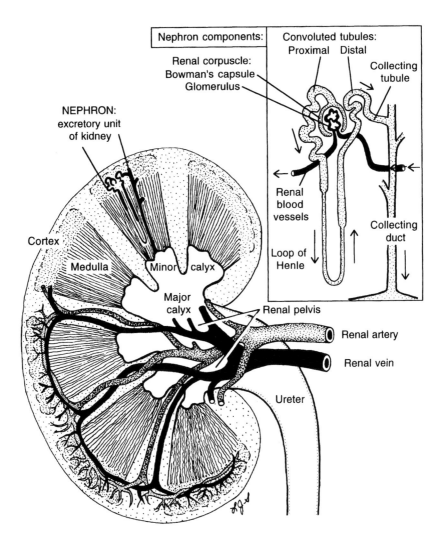

Figure 14-2
Mature kidney components.

Ureters, bladder, and urethra

The ureter, bladder, and urethra are all collecting elements (see Fig. 14-3). The ureters carry the urine from each kidney to the urinary bladder. A single urethra then carries the urine to the outside. The urethra is the one component of the urinary system whose final development and location differ in the male and female, so some of the details of its formation will be discussed in the chapter on reproductive system development (Chap. 15). The ureters and bladder are also lined by transitional epithelium. Surrounding this lining are thick walls formed by multiple layers of smooth muscle held together by connective tissue, particularly prominent in the bladder. The urethra is lined by a mélange of epithelial types, ranging from transitional to stratified squamous—the epithelium characteristic of structures close to or on the outside of the body.

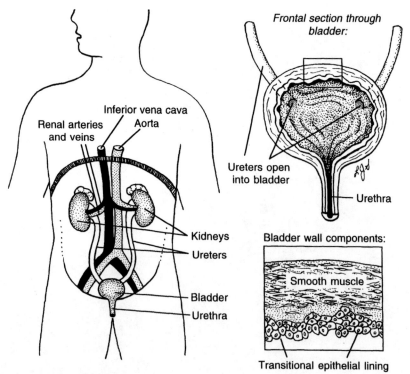

Figure 14-3
Mature urinary system components.

EMBRYONIC DEVELOPMENT OF THE KIDNEYS

As if the development of the urinary system weren't complicated enough, three successive pairs of kidneys form during embryonic development in all higher vertebrates (including humans). They are named, in sequence, the *pronephros*, *mesonephros*, and *metanephros*. The metanephros forms the final and definitive adult kidney. This apparently redundant series of developments is not a scheme to drive students of embryology over the edge. Rather, it is the result of the evolutionary history of the kidney. The good news is that the kidney reinvented itself by using the same raw material, the intermediate mesoderm (see Fig. 14-4). So why is it important to know anything about the first two kidneys? Because a few of their derivatives are incorporated into the final urinary and/or genital systems.

• **Intermediate mesoderm forms all the structures of the kidneys.**   Urinary system development begins with the proliferation of the intermediate mesoderm on each side of the embryo during week 4. This rapid growth creates a bulge called the *urogenital ridge*, which protrudes into the body (coelomic) cavity between the arms of lateral plate mesoderm. The three pairs of kidneys develop in a cranial-to-caudal sequence, using this intermediate mesoderm.

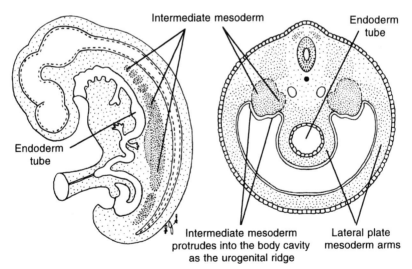

Figure 14-4
Intermediate mesoderm proliferation.

Act one: the pronephric kidney

The pronephros, or pronephric kidney, develops from the cranial end of the intermediate mesoderm (see Fig. 14-5). It is a short-lived structure (forming and degenerating during week 4), which forms only vestigial structures that never function. But the first kidney makes one contribution worth knowing about: it forms a "nephric" duct, which will become the most cranial part of the second kidney's drainage system, the *mesonephric duct*.

Act two: the mesonephric kidney

The second kidney, the mesonephros, or mesonephric kidney, forms from a long expanse of intermediate mesoderm extending most of the length of the abdominal region. It begins to form in week 4 as the pronephros degenerates. As with the first kidney, its importance lies in its components that persist and are used by the final, definitive urogenital systems: the *mesonephric tubules* and *mesonephric duct*. The mesonephric tubules are excretory elements that connect to a rapidly forming collecting duct, the mesonephric duct. This duct forms by elongation of the earlier nephric duct. It grows rapidly until it contacts and fuses with the dilated end portion of the hindgut endoderm, the cloaca, during week 4. This fusion is important to the formation of the permanent kidney. The mesonephric kidney degenerates by the end of the second month.

Act three: the permanent metanephric kidney

The permanent kidney is the result of *inductive interactions* between two different bits of intermediate mesoderm: a *ureteric bud* and a *metanephric cap*. The ureteric bud forms by sprouting from the caudal end of each mesonephric duct during week 5. The ureteric bud induces the intermediate mesoderm surrounding it to form a cluster of mesenchymal cells, called *metanephric mesoderm*, or the *metanephric cap*. The metanephric cap, in turn, induces the ureteric bud to branch repeatedly. This mutual interaction is continuous during differentiation: each bit needs the other to continue to induce it to develop.

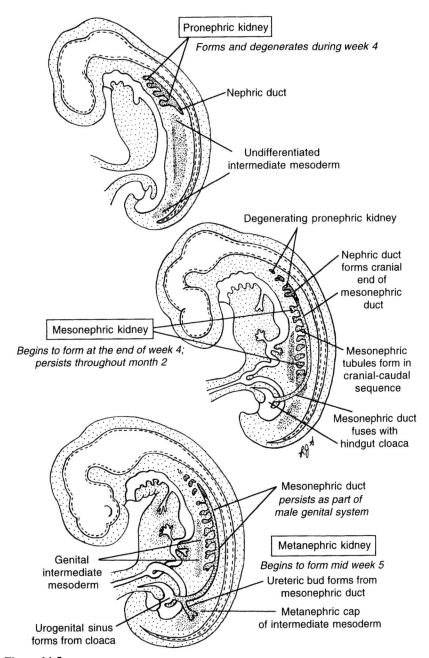

Figure 14-5
The three stages of kidney development.

• DETAILS OF DEVELOPMENT OF PERMANENT KIDNEYS.

Intermediate mesoderm forms all of the permanent kidney (see Fig. 14-6):
  The metanephric cap forms the excretory units of the kidney.
  The ureteric bud forms the collecting system of the kidney, as well as
  the ureters.

• **The collecting elements (collecting ducts, renal calyces, and renal pelvis) form first (weeks 5 to 7).**   The collecting portion is formed by the ureteric bud. The tip of the ureteric bud dilates to form the future renal pelvis. Then multiple branches bud from its margins. The first branches form 2 to 3 major calyces. Each calyx then goes through 12 or more generations of divisions. The early divisions will eventually fuse to form the minor calyces. The final divisions form the collecting ducts, whose tips interact with the metanephric cap to induce the excretory elements. The collecting elements continue to divide and mature while the excretory portion is being induced.

• **The excretory elements or nephrons form next (beginning in week 10).** The excretory elements are formed by the metanephric cap. First, its mesenchymal cells condense to form the first portion of the nephron, Bowman's capsule. (The glomerular capillaries it surrounds are formed by lateral plate mesoderm, which is induced to grow in and form blood vessels. These vessels connect to branches of the dorsal aorta, the future descending aorta.) The metanephric cap then forms all the epithelial excretory tubules leading away from Bowman's capsule, in proximal-distal sequence. Nephrons continue to be formed throughout fetal life. At least 15 successive generations form, each closer to the cortical surface than the last. Their numbers are established by birth, but nephrons continue to mature into the newborn period.

• **The fusion of the excretory and collecting portions is essential.**   To establish a functional tubular network in the kidneys, the collecting tubules must fuse with the distal convoluted tubules of the excretory portion. Fusion of two separately generated epithelial tubes to create one long one is an unusual embryonic process.

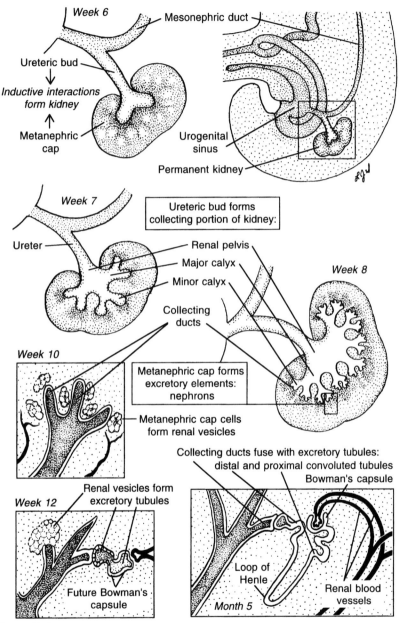

Figure 14-6
Development of the permanent kidney or metanephros.

• **The kidney changes its position during development.**   The metanephric kidney initially develops in the caudal or pelvic region of the coelomic cavity (see Fig. 14-7). But its final position is in the cranial portion of the abdominal cavity, just under the adrenal (*supra*renal) gland. Part of this change is due to actual movement cranially, made possible when the mesonephric kidneys begin to degenerate during week 6. But the apparent extensive migration required to reach its final position is part illusion, created by the extensive expansion of the body and its coelom caudal to the kidney.

Anomalies in final position of the kidneys are called *ectopic kidneys.*

Kidneys may fail to ascend to their proper location, either unilaterally or bilaterally, resulting in an ectopic pelvic kidney (*ectopic* refers to any abnormally located structure) (see Fig. 14-7). This may be caused by the kidney getting "hung up" on the umbilical arteries, which arise in the pelvis from the common iliac arteries. Ectopic kidneys are completely normal in their functioning, but their location could present a surprise to a physician not aware of such possibilities. More commonly, the kidneys may fuse with each other as their lower poles come in contact during ascent. This not only creates a single horseshoe (shaped) kidney, but this kidney also is ectopically located. It cannot complete its ascent, because it cannot move past the inferior mesenteric artery arising in the midline from the aorta. This type of kidney also is normal in its functioning.

Congenital defects can occur in kidney formation, resulting in either *renal agenesis* or *polycystic kidneys.*

Defects can occur in induction or subsequent development of the meta-nephric kidney components (see Fig. 14-7). Some are asymptomatic, while others are fatal. Unilateral (or, rarely, bilateral) *renal agenesis* can occur, which means that the kidney fails to form. This is most likely due to early degeneration of the ureteric bud, or failure of the formed metanephric elements to induce each other to differentiate. Bilateral agenesis is always fatal, but unilateral agenesis is often asymptomatic. In addition, polycystic kidneys can develop when either excretory or collecting elements fail to form or when they fail to connect with each other and degenerate. Functionless, fluid-filled cysts form in the place of nephrons. This (largely) genetic set of disorders may be due to failure of inductive interactions between any of several metanephric components. Milder forms which involve only part of one kidney may not be apparent until adulthood, while more severe forms may involve virtually all renal tissue in one or both kidneys.

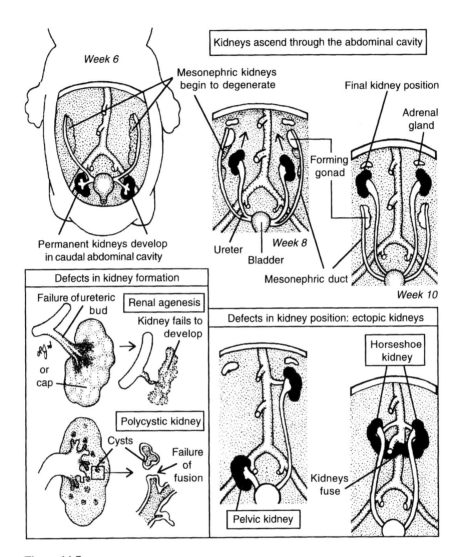

Figure 14-7
Final position of the kidney and congenital defects in kidney formation.

Blood supply changes to the kidneys during development

The definitive kidneys are supplied by renal arteries and veins (see Fig. 14-8). The renal veins and the portion of the inferior vena cava into which they drain form from subcardinal veins. The renal arteries form as lateral branches of the dorsal aorta, which becomes the definitive descending aorta.

Anomalies in formation of arterial supply lead to accessory renal arteries.

During the ascent of the kidneys, several renal arteries supply the kidney in sequence. Normally, the first renal arteries degenerate as the new ones form cranial to them. If these first arteries persist, multiple or accessory renal arteries may remain. Usually the extra arteries supply only parts of the kidney. It is important for clinicians to be aware that such anomalous arteries can be formed.

Onset of function in the fetal kidney

Kidney function begins at the start of the second trimester, but does not reach mature status until after birth. The real work of the kidney is achieved in the fetus by sending wastes in the fetal blood through the umbilical vessels to cross the placenta. Nevertheless, the permanent fetal kidney does do some filtering of the blood which is delivered to it, processing it into very dilute urine. This is excreted into the amniotic sac surrounding the fetus. The fetus swallows reflexively, drinking in its amniotic fluid, which is absorbed by the gut and transported by the circulation back to the kidney. (Think about that a minute and you will probably never forget that the kidney has some level of function prior to birth.) This filtering is not necessary for elimination of embryonic waste. So why does it occur? Most importantly, the filtrate is a major source of amniotic fluid. Also, it may be a "trial run," which in some way facilitates further kidney maturation.

Newborn kidneys are functionally and structurally immature. They are functionally limited in that they cannot concentrate urine well or excrete large volumes of fluid. This is due in large part to the fact that structural differentiation continues after birth. Nephrons do not mature in the outer cortical region of the kidney until after birth.

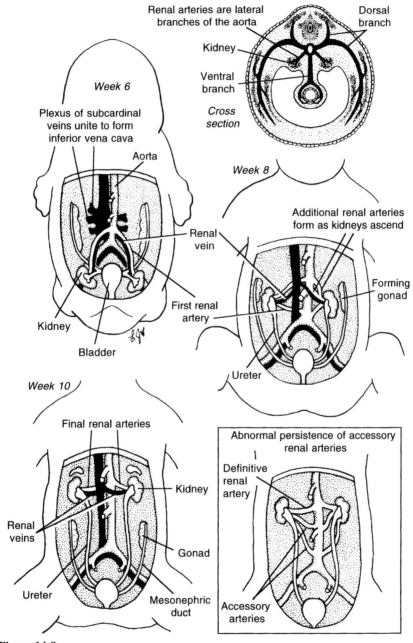

Figure 14-8
Changes in blood supply of the kidney and anomalous formation of accessory arteries.

EMBRYONIC DEVELOPMENT OF URETERS, BLADDER, AND URETHRA

Development of ureters

The ureters, which drain the kidneys to the bladder, are formed completely from intermediate mesoderm (see Fig. 14-9). The most proximal part of the ureteric bud forms the transitional epithelium lining each ureter. The supporting connective tissue and smooth muscle of their walls are formed by the intermediate mesoderm of the metanephric cap. As has already been described, the distal portions of the ureteric buds form the collecting structures within the kidneys, the renal pelvis and renal calyces which drain into the ureters.

Development of bladder and urethra

The terminal structures of the urinary system, the bladder and urethra, are formed by a portion of the hindgut endoderm and the splanchnic lateral plate mesoderm, which surrounds all endoderm (see Fig. 14-9). Mesoderm forms what it usually does in other internal organs: the connective tissue, smooth muscle, and blood vessel components. Endoderm forms the epithelial linings of the bladder and urethra. The specific region of endoderm involved is the cloaca.

How does the endoderm tube become involved in forming the lining of the terminal portions of the urinary and genital systems? To answer this, we need to take a closer look at the cloaca and its derivatives. Before the urinary system forms, the terminal portion of the hindgut endoderm dilates to form the cloaca early in week 4. The cloaca is then divided into two chambers by ingrowth of a urorectal septum: the *anorectal canal* and the *urogenital sinus*. Both are separated from the exterior only by a cloacal membrane, which soon breaks down. The anorectal canal forms the epithelial linings of the terminal portions of the gastrointestinal tract, the rectum and anus.

The urogenital sinus is the more cranially located of the cloacal chambers. It becomes connected to the rest of the urinary system right from the start, when the mesonephric ducts contact and open into the urogenital sinus during week 4. The ureteric bud then arises from the mesonephric duct, close to this junction. The endoderm of the urogenital sinus gives rise to the epithelial lining of the urinary bladder and most of the urethra. The splanchnic mesoderm, which surrounds the endoderm tube, then forms the mesodermal component of the organs.

• **Final location of the ureter openings into the bladder.** The mesonephric ducts open into the dorsal wall of the urogenital sinus at a point which will become the posterior bladder wall. As the bladder grows, its expanding wall incorporates first the mesonephric ducts and then their ureteric buds, resulting in

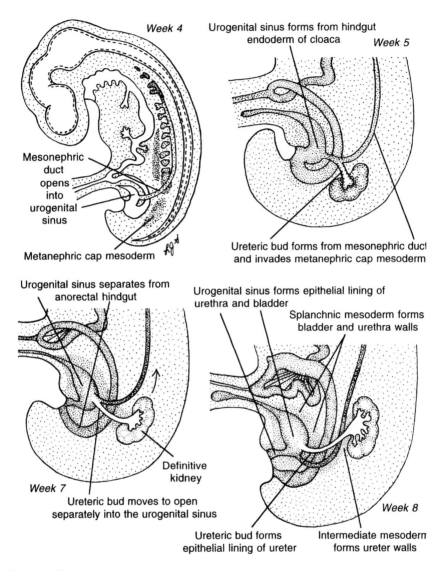

Figure 14-9
Development of ureters, bladder, and urethra.

these structures opening separately into the bladder. The ureters subsequently migrate to enter at a more cranial location than the mesonephric ducts. The mesonephric ducts will persist if the embryo is a male (more about this in Chap. 15 describing the reproductive system).

CONGENITAL DEFECTS OF THE URINARY SYSTEM

In addition to defects in kidney formation or position already covered on page 338, congenital defects can occur in the formation of ureters, bladder, and urethra (see Fig. 14-10).

• **The relationship of the embryonic allantois to congenital defects of the bladder at the urachus.**   The allantois is important for several reasons relevant to human embryology. With respect to the urinary system, the allantois can be the source of congenital defects. The allantois is an outgrowth of the urogenital sinus into the yolk sac stalk (or forming umbilical cord). It is an evolutionary holdover, which arose as a reservoir for excretory products in lower vertebrates such as birds, whose embryos have no placenta to use as a "toxic waste dump." In mammals, its lumen becomes obliterated during embryonic development. It turns into a ligament called the *urachus*, which connects the ventral surface of the bladder to the ventral body wall at the umbilicus. This ligament is called the *median umbilical ligament* in the mature body.

• **Abnormal persistence of urachal structures can occur.**   In some cases, the urachus lumen does not close completely, and urachal *fistulas*, *cysts*, or *sinuses* are formed. Cysts are blind fluid-filled structures located within the urachal ligament. Fistulas and sinuses are long open channels within the urachal remnant, which can cause urine to leak out of the body if they remain in continuity with the bladder.

• **Defects in formation of the ventral body wall can cause exstrophy of the bladder.**   This is a rare defect in which the ventral body wall overlying the bladder fails to close, largely because of a failure of sufficient mesoderm to migrate into the region to form connective tissue support for the ectodermal epithelial covering. The lower abdominal wall remains open. As a consequence, the ventral bladder wall is usually incompletely formed, so that the bladder cavity is exposed directly to the exterior of the body. This is a serious defect that results in total urinary incontinence.

• **Defects in ureter formation can result in multiple or split ureters.**   These defects may be caused by either premature or extra splitting of the ureteric bud. Each bud may then give rise to a separate ureter and renal pelvis and even induce formation of an additional kidney. Problems arise in cases in which the extra ureter opens into the urethra or the vagina (ectopic openings). (How this happens is best explained in Chap. 15.)

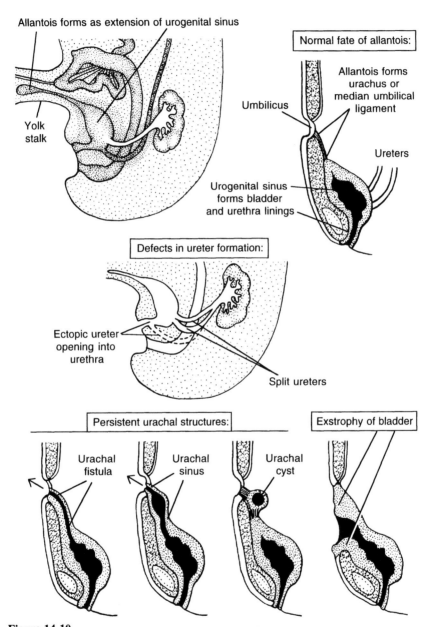

Figure 14-10
Defects in formation of the bladder and urethra, and the relationship of the allantois to some of these defects.

REPRODUCTIVE SYSTEMS

·

·   ·   ·   ·   ·   ·   ·   ·   ·   ·   ·   ·

The reproductive systems consist of gonads which produce eggs in the female and sperm in the male, and a series of tubes which transport those sex cells. In the male, the tubes carry the sperm out of the body via the urethra, which is shared with the urinary system. In the female, the egg is transported as far as the uterus if it is fertilized. Here it implants and begins development. Sperm enter the female reproductive system through the vagina, and from there move past the cervical opening into the uterus. Thus, the reproductive system contains two separate sets of organs in males and females. However, study of the embryonic development of these systems is somewhat simplified by the fact that they both originate from a common set of embryonic structures that can develop along either male or female pathways, depending on the genetic and hormonal instructions they receive. Most of the reproductive system structures are derived from one source, the intermediate mesoderm, just as are most urinary system structures.

COMMON ORIGINS OF UROGENITAL SYSTEMS

The seeds of the reproductive system are planted during the origins of the urinary system, whose development is described in Chap. 14. In this chapter you will see how the reproductive system develops from the same combination of germ layer derivatives that form the urinary system and how some reproductive system structures are formed by a "friendly takeover" of early urinary structures.

Sex selection

This is the only system that can follow either of two paths. However, this does not mean that you will have to learn two completely different sets of early embryonic precursor structures. Rather, both male and female reproductive organs are formed from a single, "unisex" set of primordial reproductive structures. These structures are referred to as indifferent stage structures. (This makes it sound a little as if the developing sex organs don't care which sex they become. However, they are waiting for their marching orders.)

> The sex chromosome complement directs the formation of the sex organs of one sex: if there is a Y chromosome on the premises, the embryo will become a male; if not, it will become a female.

COMPONENTS OF MATURE REPRODUCTIVE SYSTEMS

The *male* reproductive system consists of paired *testes*, which produce sperm in seminiferous tubules, and deliver them to a series of ducts that carry them out of the body (see Fig. 15-1). Intratesticular ducts (straight *rete testis* and *efferent ductules*) enter the coiled tubules of the *epididymis*, which each lead into a thick-walled *vas deferens*. Both vas deferens enter the single midline *urethra*, which carries both sperm and urine. Accessory sex organs are also formed along the way: paired *seminal vesicles*, and a single midline *bulbourethral gland* and *prostate*. All contribute to the seminal fluid which is ejaculated with the sperm. The external genitalia consist of the *penis*, which contains the penile urethra and erectile tissue, and the paired *scrotal sacs*, which house the testes.

In the *female* reproductive system, bilateral ovaries are anchored to the dorsal body wall by the broad ligaments and to the uterus by ovarian ligaments (see Fig. 15-1). *Uterine* (or *fallopian*) *tubes* cup their open ends (fimbria) around each ovary, scoop up ovulated eggs, and carry them toward the *uterus*. If the egg is fertilized, it will implant in the lining of the uterine cavity. If not, it will continue through the narrow uterine cervical opening into the *vagina*. The external geni-

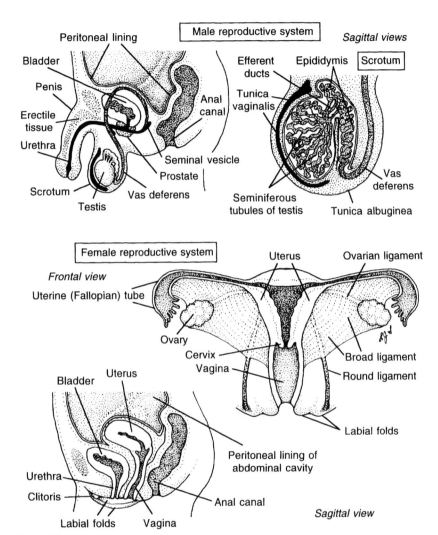

Figure 15-1
Mature male and female reproductive systems.

talia in the female consist of the *clitoris* and *labial folds*, which surround the vaginal opening. The uterus is connected to the labial folds by the round ligament.

The internal structures of the reproductive systems are *retroperitoneal*, that is, they are located behind the peritoneal lining of the pelvic region of the body cavity.

GERM LAYER ORIGINS OF THE REPRODUCTIVE SYSTEM

Structures formed at the indifferent stage

The male and female reproductive systems are indistinguishable from each other during weeks 5 and 6, when the indifferent stage structures are formed. The process of converting these indifferent structures into sex-specific organs begins in week 7, but then extends over the first several months of fetal development. These "indifferent" structures have names that for the most part aren't very helpful in deciphering their fates.

The "*sex cords*" are the precursors to the gonads. *Genital ducts* and the *urogenital sinus* form all the other internal sex organs. Finally, *genital tubercles* and *swellings* are the precursors to the external genitalia.

• **Which germ layers give rise to each of these precursors?**   The reproductive system is formed by the same combination of germ layer derivatives that form the urinary system: intermediate mesoderm forms all tissues of most of the organs, with a large dash of endoderm and splanchnic lateral plate mesoderm forming the terminal structures of the system (see Fig. 15-2).

• **Intermediate mesoderm forms the sex cords and genital ducts leading directly away from them.**   This means that the intermediate mesoderm forms the gonads and ducts leading away from them. As in the urinary system, this mesoderm forms the epithelial linings of these organs, as well as the typical mesoderm components in the walls: the connective tissues and smooth muscle.

• **Urogenital sinus endoderm and its splanchnic mesoderm give rise to the more distal parts of the reproductive system, as well as part of the external genitalia.**   As in the urinary system, there is a dividing line at which the intermediate mesoderm-derived organs unite with organs derived from the urogenital sinus endoderm. (Here's a brief recap of its formation as described in Chap. 14: the terminal part of the hindgut endoderm dilates to form the cloacal region. This is divided by a septum into the anorectal canal and the urogenital sinus.) The urogenital sinus forms the epithelial lining of most distal (terminal) elements of the internal reproductive organs, as well as of the external genitalia. Also, as is the

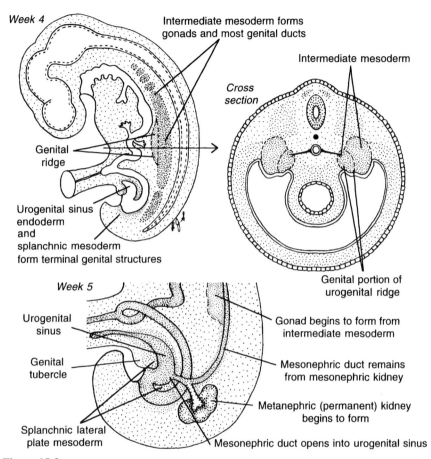

Figure 15-2
Germ layer origins of reproductive systems.

case in the urinary system, these organs' mesoderm derivatives are formed by the mesoderm that surrounds the entire endoderm tube, the splanchnic lateral plate mesoderm.

• **Genital tubercles and swellings form the external genitalia.**   The external genitalia are formed by several swellings and folds formed by surface ectoderm and underlying somatic (body wall) mesoderm which surround the opening of the urogenital sinus to the ectoderm.

DEVELOPMENT OF GONADS

Indifferent stage of development

• **Intermediate mesoderm forms all gonadal tissues.**   The gonads develop first, and their development determines what happens next. The intermediate mesoderm forms a longitudinal urogenital ridge from which both urinary and genital organs arise (see Fig. 15-3). The medial portion of each urogenital ridge proliferates to form a distinct genital ridge, which bulges into the body (coelomic) cavity during week 5. These ridges consist of surface epithelium (called the *coelomic epithelium* because it faces the coelomic cavity) and an underlying region of loose mesenchyme. The coelomic epithelium of the ridge proliferates and forms primitive sex cords. These epithelial cords grow into the underlying ridge mesenchyme. Thus, sex cords initially form in both the outer cortex and inner medulla of the genital ridge. The sex cords, in conjunction with the ridge mesenchyme surrounding them, will differentiate into all the components of the gonads. The indifferent stage of reproductive system development extends from week 5 to week 6.

• **Germ cells migrate into the gonads from their site of origin in the yolk sac endoderm (hypoblast).**   Primordial germ cells originate from the extraembryonic yolk sac endoderm (which was formed by the original hypoblast—and you thought you had heard the last of the hypoblast). The germ cells infiltrate the genital ridge by migrating from the walls of the yolk sac into the splanchnic mesoderm surrounding the hindgut, and from there into the dorsal body wall via the mesoderm stalk connecting the gut to the dorsal body wall (the forming dorsal mesentery). Germ cell infiltration must occur by week 6 for the sex cords to begin their differentiation. Germ cells will differentiate into *oogonia* in the female and *spermatogonia* in the male.

> Germ cells must enter the gonadal precursors for *both* the gonads and germ cells to develop any further. The germ cells and gonadal precursors literally "egg each other on" to differentiate. This is a prime example of *mutual induction*.

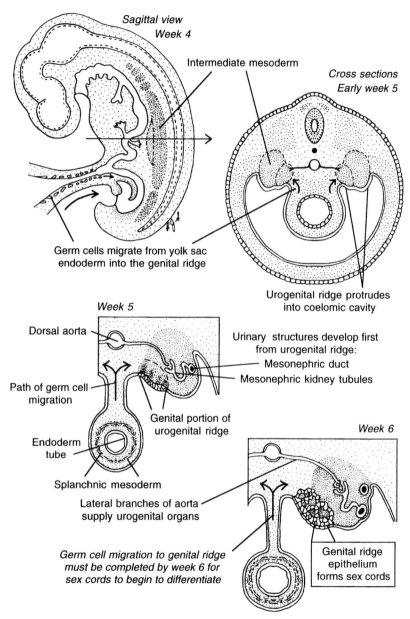

Figure 15-3
Indeterminate stage of gonad formation.

Sex-specific development of the gonads

• **This stage of gonad development depends on the embryonic genotype: the presence of a Y chromosome (see Fig. 15-4).**   Differentiation of all parts of the reproductive system along either the male or female line depends on the presence or absence of the Y chromosome in the cells of the forming gonad (which, presumably, contain the same genotype as all other cells of the body). The products of genes located on the Y chromosome induce testis development; in their absence, an ovary develops. Sex-specific differentiation begins in week 7.

• **What genes on the Y chromosome direct testis induction, and how do they do it?**   This question has been under intensive investigation for a generation. Researchers have determined that at least one gene on the Y chromosome is required for the initial differentiation of the genital ridge tissue into a testis. This gene has been dubbed the *s*ex determining *r*egion gene on the *Y* chromosome, or *Sry*. The Sry gene product is made only in individuals with the Y chromosome, and then only in cells of the genital ridge at the stage preceding initial sex-specific differentiation. It encodes a protein that appears to act as a "master switch" which is essential to activating other target genes. Those other genes are now being identifed, but their gene products and mechanisms of action remain unknown.

• **Subsequent sex-specific differentiation of all reproductive organs is induced by hormones.**   The male phenotype develops in response to the presence of male hormones which are produced by the testis while it is first differentiating. Development of the male phenotype refers to differentiation of sex organs as male organs. The female phenotype develops *in the absence of* male hormones: that is, it is the "default" condition. However, it should be realized that female hormones derived from the placenta (estrogen and human chorionic gonadotropin) are present in both male and female embryos and play a baseline role in the development of both sexes. Finally, it is important to understand that genetic sex, or *genotype*, can be overridden by "environmental factors," which counteract intrinsic hormonal signals.

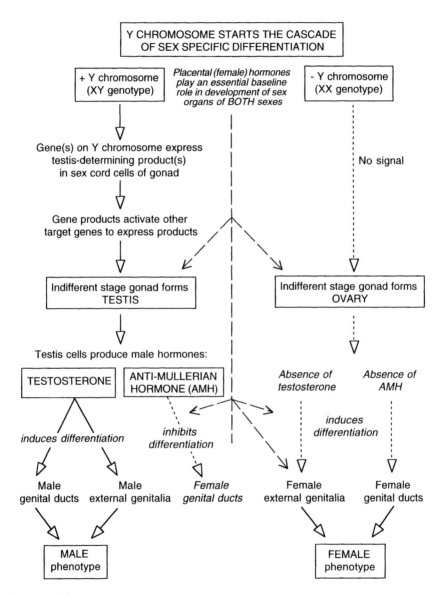

Figure 15-4
Summary of factors regulating sex selection.

• **TESTIS DIFFERENTIATION**   In the male, testis formation begins in week 7 with proliferation of the inner, or *medullary*, *sex cords* and regression of the cortical cords (see Fig. 15-5). The proliferation of sex cords in both sexes requires infiltration by the migrating germ cells. The medullary cord proliferation in the male also requires exposure to products of the Sry gene on the Y chromosome. During month 3, the medullary cords form the *seminiferous tubules* of the testis, as well as the network of tubes (the rete testis) into which the seminiferous tubules drain. The cortical cords degenerate and are replaced by a thick outer fibrous capsule around the testis called the *tunica albuginea*. All the tubular structures of the testis remain largely solid cords of cells prior to puberty.

Two important cell types form in the testis from its intermediate mesoderm: the *Sertoli* cell and the *Leydig* cell. Sertoli cells form the walls of the seminiferous tubules. They become the nurse or support cells for sperm development. During early development of the testis, they secrete *müllerian inhibiting substance* (*MIS*), a glycoprotein hormone in the transforming growth factor β (TGFβ) family. Müllerian inhibiting substance plays a role in differentiation of the Leydig cells. These cells differentiate from the intermediate mesoderm between the medullary cords. They secrete testosterone and its derivative dihydrotestosterone, which are essential for differentiation of all components of the male reproductive system, including commiting the germ cells to the spermatogonia line. This commitment includes inhibiting the onset of meiosis (in contrast to what happens in the female). Testosterone and MIS are essential for the next phase of male development: the induction of sex-specific differentiation of the genital ducts (see next section). In summary, the origins of the three cell types in the testis are the following:

Sertoli cells: intermediate mesoderm of medullary sex cords
Leydig cells: intermediate mesoderm surrounding sex cords
Spermatogonia: primitive germ cells from yolk sac endoderm

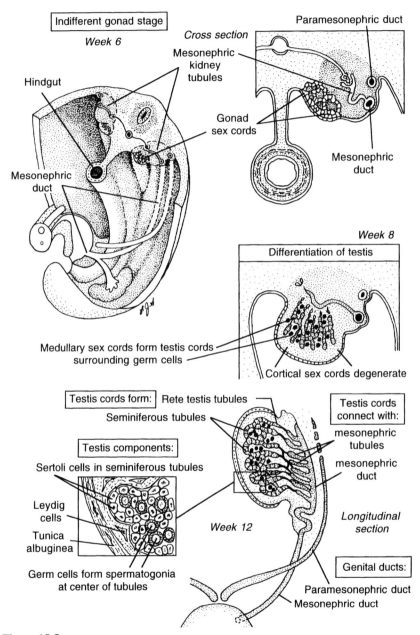

Figure 15-5
Testis differentiation.

• **OVARY DIFFERENTIATION**   In the female, the *cortical cords* become highly developed beginning in week 7 and extending through month 3 (see Fig. 15-6). The medullary cords regress and are replaced by vascular and connective tissue stroma. Instead of the cortical cords remaining epithelial tubes, they split up and their cells move to surround individual germ cells that have migrated into the gonad. The cortical cords thus become the ovarian follicular cells, which perform a support cell function in the mature ovary similar to that performed by the Sertoli cells in the testis. Follicular cells begin their work directing germ cell development during embryonic life. They contact germ cells in the ovaries and, in the absence of testosterone, direct the germ cells to begin to differentiate into *oogonia*. Follicular cells permit the onset of meiosis, but then stop it in its tracks. Partial development of germ cells during fetal life, which is an important feature in the female, is covered at the end of this chapter. Follicular cells secrete female hormones, principally estrogen, throughout embryonic and fetal life. Estrogen is essential for development of external genitalia. Estrogen and other hormones present in the embryo are also derived from the placenta throughout development. In summary, the origins of the cell types in the ovary are the following:

Follicular cells: intermediate mesoderm of cortical sex cords
Oogonia: primitive germ cells from yolk sac endoderm

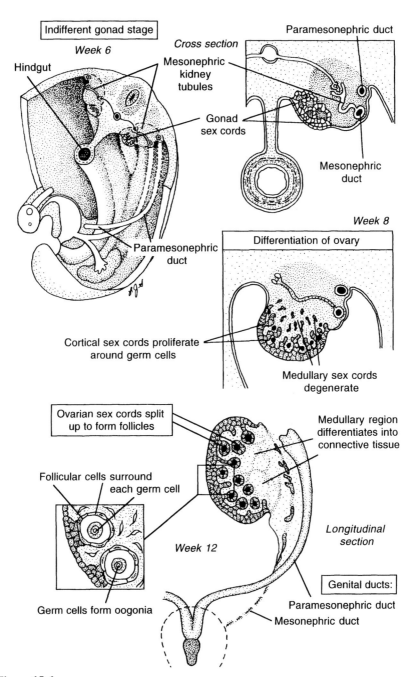

Figure 15-6
Ovary differentiation.

DEVELOPMENT OF OTHER INTERNAL REPRODUCTIVE ORGANS

> Genital ducts form the proximal reproductive organs, while the more distal ones are formed by the urogenital sinus and surrounding splanchnic mesoderm.

Indifferent stage

• **Two pairs of genital ducts form in both sexes (see Fig. 15-7).** These ducts are formed by intermediate mesoderm of the genital ridge. Both pairs of ducts begin proximally in the area of the gonads and terminate distally on or near the urogenital sinus. When they are formed, they will to be able to carry the gametes away from the gonads toward their ultimate destinations. In the male, this means exit from the body. In the female, this means implantation part way along the path in the uterine wall.

• **Mesonephric (Wolffian) ducts form first.** Recall that these ducts arise as the "drainage channels" of the transient mesonephric kidneys and become appropriated by the reproductive system. They grow toward and then open into the urogenital sinus. (This makes sense if you recall from Chap. 14 that the urogenital sinus later forms the bladder and urethra linings.) Since the urinary system gets a head start on the reproductive system, the mesonephric ducts are already in place by week 6 when the sex cords of the primordial gonads begin to form. The mesonephric ducts leave no significant derivatives in the urinary system; the only reason you need to concern yourself with them is that they form important structures in the male reproductive system.

• **Paramesonephric (Müllerian) ducts form next.** These ducts form lateral to the mesonephric ducts, hence the name *paramesonephric*. The cranial ends are open to the pelvic cavity. As the ducts grow caudally, they come together in the midline, crossing over the mesonephric ducts. The paired ducts grow toward the posterior wall of the urogenital sinus. A swelling forms in the wall of the urogenital sinus under the end of these ducts, which is called the *Müllerian*, or *genital, tubercle*. Whether actual contact occurs depends on the sex that develops.

Sex-specific differentiation of genital ducts

Hormones direct the persistence of only one duct system in each sex during month 3. This is the key to formation of different internal sex organs in each sex.

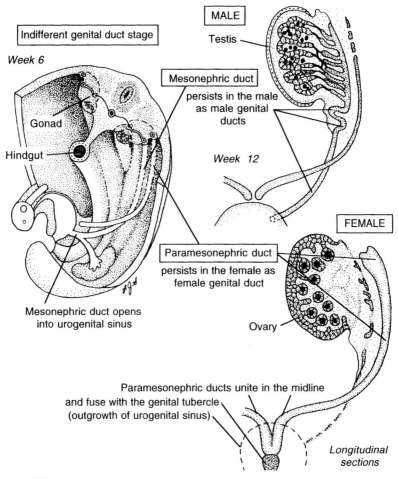

Figure 15-7
Different genital ducts survive in each sex.

In the male, the mesonephric ducts persist and the paramesonephric ducts regress. In the female, this is reversed: the paramesonephric ducts persist, while the mesonephric ducts regress.

The difference is due to the presence of the Y chromosome in the genetic male embryo and the chain of hormonal signals its Sry (sex-determining region) gene sets in motion.

Male differentiation of internal reproductive organs

All parts of the male reproductive system require the presence of the Y chromosome, and the male hormones that are produced as a result of its presence. Leydig cells secrete testosterone, which causes persistence of the mesonephric ducts (see Fig. 15-8). Sertoli cells secrete MIS which actively causes regression of the paramesonephric (Müllerian) ducts.

• **The mesonephric ducts connect with the testis ducts at their proximal ends and with the urogenital sinus at their distal ends.**   The mesonephric ducts and tubules form the ducts through which the sperm travel in their search for a mate. The proximal ends of some of the mesonephric tubules are transformed into intratesticular efferent ductules into which the seminiferous tubules and rete testis drain. The mesonephric ducts into which these mesonephric tubules originally emptied form the ducts or tubules outside the testis: the epididymis and ductus deferens (or vas deferens). In addition, outpocketings from each vas deferens form the seminal vesicles (which are therefore formed by intermediate mesoderm).

• **The terminal internal reproductive organs are formed by urogenital sinus endoderm and its surrounding splanchnic mesoderm.**   Early in their development, the mesonephric ducts open into the urogenital sinus as part of their role as transient ureters. When this terminal portion becomes transformed into the vas deferens, their openings into the urogenital sinus move away from the portion that becomes the bladder and open into the distal part of the urogenital sinus, which forms the urethral lining. Thus, in the male, the urethra is both the final internal reproductive structure and urinary structure. All connective tissue and smooth muscle components of the urethra are formed by splanchnic mesoderm, which surrounds all parts of the endoderm tube. The prostate and bulbourethral glands later form as buds from the urethra just after its point of origin, which means that they are formed by endoderm and its surrounding splanchnic mesoderm.

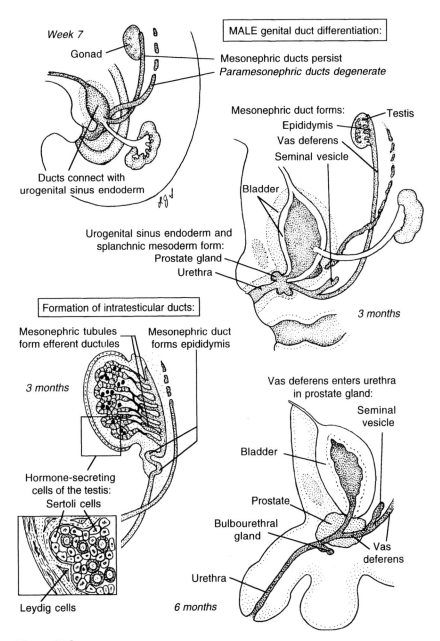

Figure 15-8
Development of male internal reproductive organs.

Female differentiation of internal reproductive organs

The female reproductive tract forms in the absence of the Y chromosome, its induction of the testis, and its subsequent hormone production. This means that a female reproductive tract also forms if gonads are absent. The female system forms from the paramesonephric ducts, which are retained in the absence of the inhibiting factor MIS. The mesonephric ducts regress in the absence of testosterone. The paramesonephric ducts form the lining of the *uterine* (or *Fallopian*) *tubes*, which remain open cranially into the abdominal cavity (see Fig. 15-9). This opening permits the tubes to scoop up eggs once they begin to be released from the ovary at puberty. The caudal ends of these ducts grow medially and fuse together in the midline to form the epithelial lining of the uterus and upper portion of the *vagina*. The connective tissues and substantial smooth muscle of the walls are formed by intermediate mesoderm surrounding these ducts. This involves a rather considerable transformation from a slender duct to organs with thick muscular walls and dilated lumens.

The vagina is the transition point in the female system between intermediate mesoderm and endoderm. The lower portion of the vagina is formed by an outgrowth of the urogenital sinus, which connects with the lower end of the fusing paramesonephric ducts. This unusual fusion of outgrowth from two different germ layer derivatives occurs when the paramesonephric ducts contact the urogenital sinus and induce an outgrowth from its tip (the *vaginal plate*). The epithelial lining and cavity of the lower portion of the vagina is then formed by growth and hollowing out (or canalization) of the vaginal plate, which does not begin until month 5. This connects the upper and lower portions of the vagina. The surrounding splanchnic mesoderm forms the connective tissue and smooth muscle walls. Subsequent development moves the vaginal opening from the terminal or urethral part of the urogenital sinus directly to the exterior. (This will be clearer after reading the section on development of external genitalia.)

Incomplete fusion of the uterine tubes can result in partial or complete duplication of the uterus (typically called a *bicornuate uterus*), as well as atresia of the cervical opening of the uterus into the vagina. In addition, if the vaginal plate does not form from the urogenital sinus, this results in atresia of the lower portion of the vagina.

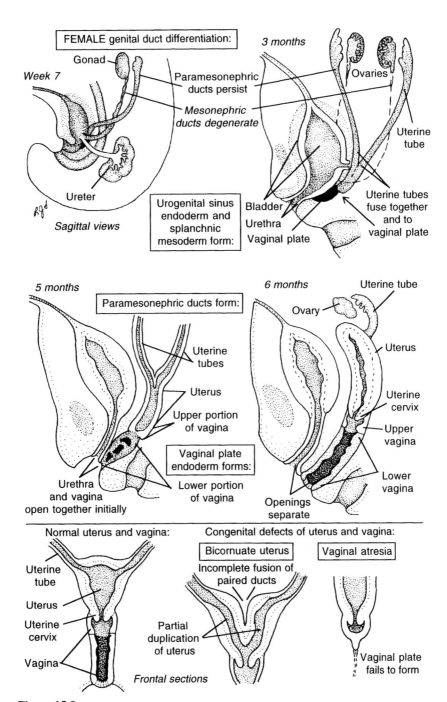

Figure 15-9
Development of female internal reproductive organs, and congenital defects in their development.

DEVELOPMENT OF EXTERNAL GENITALIA

Sexually indifferent stage

External genitalia form from the mesoderm and overlying ectoderm that surround the future cloacal opening. The proliferating mesoderm forms swellings (cloacal folds) around the common cloacal membrane at week 3 (see Fig. 15-10). At their ventral end (that is, the end closest to the ventral, or abdominal, surface of the body), the cloacal folds unite to form the genital tubercle. Genital swellings form lateral to the cloacal folds. When the cloaca is divided internally into the urogenital sinus and anorectal canal during week 6, the external cloacal folds are divided into the urethral or urogenital folds and anal folds. The cloacal membrane is also divided into the urogenital and anal membranes. These membranes will shortly break down, creating exit points for the urinary and reproductive systems, as well as the digestive system. The reason for distinguishing between these structures is that each forms specific components of the external genitalia.

Sexual differentiation stage

While much sex-specific differentiation of external genitalia occurs between weeks 7 and 12, the external genitalia still appear similar in structure through this period. Continued development through month 6 forms the male and female external genitalia.

• **Male differentiation requires testosterone.** The *phallus*, or penis, forms from the genital tubercle and urethral folds. The genital tubercle enlarges under control of androgens from the testis (dihydroxytestosterone). The *penile urethra* running through its center is formed mostly from the endoderm of the urogenital sinus. Elongation of the phallus causes a long urethral groove to form from the opening of the urogenital sinus. The urethral folds on either side fuse and encompass the urethral groove, forming the penile urethra. The terminal part of the penile urethra (in the glans penis) forms from ectoderm dragged into the interior, as happens at all body openings. The erectile tissues within the penis are formed from mesoderm of the urethral folds. The more lateral genital swellings enlarge to form the walls of the *scrotum*, into which the testis will be drawn.

Defects that can occur in this process include *hypospadias*: abnormal urethral openings along the line of fusion of the urethral folds.

• **Female differentiation requires estrogen (from the placenta).** Initially the vagina and urethra open into a common chamber formed from the urogenital

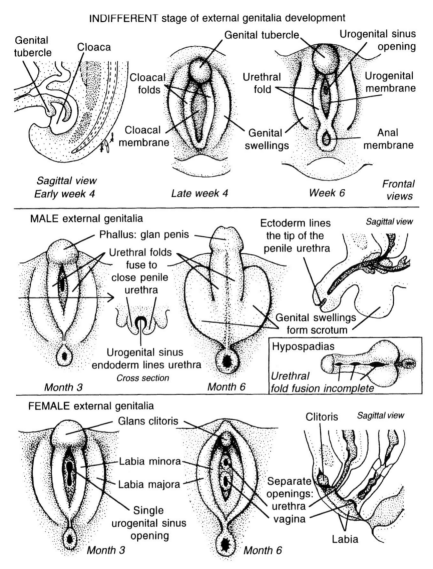

Figure 15-10
Differentiation of external genitalia.

sinus: the *vestibule*. With development, their openings become separated. The urethral folds form the *labia minora* surrounding both openings, while the genital swellings form the *labia majora*. The *clitoris* forms from the genital tubercle in the female.

Descent of gonads occurs in both sexes

In both sexes, the gonads are retroperitoneal, and all descent occurs in that position (see Fig. 15-11). In both sexes a *gubernaculum* ligament forms, which assists this descent. It attaches to the gonad proximally, and to the genital swellings distally. In both sexes the peritoneal lining of the body cavity grows out of the body cavity along the path of the gubernaculum, forming an *inguinal canal* in the process.

• **Descent of the testis into the scrotum is required for normal function.** The testes descend to their final location outside the body cavity in the scrotum beginning in month 3. This results in the mature arrangement of the testes, male ducts, and ureters, and provides the testes with the proper (lower) temperature for sperm development. It is initially attached to the dorsal, or posterior, abdominal wall by the dorsal mesentery. The testis descends along the gubernaculum, a mesenchyme band that grows from the caudal pole of the testis toward the developing scrotal swelling outside the ventral body wall. The coelomic epithelial lining, or *peritoneum*, evaginates into the scrotum along the growing gubernaculum, forming the *process vaginalis*. It surrounds the testis as it descends. The peritoneum encounters all abdominal wall components in its march and pushes them ahead of it, forming the inguinal canal. The inguinal canal connection with the peritoneum is normally obliterated, leaving a *tunica vaginalis* to surround the testis in the scrotal sac.

Defects of descent include *cryptorchism* (undescended testis). Defects of formation of the inguinal canal include *congenital hernia* of abdominal contents into a persistent canal, as well as *hydrocele* (fluid-filled cysts along the inguinal canal route).

• **Descent of the ovaries occurs within the body cavity, forming the ligaments of the ovaries and uterus in the process.**   A gubernaculum forms in the female, but doesn't shorten as in the male. As the ovaries descend caudally within the pelvic cavity, they carry their mesenteric coverings out into peritoneal folds. These movements create the ligaments of the ovary and uterus out of the gubernaculum. These include the broad ligament, within which the ovary descends, the round ligament of the ovary or ovarian ligament (connecting the ovary to uterus), and the round ligament of the uterus (connecting the uterus to the labial fascia).

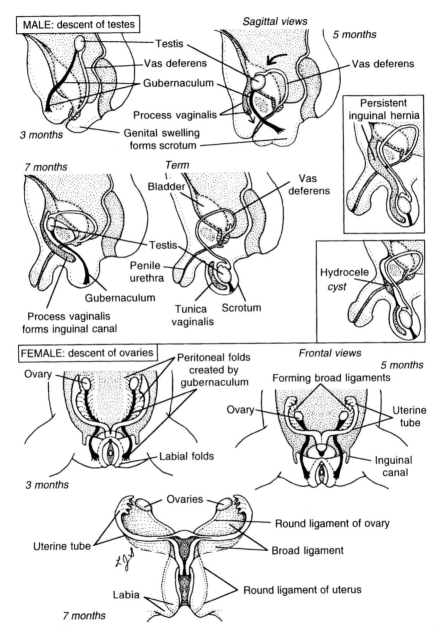

Figure 15-11
Descent of the gonads, and defects in descent.

PRODUCTION OF GAMETES IN THE FETUS AND AFTER PUBERTY

• **Secondary sexual characteristics develop at puberty.**   Another unique feature of the reproductive system is that there are two phases to its development. The primary sex organs are formed during embryonic development, but secondary sexual features appear only at puberty. The only feature of sexual maturation that we will concentrate on here is the onset of production of gametes in both sexes, since some steps in this process occur during fetal life (see Fig. 15-12). The differences in male and female gamete development are striking in this timing.

In the male embryo, testosterone (produced by Leydig cells from the earliest stages of formation of the testis) causes the germ cells to become committed to the spermatogonia lineage shortly after they invade the forming testis. It also suppresses any further differentiation, but permits a process of continual mitosis that continues throughout life. The onset of differentiation of spermatogonia commences only at puberty. At this time, the seminiferous tubules and ducts leading out of the testis also become patent and the Sertoli cells mature. Differentiation proceeds by waves of mitosis in subpopulations of spermatogonia. Some of these dividing cells then enter meiosis and proceed continuously through the process of meiosis and sperm cell maturation in about 60 days.

In the female embryo, the germ cells become commited to the oogonia lineage in the absence of testosterone. The baseline levels of placental hormones (principally estrogen) direct this commitment. This also causes the oogonia to undergo intense mitosis through month 5 of fetal life, by which time a maximum of several million oogonia will be created. After this point, oogonia continually undergo atresia, so that by birth only thousands of potential gametes remain. The most significant difference between the male and female is the different timing of gametogenesis. Oogonia begin the process of meiosis by about month 4 of fetal development. By month 7, almost all oogonia are transformed into primary oocytes, surrounded by flat follicular cells forming primordial follicles. They remain in this stage until just before ovulation, when the follicular cells mature into primary follicles and meiosis resumes.

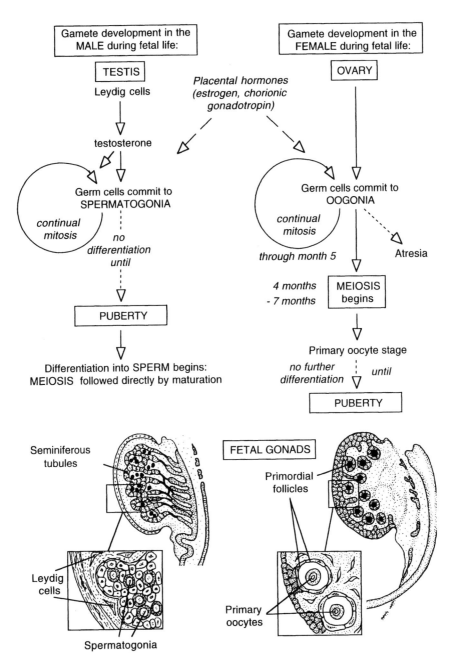

Figure 15-12
Development of gametes.

· C H A P T E R · 16 ·

ENDOCRINE SYSTEM

·

· · · · · · · · · · · ·

The endocrine system comprises a series of organs called *glands* that secrete *hormones* into the bloodstream for distribution throughout the body. Hormones are signaling molecules that trigger changes within target cells by interacting with specific receptors on the cells. Hormones are secreted in response to both neuronal signals and other circulating hormones. In fact, there is such extensive mutual interaction between endocrine glands and the nervous system that they form a functional *neuroendocrine* system.

Endocrine organs originate from all embryonic germ layers. However, they all develop in largely the same way. Development of all endocrine organs is described in this chapter, but particular attention is paid to those organs that have not been previously described.

ORGANS OF THE ENDOCRINE SYSTEM

Organs of the endocrine system are formed throughout the body from the head to the abdominal cavity. They consist of the *pituitary* and *pineal* glands in the head, the *thyroid* gland and *parathyroid* glands in the neck, and the *adrenal* gland in the abdominal cavity. In addition, several organs contain endocrine tissues within them. These include the *islets of Langerhans* in the pancreas, *enteroendocrine* cells distributed along the gastrointestinal tract lining, and cells in the *ovaries* and *uterus* in the female and the *testes* in the male. Finally, the *placenta* is a temporary but important endocrine organ.

• **All endocrine glands are structured in basically the same way (see Fig. 16-1).**   Their functional cells are groups of epithelial cells that manufacture and secrete specific hormones. The secretory cells are closely surrounded by a rich blood vasculature that picks up the hormones for distribution throughout the body. Connective tissue holds the epithelial groups together and provides a supporting framework for entry of the blood vessels and nerves. In most cases, the gland is covered by a prominent connective tissue sheath that often extends into the substance of the glandular tissue at intervals to form septa.

• **The structural arrangement of endocrine cells within other organs can take several forms.**   Some endocrine cells form nests that sit close to blood vessels (islets of Langerhans). Others are contained within the epithelial lining of organs (gastrointestinal tract) or scattered within the connective tissue stroma of organs (testes and ovaries).

• **It is important to distinguish between endocrine and exocrine glands.** The functional cells of both types of glands are epithelial cells that secrete products. Both types of glands exist as independent organs and as components of other organs. The major differences between the two are the functional differences in their secretory products and the structural differences in their methods of secretion. Endocrine glands are *ductless* glands that secrete hormones into surrounding blood vessels. Exocrine glands secrete primarily enzymes. They secrete their products into a central lumen, and from there into epithelial-lined ducts. The ducts open into the lumen of an organ, or onto the surface of the body. Major exocrine glands include the salivary glands, pancreas, gallbladder, sweat glands of the skin, and mammary glands in the female.

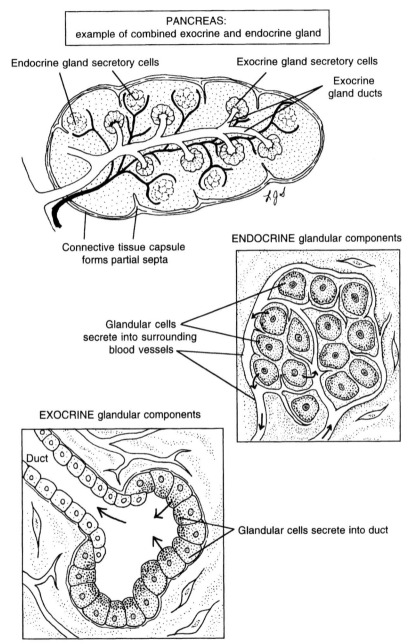

Figure 16-1
The structure of endocrine glands and their comparison to exocrine glands.

EMBRYONIC DEVELOPMENT OF ENDOCRINE GLANDS

All endocrine glands begin to form by proliferation of an existing epithelium (see Fig. 16-2). The major variable in their development is the germ layer of origin of this epithelium. As you will see in the accounts that follow, all three germ layers give rise to endocrine tissue. The epithelium proliferates in response to specific signals from surrounding mesoderm. It forms a bud that sprouts into the surrounding mesoderm and branches in a specific pattern to form the appropriate epithelial morphology for that organ. The cells at the distal ends of these epithelial buds will differentiate into glandular secretory cells. The surrounding mesoderm cells are then recruited to form the connective tissue and vascular components of the gland. This is one of many examples of epithelial-mesenchymal interactions required for embryonic development.

Both endocrine and exocrine glandular structures begin to form in basically this same way. The distinction between endocrine and exocrine glands begins to develop when the epithelial cells connecting the secretory cells to the originating epithelium begin to atrophy in developing endocrine glands, eliminating the connection to the epithelial surface. This newly isolated nest of secretory epithelial cells is then surrounded by proliferating blood vessels that will carry their secretions away. By contrast, in forming exocrine glands, the epithelial cells that connect the glandular cells to the originating epithelium persist and become specialized as ducts. Since exocrine glands always remain connected directly to the epithelium from which they originated, their origins are easy to determine.

• **The timing of structural development precedes the onset of function of endocrine glands in the fetus.** Endocrine cells begin to form in week 4 and continue to proliferate into month 2. The secretory cells continue to differentiate into the start of the fetal period in month 3. As they differentiate, the endocrine cells develop the capacity to produce hormones, but secrete little or no hormone in most cases for several more months. The major exceptions are the fetal pituitary and reproductive organs, which secrete some hormones in months 3 and 4. The pituitary hormones stimulate proliferation of most other endocrine glands, and sex hormones are required for development of reproductive organs.

• **A major source of hormones during the embryonic and early fetal period is the placenta.** It manufactures many hormones and activates others produced by the fetus. The hormones it manufactures duplicate the functions of most hormones produced by endocrine organs, thus providing the fetus with appropriate hormonal signals before all its own endocrine organs become functional.

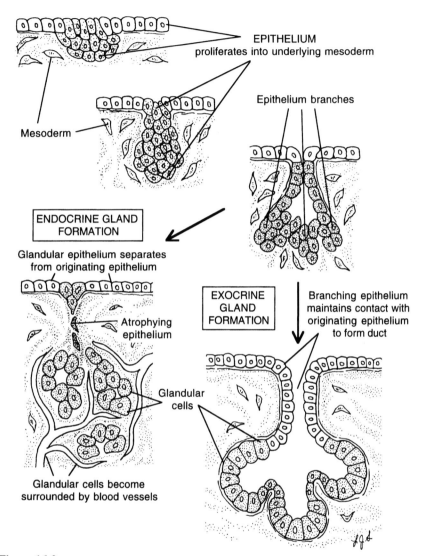

EPITHELIUM
proliferates into underlying mesoderm

Epithelium branches

Mesoderm

ENDOCRINE GLAND
FORMATION

Glandular epithelium separates
from originating epithelium

EXOCRINE
GLAND
FORMATION

Branching epithelium
maintains contact with
originating epithelium
to form duct

Atrophying
epithelium

Glandular
cells

Glandular cells become
surrounded by blood vessels

Figure 16-2
Embryonic formation of endocrine glands.

STRUCTURE AND ORIGINS OF THE PITUITARY GLAND

It is appropriate to start the discussion of endocrine organs with the pituitary gland, since most of its hormonal secretions regulate the hormonal secretions of other endocrine organs. The pituitary is a major component of the neuroendocrine system, converting neural input into hormonal output. It is formed by two components: a neural-tissue-derived *neurohypophysis* and an ectoderm-derived *adenohypophysis* (see Fig. 16-3). These regions remain anatomically and functionally distinct. Each region has a number of duplicate names that it is usually necessary to know.

• **The neurohypophysis is really an extension of the hypothalamus region of the forebrain.** It is also known as the *posterior pituitary*, or *pars nervosa*. Its connection to the hypothalamus forms a narrow infundibular stalk that expands distally to form the bulk of the posterior pituitary tissue. The neurohypophysis contains axonal processes of nerves whose cell bodies are located in the hypothalamus. These are secretory neurons that manufacture "releasing factors" that are carried down the axons to their terminals in the posterior pituitary. They are stored in the nerve terminals until an action potential causes their release, much as classic neurotransmitters are released. However, most of these factors are picked up by the capillary network supplying the posterior pituitary and carried via portal veins to a second plexus of capillaries supplying the anterior pituitary. Here the factors act as hormones to stimulate (or inhibit) the release of hormones by specific endocrine cells. The factors are named for the hormones whose secretion they regulate.

The posterior pituitary also releases two hormones directly into the circulation from the axons of separate hypothalamic nerves. *Vasopressin*, or *antidiuretic hormone*, increases reabsorption of water in the kidney. *Oxytocin* initiates the birth process by causing smooth muscle contraction in the uterine wall.

• **The adenohypophysis is the endocrine portion of the pituitary.** It is also known as the *anterior pituitary*, or *pars distalis*. The portion that wraps around the infundibular stalk forms the *pars tuberalis*, while the portion that lies adjacent to the pars nervosa forms the *pars intermedia*. The anterior pituitary releases a number of hormones that are picked up by an extensive capillary bed and carried from there throughout the body. Pituitary hormones are "tropic" hormones, meaning that they stimulate growth and development of target organs. In most cases, pituitary hormones act by stimulating release of other hormones by target organs, as is reflected in their names: *adrenocorticotropin, thyroid stimulating hormone*, and *gonadotropins*. Two pituitary hormones have direct effects on targets: *somatotropin*, or *growth hormone*, stimulates bone development; and *prolactin* stimulates mammary gland secretion.

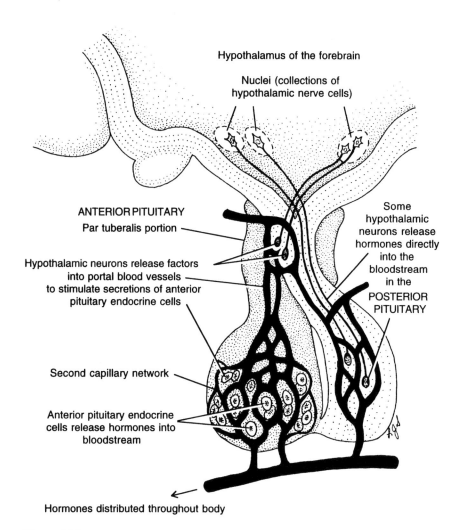

Hypothalamus of the forebrain

Nuclei (collections of
hypothalamic nerve cells)

ANTERIOR PITUITARY
Par tuberalis portion

Hypothalamic neurons release factors
into portal blood vessels
to stimulate secretions of anterior
pituitary endocrine cells

Some
hypothalamic
neurons release
hormones directly
into the
bloodstream
in the
POSTERIOR
PITUITARY

Second capillary network

Anterior pituitary endocrine
cells release hormones into
bloodstream

Hormones distributed throughout body

Figure 16-3
Pituitary structure.

Development of the pituitary gland

• **Pituitary development involves interaction of neuroectoderm and ectoderm lining the roof of the mouth (see Fig. 16-4).** The neurohypophysis arises as an evagination of the floor of the forming diencephalon portion of the forebrain beginning in week 3. It retains its connection to the brain. The secretory neurons of the posterior pituitary develop within the hypothalamus and extend their axons into the posterior pituitary outgrowth during month 3.

The adenohypophysis arises from an outpocketing of the ectoderm that forms the epithelial lining of a portion of the roof of the mouth. (Why is ectoderm found inside the mouth? The boundary between ectoderm and endoderm is pulled to the interior of the mouth cavity after the two germ layers meet and fuse in week 3.) This oral ectoderm thickens, proliferates, and grows cranially to form a structure called *Rathke's pouch* beginning in week 4. By the end of month 2, a constriction forms at the base of Rathke's pouch separating it from the oral ectoderm. The original lumen of the pouch usually persists as a small sac within the anterior pituitary.

• **Onset of pituitary function in the fetus.** Anterior pituitary cells produce the first hormones in month 3, but do not release most of them until several months into fetal development. Posterior pituitary factors begin to be released about the same time and may be responsible for this upturn in secretion. Most of the functions of pituitary hormones in stimulating development of other fetal organs are performed by circulating hormones derived from the placenta prior to the onset of pituitary secretion. The vascular portal system that transfers these factors to the anterior pituitary becomes fully formed at the end of month 3.

STRUCTURE AND ORIGINS OF THE PINEAL GLAND

The pineal gland is a small gland that projects from the roof of the third ventricle in the brain (see Fig. 16-4). Cords of endocrine cells are surrounded by blood vessels and partially separated by connective tissue septa, which carry sympathetic innervation to pineal cells. Pineal cells secrete *melatonin* in response to sympathetic nervous stimuli, which is involved in maintaining circadian rhythms.

The pineal gland develops as an outgrowth of the neuroectoderm of the diencephalon portion of the forebrain beginning in week 3, in much the same manner as the neural portion of the pituitary gland develops.

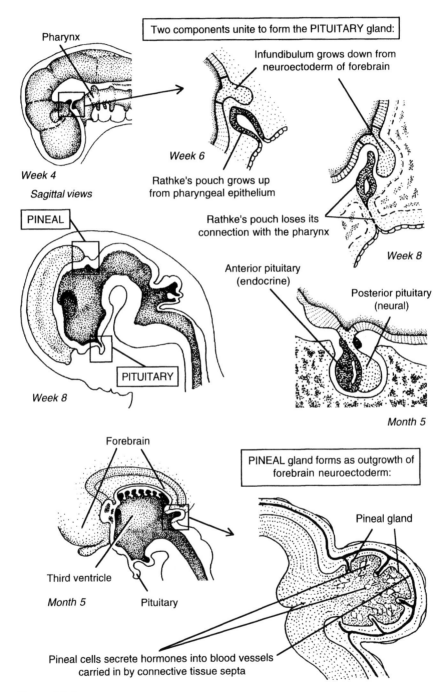

Figure 16-4
Pituitary embryogenesis, and pineal gland structure and embryogenesis.

STRUCTURE AND ORIGINS OF THE THYROID AND PARATHYROID GLANDS

The thyroid and parathyroid glands are formed in the neck from tissues that are derived largely from the pharyngeal arches (see Fig. 16-5). The thyroid gland forms in the midline ventral to the laryngeal cartilage. It contains two lobes connected by a narrow central isthmus. Four separate parathyroid glands (two superior and two inferior) form on the dorsal surface of the thyroid gland. They are usually embedded within the connective tissue capsule of the thyroid gland.

• **The thyroid gland contains two types of endocrine cells that secrete thyroid hormone and calcitonin.** The organization of the thyroid gland at first appears to suggest an exocrine gland, with epithelial cells forming spheres surrounding central lumens. However, these structures, which are called *follicles*, are actually blind storage spaces for *thyroid hormone* secreted by the epithelial cells forming the follicular walls. When signaled, the follicular cells remove the stored hormone, process it, and release it into the network of surrounding blood vessels. Thyroid hormone is essential for growth and metabolism.

Thyroid follicles are surrounded by *parafollicular* cells, also called *C cells*. These cells secrete calcitonin, a hormone that is involved in regulating both bone density and blood calcium levels.

• **The organization of the parathyroid glands is typical of endocrine organs.** In these small glands, clusters of epithelial cells called chief cells secrete *parathyroid hormone* into surrounding blood vessels. The glands consist of clumps of endocrine cells, blood vessels, and small amounts of connective tissue.

Together, parathyroid hormone and calcitonin regulate bone density and blood calcium levels. Parathyroid hormone increases bone matrix resorption by osteoclasts, increasing circulating blood calcium levels. Calcitonin inhibits bone matrix resorption, decreasing blood calcium levels.

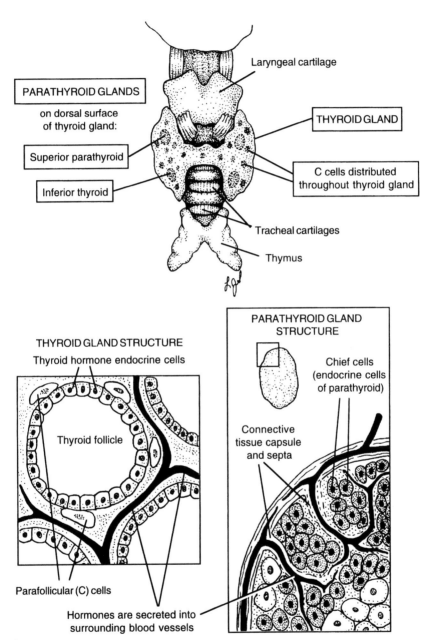

Figure 16-5
Thyroid and parathyroid gland structure.

Development of thyroid and parathyroid glands

• **Endocrine cells of the thyroid and parathyroid glands are formed from pharyngeal endoderm (see Fig. 16-6).** The full range of both pharyngeal endoderm derivatives and pharyngeal arch derivatives is covered in Chap. 10. The connective tissues and blood vessels of these glands are derived from both neural crest and mesoderm that form the core of the pharyngeal arches and the forming tongue and migrate along with the endoderm.

• **Thyroid endocrine cells originate from an outgrowth called the *thyroid diverticulum*.** This epithelial outgrowth of the endoderm covering the ventral midline of the forming tongue extends down through the substance of the tongue. It extends past the hyoid bone and thyroid cartilage into the neck, where its terminal portion proliferates to form epithelial follicles in month 2. The connecting diverticulum normally regresses, separating thyroid tissue from its originating epithelium.

Abnormal persistence of portions of the thyroglossal duct can result in two types of defects. Nests of *ectopic* thyroid tissue can differentiate from remnants along the path of the thyroglossal duct, most typically within the tongue. In other cases, parts of the duct remain as *thyroglossal cysts* or *fistulas* along the path of the duct.

• **Parafollicular C cells of the thyroid originate bilaterally from the endoderm of the fourth pharyngeal pouches.** These cells separate from the pouches and migrate ventrally and caudally to the midline, where they invade the forming thyroid gland. They form small nests surrounding the thyroid follicles. There is some conflict as to whether the neural crest cells surrounding the endoderm in the fourth pharyngeal arches form these endocrine cells as well.

• **The parathyroid glandular tissue is formed from the dorsal portions of pharyngeal pouches 3 and 4.** The endoderm cells separate from the pouches and migrate as epithelial clusters caudally and toward the midline, where they settle on the dorsal surface of the thyroid gland in four separate clusters. The superior parathyroid cells originate from pouch 4 and hitch a ride on the migrating thyroid tissue. The inferior parathyroid cells hitch a ride on the thymus cells that also originate from pouch 3 and then follow a separate path.

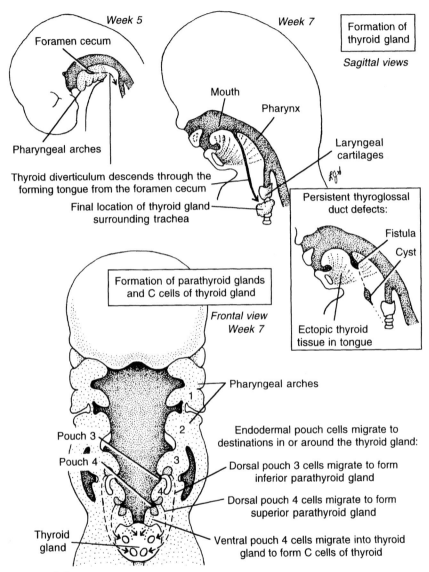

Figure 16-6
Thyroid and parathyroid gland embryogenesis.

• **Onset of thyroid and parathyroid function in the fetus:** Thyroid hormone is one of the first hormones secreted by fetal endocrine glands. Thyroid hormone is secreted from the end of month 3. During the fetal period it directs growth and development, particularly of the nervous system. Onset of parathyroid and parafollicular cell endocrine function occurs much later in fetal life.

STRUCTURE AND ORIGINS OF THE ADRENAL GLAND

The adrenal glands, or *suprarenal* glands, are bilateral glands named for their location close to (*ad*) or cranial to (*supra*) the renal organs, or kidneys (see Fig. 16-7). Each adrenal gland is organized into two separate regions, an outer *cortex* and an inner *medulla*. Both regions are organized as typical endocrine tissue, with cords of epithelial secretory cells surrounded by networks of capillaries. In the cortex, the cords run radially from the periphery toward the center of the organ. Different regions or zones of the cortex secrete specific hormones. These include *corticosteroids*, or steroid hormones; *mineralocorticoids*, which regulate water and ion balance; *glucocorticoids*, which regulate glucose metabolism; and small quantities of *androgens*, or male sex hormones.

The adrenal medulla secretes hormones in response to stress-induced nervous stimulation from preganglionic sympathetic autonomic nerves. These *catecholamine* hormones are identical to the neurotransmitters secreted by secondary or postganglionic nerves in the autonomic chain. They cause blood vessel constriction and an increase in heart rate.

Different germ-layer origins of the two portions of the adrenal gland

• **The adrenal cortex originates from mesoderm, while the medulla develops from neural crest cells.**   Neural crest cells migrate into the intermediate mesoderm at the cranial end of the forming abdominal cavity during week 6. Here they rapidly become surrounded by mesoderm cells derived from the intermediate mesoderm lining the body cavity. (All other intermediate mesoderm forms structures of the urogenital systems; see Chaps. 14 and 15.) The adrenal cortex forms in two stages, both derived from the same mesoderm. The fetal cortex is actually bigger than the definitive cortex that replaces it. It secretes forms of steroid hormones that are converted in the placenta into active steroids from month 3 until birth. The fetal cortex regresses after birth. The definitive cortex begins to differentiate late in fetal life, but is not fully formed until the third year of life.

• **The adrenal medullary cells differentiate into endocrine cells under direction of signals from the cortical mesoderm.**   Neural crest often receives its final commitment instructions at its destination site. In other parts of the embryo, these crest-derived cells would differentiate into postganglionic (secondary) sympathetic neurons. Here they become innervated by preganglionic sympathetic neurons and release, as hormones, the same catecholamines that are used as neurotransmitters by secondary sympathetic neurons.

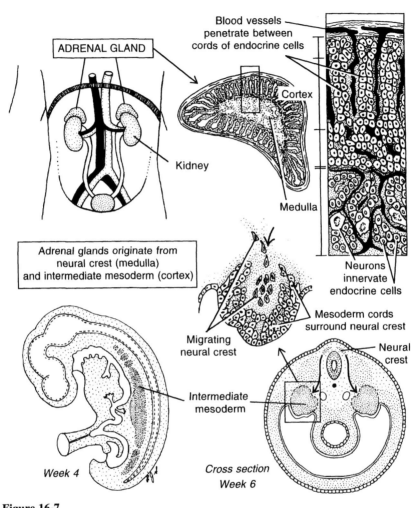

Figure 16-7
Adrenal gland structure and embryogenesis.

Adrenal hyperplasia, or overdevelopment of the fetal cortex, causes female *pseudohermaphroditism*, in which external genitalia become masculinized in female fetuses due to excessive androgen production by the fetal cortex. Progestins administered to prevent spontaneous abortion can cause similar abnormalities.

STRUCTURE AND ORIGINS OF ENDOCRINE TISSUES CONTAINED WITHIN OTHER ORGANS

Structure and formation of the endocrine pancreas

The pancreas combines exocrine and endocrine glandular secretory functions in one organ (see Fig. 16-8). Its exocrine secretions are mostly digestive enzymes that are secreted via the pancreatic duct into the lumen of the small intestines. Its endocrine secretions include the hormones *insulin, glucagon,* and *somatostatin,* which are all involved in regulating blood glucose levels and its entry into cells. The endocrine cells are scattered throughout the pancreas in clumps called *islets of Langerhans.* Each hormone is manufactured by different cells, which are mixed within each islet. They secrete their hormones into surrounding blood vessels in response to parasympathetic autonomic innervation and in response to circulating hormones, including those released by enteroendocrine cells in the small intestines.

• **Both the exocrine and endocrine secretory epithelial cells are derived from an outgrowth of the midgut endoderm into surrounding mesoderm.**   The formation of both portions of the gland was described in Chap. 12. Epithelial outgrowths from the endoderm tube form dorsal and ventral pancreatic buds in week 5. The proximal portions of these buds migrate toward each other and fuse to form a common duct for the exocrine secretions during month 2. The distal outgrowths of the endoderm buds branch repeatedly to form both the exocrine and endocrine secretory cells also during month 2. Most buds form exocrine cells that remain connected to the main buds. Other groups of cells that form from the distal ends of some buds separate from the buds and clump together to proliferate and differentiate into the endocrine cells.

• **Onset of endocrine pancreas function.**   The endocrine cells begin to differentiate during month 3. They become mature functionally and begin to secrete glucagon and insulin by the end of month 5 and, later during the fetal period, somatostatin. These hormones play a role in directing growth of the fetus. Prior to their secretion, placental hormones assume their growth-promoting role.

Ectopic pancreatic endocrine tissue can be found along the digestive tract, most commonly in the wall of the stomach and duodenum.

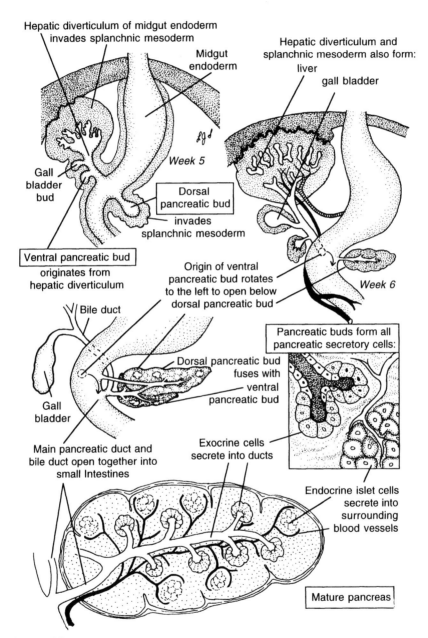

Figure 16-8
Endocrine pancreas structure and embryogenesis.

Structure and origins of enteroendocrine cells of the gastrointestinal tract

A diffuse system of endocrine cells is spread throughout the epithelial lining of the gastrointestinal tract (see Fig. 16-9). These cells are called *enteroendocrine cells*, because of their gastrointestinal, or *enteric*, origins. The cells are located at the base of glands in the walls of the stomach and small intestines. These glands are mixed glands, comprised mostly of exocrine cells that secrete their products via short ducts into the lumen of the gastrointestinal tract. Even though enteroendocrine cells sit side by side in glands with exocrine cells, they secrete products in opposite directions. Exocrine cells secrete across their apical surfaces into the lumen of the duct, while endocrine cells secrete across their basal surfaces into the underlying extracellular matrix. These cells release a variety of hormones that activate other secretory cells of the gastrointestinal tract via both *paracrine* and *endocrine* effects. Paracrine secretions affect only local cells via diffusion through the extracellular matrix, while endocrine secretions diffuse into the bloodstream for broad dissemination. Hormones released by enteroendocrine cells in the stomach and small intestines stimulate secretion of digestive enzymes by both the small intestinal glands and the exocrine pancreas, as well as insulin and glucagon by the pancreatic endocrine cells. Other secretions regulate acid secretion in the stomach and bicarbonate ion release from the pancreas to counter the acid. Several others help regulate motility of intestinal smooth muscle.

• **Development of enteroendocrine cells.**   Gastrointestinal tract glands form as buds from the endoderm tube during month 2 at the same time the other components of the tract are differentiating. Glands are induced to form with different specific configurations and containing specific combinations of cell types in each region of the endoderm tube under the direction of the surrounding splanchnic lateral plate mesoderm. All cells have differentiated within the epithelial lining of the gastrointestinal tract by month 6. However, there is a wide range of onset of functional maturation later in life, since there are no major digestive functions during fetal life.

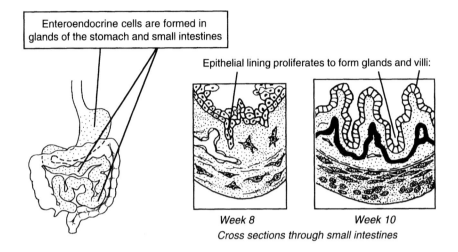

Enteroendocrine cells are formed in glands of the stomach and small intestines

Epithelial lining proliferates to form glands and villi:

Week 8   *Week 10*

Cross sections through small intestines

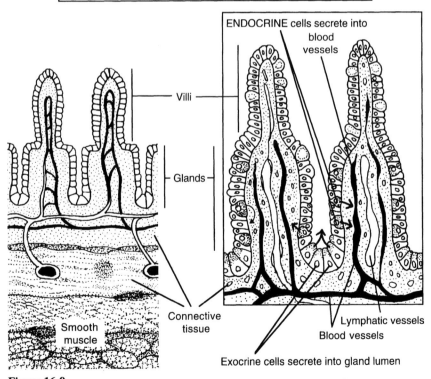

Epithelium lining the GI tract differentiates into multiple cell types:

ENDOCRINE cells secrete into blood vessels

Villi

Glands

Smooth muscle

Connective tissue

Lymphatic vessels

Blood vessels

Exocrine cells secrete into gland lumen

Figure 16-9
Development of enteroendocrine cells.

Structure and origins of the endocrine components of the sex organs and placenta

The ovaries and uterus in the female and testes in the male contain endocrine cells. Endocrine cells in both male and female reproductive organs differentiate and begin to secrete hormones during fetal development. Some of these hormones are essential for embryonic and fetal development of the reproductive structures. Endocrine cells of the reproductive system are unique in that they then become inactive after birth and are reactivated only when puberty is reached.

• **All endocrine tissues of the reproductive organs are formed from the same intermediate mesoderm that forms the reproductive organs (see Fig. 16-10).** As described in Chap. 15, the reproductive organs develop from a common set of precursor structures that only begin to differentiate along male or female lines in week 6. Hormones present in the embryo are essential to the direction that differentiation takes.

• **The placenta is a regulator of fetal development.**   Placental hormones are essential, first for maintenance of the placenta and pregnancy and then for fetal development. In the first two months of pregnancy, the syncytiotrophoblast layer of the placenta produces *progesterone* and *estrogen* that directly maintain the pregnancy. It also produces *chorionic gonadotropins* that act like pituitary gonadotropins to maintain estrogen and progesterone output of the ovarian cells of the corpus luteum, which is essential for long-term maintenance of the pregnancy. The placenta continues to produce hormones throughout pregnancy.

Placental hormones are also essential for development of the fetal reproductive systems. Placental *corticotropin-releasing factors* and *chorionic gonadotropins* take the place of pituitary versions of these hormones in directing development of fetal reproductive organs. Placental hormones also include equivalents of most other hormones released from the pituitary gland. The placenta also converts hormones from some fetal glands to active forms. Later, endocrine cells in the fetal gonads and pituitary take over from the placenta.

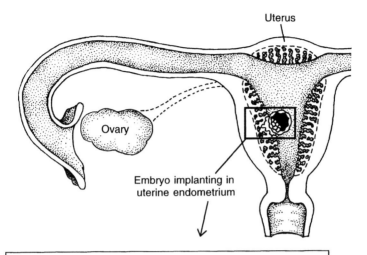

Uterus

Ovary

Embryo implanting in
uterine endometrium

The embryo forms part of the PLACENTA from its trophoblast layer:

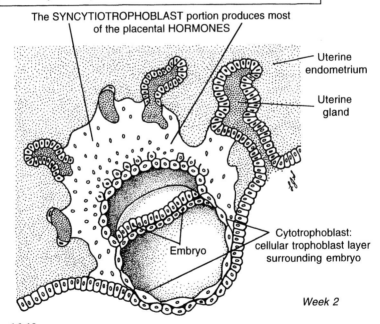

The SYNCYTIOTROPHOBLAST portion produces most
of the placental HORMONES

Uterine
endometrium

Uterine
gland

Embryo

Cytotrophoblast:
cellular trophoblast layer
surrounding embryo

Week 2

Figure 16-10
Development of placental endocrine cells.

• **Development of endocrine cells in the female reproductive system (see Fig. 16-11).** In the adult ovary, both the follicular cells and theca interna cells surrounding the oocyte function as endocrine cells. Together, they secrete estrogen and progesterone in a cyclic fashion which directs both oocyte maturation and development of the uterine lining in preparation for possible implantation. This cyclic release is coordinated by two *gonadotropin* hormones released from the pituitary, *follicle-stimulating hormone* and *luteinizing hormone*.

In the female fetus, gonadal development is slow. Follicular cells become recognizable around primitive oocytes during month 4, and by month 5 follicular development is underway. Estrogens derived from the placenta and developing adrenals provide the stimulus for development of all female reproductive organs.

• **Development of endocrine cells in the male reproductive system (see Fig. 16-11).** Two separate cell types in the adult testis are endocrine cells. They are the *Sertoli* cells in the seminiferous tubules that surround and "nurse" the development of the sperm and the *interstitial cells of Leydig*, which lie in the connective tissue spaces between seminiferous tubules. Pituitary gonadotropins cause each of these endocrine cells to release specific hormones after puberty. Follicle-stimulating hormones (FSH) causes Sertoli cells to release *androgen binding proteins*. These protein hormones find and concentrate androgens within the seminiferous tubules and feed back to the pituitary to inhibit its FSH secretion. *Luteinizing hormone* stimulates Leydig cells to secrete *testosterone* essential for sperm development and maintenance of secondary sex characteristics.

During embryonic and fetal development, placental versions of pituitary gonadotropins stimulate development of both male reproductive organs and the endocrine cells within them. The indeterminate gonad develops seminiferous tubules containing Sertoli cells under direction of placental chorionic gonadotropins. Sertoli cells then secrete *Müllerian-inhibiting substance* (MIS), a hormone that acts to shape the genital duct system by causing regression of embryonic Müllerian ducts in the male fetus during month 3. (These ducts form female reproductive structures without this inhibitory signal.) Leydig cells develop later, beginning in month 3, in response to MIS. The placental chorionic gonadotropins then stimulate the Leydig cells to secrete testosterone until months 4 to 5 of fetal development, when the Leydig cells become inactive until puberty.

Testosterone secretion by fetal Leydig cells is essential for development of all male reproductive system structures.

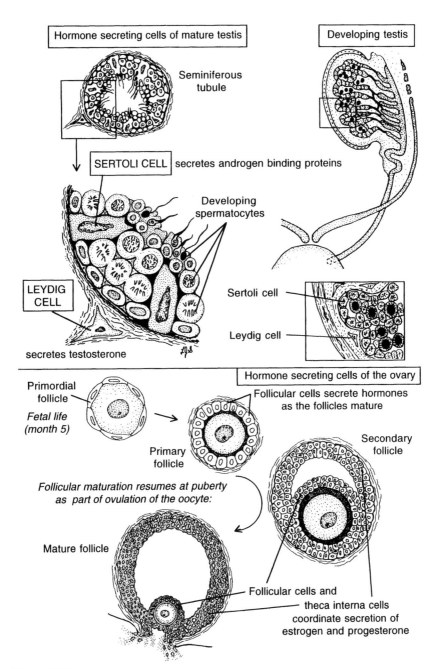

Figure 16-11
Development of male and female reproductive system endocrine cells.

HEMATOPOIETIC SYSTEM

·

· · · · · · · · · · · ·

The hematopoietic system consists of organs and the cells they produce that circulate in the vascular system. The primary organs of the system are the bone marrow and thymus, while secondary organs include the lymph nodes and spleen, as well as lymphoid nodules within the walls of a number of organs. Two major lines of cells are formed by hematopoiesis, the myeloid lineage and lymphoid lineage. The cells of the lymphoid lineage are the principal players in the immune response of the individual. It is beyond the scope of this chapter to detail all the steps in hematopoiesis or in development of the immune response. These phenomena begin in the embryo, but continue throughout the life of the individual. Rather, this chapter concentrates on the development of the organs of this system and on the origins of hematopoietic stem cells.

COMPONENTS OF THE MATURE HEMATOPOIETIC SYSTEM

The hematopoietic system provides a continual supply of circulating blood cells throughout the life of the individual. Most have a relatively short life span, ranging from days to months, so they must be constantly replaced by differentiation from stem cells. This process, called *hematopoiesis*, occurs in several primary or central hematopoietic organs, from which cells then seed peripheral organs.

• **What are stem cells, and why are they so important in this system?**   Stem cells are *undifferentiated* but *committed* cells that provide a continual, self-renewing source of new cells throughout life. In the hematopoietic system, stem cells remain *pluripotent*. This means that each stem cell can give rise to any of the hematopoietic cell types. Stem cells exist in a few other systems, but they are committed to a single fate (osteoprogenitors in bone, chondroblasts in cartilage, satellite cells in skeletal muscle, and spermatogonia in the testes).

Cells of the hematopoietic system

• **The cells of the hematopoietic system can be divided into the myeloid lineage and lymphoid lineage (see Fig. 17-1).**   The myeloid lineage includes the erythroid lineage, or red blood cells that carry oxygen in the blood, and a number of "white" blood cells. These include the *granulocytes*, named for the specific granules in their cytoplasm. Each of the granulocytes (neutrophils, eosinophils, and basophils) plays a specific role in defense of the body. The myeloid lineage also generates *megakaryocytes*, which fragment to form *platelets* that enter the circulation to play an essential role in blood clotting. Finally, the myeloid lineage includes *monocytes*, which differentiate into *macrophages* in the connective tissues. Macrophages are important as scavengers of debris and antigenic substances in the body.

• **Cell types in the lymphoid lineage are involved in the immune response.** The lymphoid lineage produces T lymphocytes, which direct *cell-mediated immunity*, and B lymphocytes, which mediate the *humoral immune response* by producing specific antibodies. Both T cells and B cells proliferate when they encounter an antigenic source, producing activated lymphocytes, which launch an immune reaction, and memory cells, which react rapidly to a second exposure. Macrophages facilitate the immune reaction by phagocytosing substances and then "presenting" them to lymphocytes as antigens to generate an immune response.

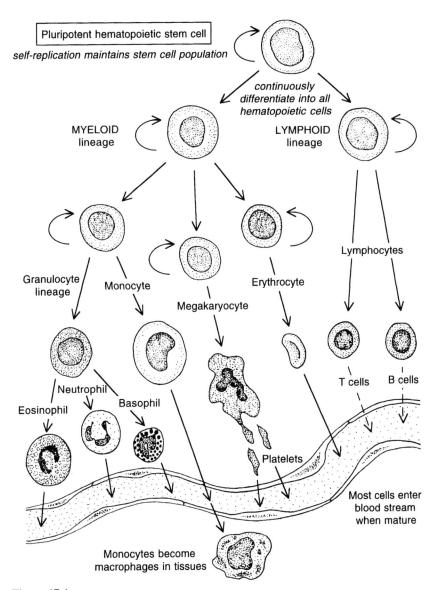

Figure 17-1
Cells of the hematopoietic system.

Organs of the hematopoietic system

In the adult, the central or primary hematopoietic organs are the *bone marrow* and the *thymus* (see Fig. 17-2). Cells generated here continuously enter the circulation to seed the secondary organs of the system.

- ## CENTRAL ORGANS: BONE MARROW AND THYMUS
- **The bone marrow is the home of pluripotent stem cells throughout life.** It is the site of a continuous production of all cells of the myeloid lineage. It is also the primary site of continuous B-cell generation (*B* can stand for bone marrow origin). By contrast, while the bone marrow generates T-cell progenitors, they must first migrate to the thymus for commitment and differentiation to occur (hence the *T*, which stands for thymus generated).

Bone marrow is one of the largest organs in the body. It is found in the central cavities of long bones and between the spicules of bone in the flat bones (principally vertebral bodies, sternum, ribs, cranium, and pelvis). In newborns, all marrow is active; later in life only some bones retain active marrow. Active marrow regulates hematopoiesis by the release of cytokines or growth factors from its meshwork of supporting stromal cells. These factors act as "colony-stimulating factors" to stimulate stem cells to produce colonies of the required cell types. When cells mature, they enter large sinusoidal blood vessels in the marrow cavity and from there enter the body circulation.

- **The thymus is the home of T cells, which must mature here before seeding other peripheral lymphoid organs.** Thymic progenitors, or *thymocytes*, enter the thymus from the bone marrow. The thymus forms in the mediastinum or dorsal part of the thoracic cavity behind the sternum. Connective tissue septa partially divide the organ into lobules and distribute blood vessels and efferent (outgoing) lymphatics. Each lobule has a cortex and medulla that both contain a stromal network of elongated epithelial cells that surround developing lymphocytes. The cortex receives thymocytes and serves as their primary maturation center, with epithelial cells functioning as nurse cells. They produce cytokines and hormones that stimulate thymocyte proliferation and condition (or instruct) thymocytes to commit to the T-cell lineage and differentiate. The medulla coordinates later steps in T-cell development and releases T cells into the bloodstream.

- **The thymus exports immunocompetent but "virgin" T cells.** These T cells have developed receptors for specific antigens, so they are immunocompetent (capable of reacting to the antigen). They are "virgin" cells since they have not yet encountered the antigen.

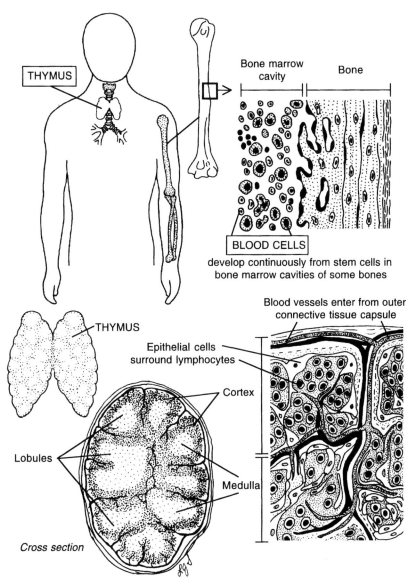

Figure 17-2
Bone marrow and thymus as hematopoietic organs.

• **PERIPHERAL HEMATOPOIETIC ORGANS**   Peripheral hematopoietic organs are primarily (but not exclusively) involved in lymphopoiesis, or the generation of mature lymphocytes, since most cells of the myeloid lineage are released mature from bone marrow. Each peripheral organ or lymphoid nodule has its own specialized role in collecting specific types of antigens for generation of an immune reaction (see Fig. 17-3).

• **Peripheral lymphoid organs are invaded by immature lymphocytes, which then proliferate and complete differentiation after exposure to antigenic stimuli.**   B cells spend most of their life within these organs, forming nodules that turn into germinal centers when B cells are activated. By contrast, some T cells remain in organs, while most circulate on continuous surveillance.

• **The spleen is an abdominal organ that filters all components of blood.**   It is the largest lymphoid tissue accumulation in the body, containing about 25 percent of the body's lymphocytes. Blood flow through the *white pulp* region constitutes the major site of initiation of the immune response against blood-borne antigens. Arteries that enter the white pulp are surrounded by periarteriolar lymph sheaths containing T cells, while B cells form nodules in the outer white pulp. Blood also percolates through the sinusoidal blood vessel network in the *red pulp* region, where particulate matter and damaged erythrocytes are removed and destroyed by macrophages.

• **Lymph nodes filter the contents of the lymphatic vessels that drain the connective tissue spaces of the body.**   Lymph nodes are found in the axilla, groin, along the blood vessels of the neck, and in the thorax and abdomen. Incoming or afferent lymphatics enter around the circumference of each node. Their contents percolate through lymphatic sinuses leading from the cortex into the medulla, where they exit via efferent lymphatics. Nodes contain both B and T cells localized in different regions.

• **Unencapsulated lymphoid tissues are the first line of defense against antigenic substances that enter the body from the outside environment.**   The gastrointestinal, respiratory, and urinary systems are all directly connected to the outside environment and are a route of entry of antigenic substances. *Tonsils* are partially encapulsated nodules lying in the connective tissue just under the epithelium lining the mouth and pharynx. Unencapsulated nodules underlie the epithelium lining other parts of the digestive tract as well. Some are very large, forming Peyers patches in the ileum, and virtually taking over the wall of the appendix at the start of the large intestines. Nodules are also found in the trachea and bronchi of the upper respiratory tract and the urinary passages of the ureters and urethra.

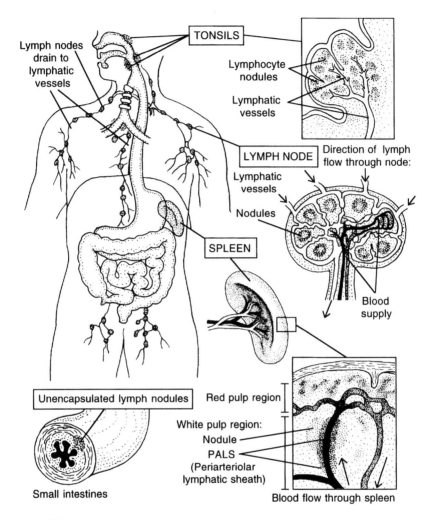

Figure 17-3
Peripheral lymphoid organs and tissues involved in initiation of the immune response.

DEVELOPMENT OF THE HEMATOPOIETIC SYSTEM

The hematopoietic system begins to develop early. The major event that necessitates this early development is that the embryo gets too large by week 3 for diffusion to continue to suffice as the source of nutrient and oxygen supply. Thus, the embryo develops a functional circulatory system during week 3, including formation of an exchange network with the maternal circulation in the placenta. While nutrients and carbon dioxide wastes can be transported dissolved in blood plasma, red blood cells are required to transport oxygen in the blood.

Development of hematopoietic cells

Hematopoiesis of red blood cells, or erythropoiesis, is thus the first order of business, followed later by development of other hematopoietic cells and organs. All other hematopoietic cells participate in some way in protection of the embryo, which is not an urgent need early in embryonic development. First, the embryo is in a somewhat (but not entirely) protected environment due to the partial barrier provided by the placenta. Second, antibodies (primarily immunoglobulin G) are actively transported across the placenta from week 10 until birth, conferring partial immunity.

All hematopoietic cells and organs are entirely derived from mesoderm, except the thymus.

• **A series of sites serve sequentially as the location of hematopoiesis during embryonic development.** These sites do not all remain sites of hematopoiesis in the adult. By month 6 a pattern similar to that of the adult is established. The origins of the stem cells that populate each newly formed hematopoietic organ is not clear in many cases.

• **Hematopoiesis begins in the yolk sac with production of red blood cells at week 3 (see Fig. 17-4).** Blood islands form within the extraembryonic mesoderm surrounding the yolk sac endoderm. The outer cells of the blood islands form endothelial walls that unite to form vascular channels. These become the vitelline vessels. Cells at the center of the islands form stem cells called *hemocytoblasts*. These pluripotent stem cells have vast proliferative capacity. While they can give rise to all blood cells types, it is not known whether they actually give rise to lymphocytes or myeloid lineage cells other than red blood cells. The yolk sac is the major source of red blood cells through week 4, but their formation continues here until week 6.

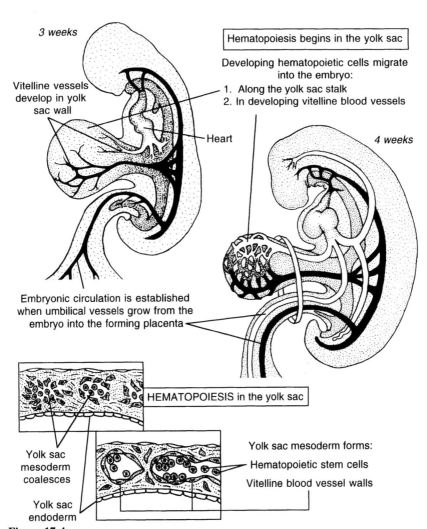

Figure 17-4
Early embryonic development of hematopoietic cells.

• **The developing liver becomes the next site of hematopoiesis (see Fig. 17-5).**
Beginning in week 5, the liver primordium becomes a site of hematopoiesis, initially using yolk-sac-derived stem cells that have seeded it. During month 2, the liver is the primary site of hematopoiesis. It remains a major hematopoietic site until month 6 and continues to play some role until birth. During its time of hematopoiesis, stem cells give rise to cells of the lymphoid and myeloid lineages. These cells seed the permanent hematopoietic organs.

• **The spleen becomes a site of fetal hematopoiesis shortly after the liver.**
The development of the spleen in the abdomen is described here in some detail, since it does not have a "home" in any other chapter (see Fig. 17-5). Its relation to abdominal mesenteries is described in Chap. 12. It begins to differentiate in week 5 from a portion of the splanchnic lateral plate mesoderm sandwiched between the layers of the dorsal mesentery (or mesogastrium) that attaches the stomach to the body wall. This mesoderm proliferates to form the connective tissue stromal framework and capsule of the spleen, as well as an extensive network of blood vessels that ramify through the organ.

The spleen becomes a site of hematopoiesis as it forms beginning in week 5. The source of its hematopoietic stem cells remains unclear, but may be the liver. The spleen remains an important site of hematopoiesis of cells of the myeloid lineage through month 7, particularly red blood cells. First T cells and then B cells invade the organ in month 5 from other origins, probably the liver and thymus. Hematopoietic centers are present until late fetal life.

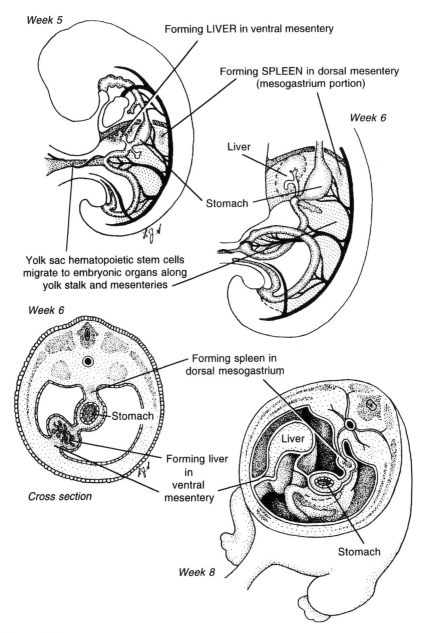

Figure 17-5
Development of the liver and spleen, and the path of hematopoietic stem cells into these organs.

Development of permanent hematopoietic organs (see Fig. 17-6)

• **Lymph nodes begin to develop in month 2.**   Lymph sacs along the path of the developing lymphatic system are transformed into groups of lymph nodes by formation of a connective tissue stromal framework beginning by week 8. Definitive nodes are present by week 10. Other mesodermal mesenchymal cells invade each lymph sac and break up its cavity into a network of lymph channels and lymph sinuses. By week 10, lymphocytes are present in lymphatics and are channeled through nodes, where they begin to take up residence. However, organized lymphoid nodules do not appear in lymph nodes until near birth. Lymphatic vasculature develops throughout the body during month 2, and drains to the nodes.

• **Tonsils are formed as partially encapsulated lymph nodules.**   They form in the walls of the pharynx just below the surface epithelium during month 2. All tonsils are covered by the endoderm lining the mouth and pharynx. The connective tissue framework is formed by mesoderm and neural crest. The tonsils consist of bilateral palatine tonsils, midline pharyngeal tonsils (commonly called *adenoids*), and lingual tonsils at the base of the tongue. The palatine tonsils form from the mesoderm and neural crest of arch 2 and are covered by endoderm of pharyngeal pouch 2. The other tonsils are formed by mesoderm surrounding the pharyngeal endoderm. Lymphocytes invade the tonsils after the framework is established. The B lymphocytes housed here secrete antibodies that defend the body against foreign organisms.

• **Bone marrow begins to be a site of hematopoiesis by month 6, as the role of the liver and spleen diminish.**   It remains a permanent hematopoietic organ from this point on. While bone tissue begins to develop at the start of month 2, formation of the first marrow cavities that can become invaded by hematopoietic stem cells does not occur until month 3 at the earliest in bones formed directly by intramembranous ossification. Endochondral ossification, or transformation of cartilage models into bones, produces marrow cavities in the more numerous long bones. This is a gradual process that begins with formation of cartilage models during month 2. Their transformation into bone begins during month 3 but continues throughout fetal life (see Chap. 7). Thus, the onset of hematopoiesis in bone marrow progresses throughout fetal life.

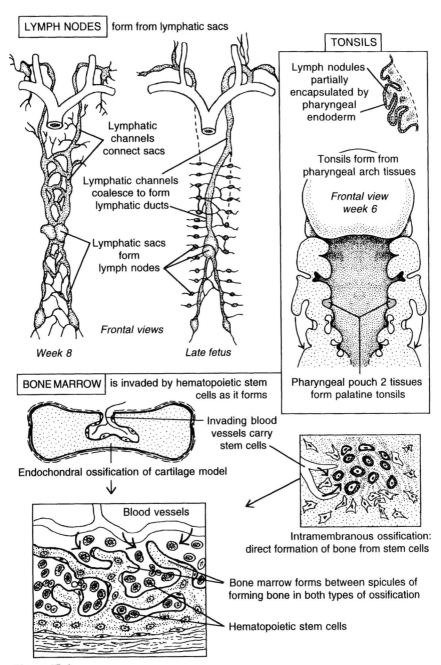

LYMPH NODES form from lymphatic sacs

Lymphatic channels connect sacs

Lymphatic channels coalesce to form lymphatic ducts

Lymphatic sacs form lymph nodes

Frontal views

Week 8

Late fetus

TONSILS

Lymph nodules partially encapsulated by pharyngeal endoderm

Tonsils form from pharyngeal arch tissues

Frontal view week 6

Pharyngeal pouch 2 tissues form palatine tonsils

BONE MARROW is invaded by hematopoietic stem cells as it forms

Invading blood vessels carry stem cells

Endochondral ossification of cartilage model

Blood vessels

Intramembranous ossification: direct formation of bone from stem cells

Bone marrow forms between spicules of forming bone in both types of ossification

Hematopoietic stem cells

Figure 17-6
Formation of peripheral lymphatic organs.

• **Thymus development.**   The thymus is distinct from other lymphoid organs in that its stroma develops from epithelial cells, not mesodermally derived connective tissue cells (see Fig. 17-7). These epithelia form a network of interdigitating cells through which maturing lymphocytes can move.

> Thymic epithelia are formed from endoderm of the third pharyngeal pouches and ectoderm of the corresponding third pharyngeal clefts.

The bilateral endodermal evaginations that form the second pharyngeal pouches become surrounded by ingrowing ectoderm from the second pharyngeal clefts (called *cervical vesicles*). Both separate from their originating epithelium, and the ectodermal vesicle surrounds the endoderm. The ectoderm is believed to give rise to the epithelium of the thymic cortex, while endoderm gives rise to the medullary epithelium. *Neural crest* from the core of pharyngeal arch 3 forms the connective tissue capsule surrounding the thymus, as well as some epithelial components and myoid cells in the medulla.

In week 6, the bilateral thymic precursors migrate into the neck and meet behind the forming sternum. The ectoderm and endoderm begin forming epithelial cords that branch repeatedly. Septa that partially divide the thymus into lobules begin to form from neural crest. Inductive interactions between the two types of epithelium, as well as with the neural crest, are necessary for thymic development. The thymus becomes divided into cortex and medulla by week 10. The organ is configured much as in the adult by month 4.

• **Circulating lymphoid cells begin to colonize the epithelial thymic rudiment.**   By weeks 9 to 10, blood-borne thymocyte precursors begin to invade the thymus, probably derived from the liver. The thymic epithelial cells secrete colony stimulating factors (CSFs) as attractants. The thymocyte precursors force apart the epithelial cells, causing them to form a spongy epithelial reticulum. In turn, the epithelial reticulum induces the thymocytes to proliferate and migrate into forming cortical and medullary regions.

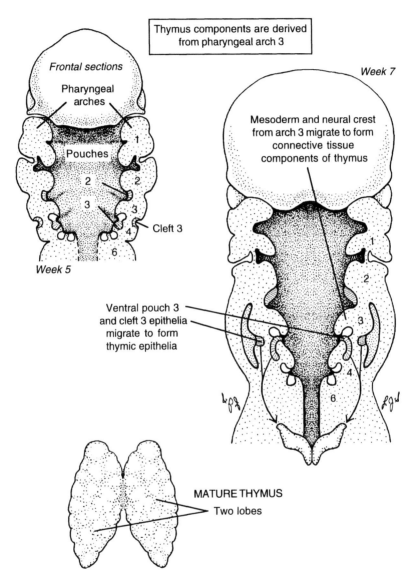

Thymus components are derived
from pharyngeal arch 3

Frontal sections

Pharyngeal
arches

Pouches

Cleft 3

Week 5

Week 7

Mesoderm and neural crest
from arch 3 migrate to form
connective tissue
components of thymus

Ventral pouch 3
and cleft 3 epithelia
migrate to form
thymic epithelia

MATURE THYMUS
Two lobes

Figure 17-7
Development of the thymus.

· C H A P T E R · 18 ·

MATURATION OF PLACENTA AND FETAL MEMBRANES

·

·   ·   ·   ·   ·   ·   ·   ·   ·   ·   ·   ·

This chapter picks up the story of development of the placenta and fetal membranes where Chap. 4 stops. The fetal membranes consist of the amnion, yolk sac, and allantois. After all the components are established, the placenta and fetal membranes must still continue to develop for the pregnancy to thrive. These developments include morphologic alterations and biochemical maturation of cells within the placenta.

REVIEW OF INITIAL EVENTS IN IMPLANTATION AND PLACENTAL FORMATION

• **Implantation and establishment of placental transfer must occur for the embryo to develop.** The embryo forms part of the placenta. Its contribution is derived mostly from the outer trophoblast layer of cells formed at the blastula stage of embryonic development (see Fig. 18-1). This trophoblast layer itself forms the *cytotrophoblast*, or cellular trophoblast layer that remains closest to the embryo, and the *syncytiotrophoblast*. The syncytiotrophoblast is in direct contact with maternal uterine tissue (endometrium). It is a syncytium or multinucleated mass formed by cells leaving the cytotrophoblast and fusing with each other. Finally, extraembryonic mesoderm forms between the cytotrophoblast and embryo proper. It is an embryonic derivative, but the precise source is a matter of dispute.

Implantation occurs as a result of the syncytiotrophoblast producing substances that erode the uterine endometrium, causing the embryo to become completely embedded within the endometrial wall. The syncytiotrophoblast also erodes the walls of maternal blood vessels and endometrial glands, forming *lacunae* (spaces) into which maternal blood and glandular secretions empty. Thus, maternal fluids are in direct contact with an embryonic tissue. Materials are transported from maternal vessels across the syncytiotrophoblast membrane into its cytoplasm from the onset of its invasion of the endometrium. These materials must then diffuse through the syncytiotrophoblast to reach the tissues of the embryo proper. This is the beginning of uteroplacental circulation.

• **These events all occur with the first three weeks of development.** The embryo begins to implant in the uterus in week 1. In week 2, fetal membranes begin to form and the embryo becomes *completely* embedded (implanted) in the uterine wall. During week 3, placental circulation begins and the extra-embryonic fetal membranes and other extraembryonic structures are well established. Thus, by week 4, embryonic organogenesis can begin in earnest due to formation of the placenta and establishment of intraembryonic circulation.

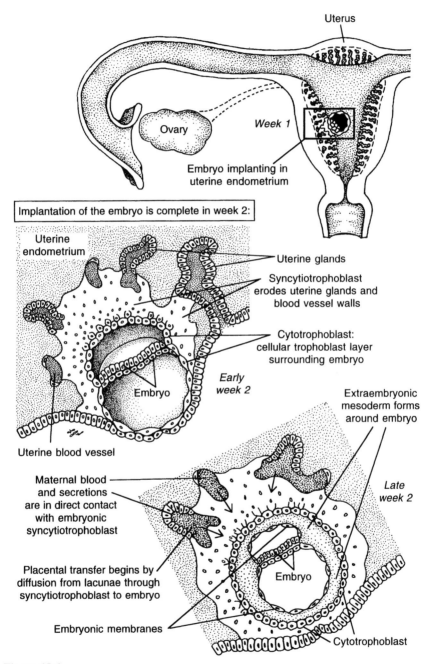

Figure 18-1
Review of implantation and initial formation of the placenta.

FORMATION OF THE MATURE PLACENTA

• **The placenta is formed by fetal and maternal contributions (see Fig. 18-2).**
The fetal part of placenta is called the *chorion*. It is formed from the trophoblast
layers and extraembryonic mesoderm. A chorionic cavity develops within the
extraembryonic mesoderm. The chorion remains connected to the fetus by a *connecting stalk* of this mesoderm that will form the core of the umbilical cord.

   The maternal part of the placenta is called the *decidua*. It is formed by elab-
oration of the portion of the uterine endometrium closest to the lumen, called the
functionalis layer. This is the layer of the endometrium that is shed during menstruation if implantation does not take place.

Development of the chorionic part of placenta

The mature structure of the placenta begins to develop during month 1. The trophoblast layers form projections that further invade the uterine endometrium.
Since these layers are the chorionic part of the placenta, they are called *chorionic
villi*. Villi develop in stages. The contents of the large spaces, or *lacunae*, that
have already formed by syncytiotrophoblast erosion of the walls of maternal
endometrial blood vessels and secretory glands are in direct contact with the outermost syncytiotrophoblast layer.

> The syncytiotrophoblast is always the outermost fetal-derived layer and,
> thus, is always the fetal derivative in direct contact with the maternal
> endometrium and its secretions.

   The initial stage of villous projection consists of syncytiotrophoblast covering a core of cytotrophoblast. These projections are called *primary villi*. They
become *secondary* villi when extraembryonic mesoderm invades to form a connective tissue core. They become *tertiary* villi in week 3 when umbilical blood
vessels invade the connective tissue core. The lacunae in which maternal blood
and secretions pool are now called *intervillous spaces*.

• **Maturation of villi occurs throughout fetal development.**   The tertiary villi
develop into *main stem villi*, which are anchored to both the fetal and maternal
sides of the placenta, and *"free" villi*, which extend from the fetal side and end
in the intervillous spaces. Chorionic tissue on the fetal side of the placenta condense into a *chorionic plate* in which main branches of umbilical vessels are distributed to all the villi. The chorionic plate becomes covered by amnion on its surface facing the amnionic cavity. During the course of pregnancy, chorionic villi

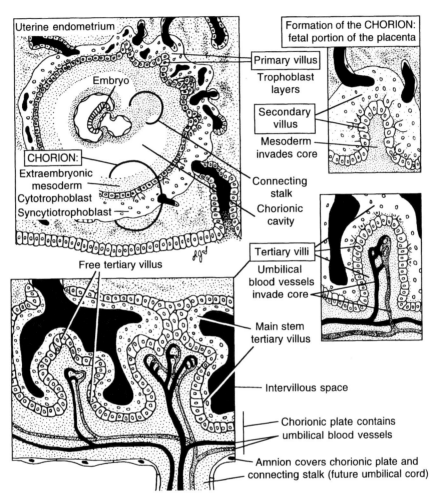

Figure 18-2
Formation of the mature placenta.

become thinner, providing a minimal barrier to diffusion, while the number of fetal capillaries within them increases. The cytotrophoblast and connective tissue core become thinned out overlying fetal capillaries, so that by the start of month 6, the fetal capillaries are separated from the maternal fluids only by the syncytiotrophoblast membranes and a thin layer of cytoplasm. This increases the efficiency of transport.

• **Transport from the placenta to the embryo prior to formation of umbilical vessels is by diffusion (see Fig. 18-3).**   Nutrients and gasses are transported from the maternal lacunar spaces into the syncytiotrophoblast. Once within the cytoplasmic syncytium, the nutrients and gasses must diffuse into embryonic germ layers during week 2. During week 3, they only have to diffuse as far as the vitelline vessels forming in the wall of the yolk sac. However, diffusion has a limited range, and a functional fetal circulatory system must be established within the embryo as well as between the embryo and placental tissues in order for development to progress beyond the three germ layers formed in week 3. As part of the fetal circulatory system, umbilical blood vessels begin to develop in week 3. It is not a coincidence that the establishment of a functional fetal-placental circulation by the end of week 3 is immediately followed by the onset of organogenesis in all systems in week 4.

• **How an obscure evolutionary holdover called the *allantois* plays a key role in formation of the umbilical blood vessels that supply the embryo.**   The allantois is an outpocketing of the endoderm of the cloaca which begins to form in week 3. It forms as an outpocketing of the part of the cloaca called the *urogenital sinus*, which forms the lining of the urinary bladder. (The development of the urogenital sinus was covered in Chap. 14.) It originates in our evolutionary ancestors as a receptacle for the wastes formed by the embryonic body before the placenta evolved in mammals. In those ancestors, the allantois becomes a prominent structure that requires blood vessels in its wall to supply its tissues. In mammals, the allantois never acquires the waste receptacle function, but the blood vessels that form in its walls become appropriated by the embryo as its umbilical blood vessels.

The allantois first grows out into the forming connecting stalk. The extraembryonic mesoderm of the connecting stalk becomes transformed into the connective tissue core of the umbilical cord. The allantois elongates along with the connecting stalk, forming a central endodermal structure around which mesodermal cells form blood islands. These blood islands coalesce to form vascular channels that grow together to form the lining of blood vessels that will form the two mature *umbilical arteries* and one *vein*.

The allantoic endoderm and surrounding mesoderm form a dense connective tissue cord called the *urachus* within the embryonic body. The urachus normally regresses. (See Chap. 14 for details of its fate.)

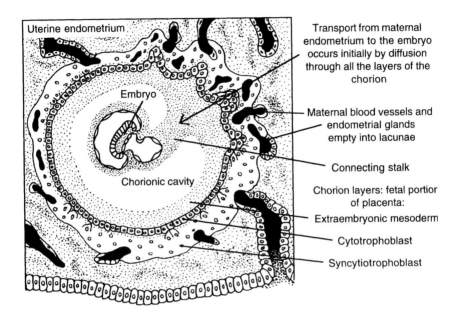

Uterine endometrium

Embryo

Chorionic cavity

Transport from maternal endometrium to the embryo occurs initially by diffusion through all the layers of the chorion

Maternal blood vessels and endometrial glands empty into lacunae

Connecting stalk

Chorion layers: fetal portion of placenta:

Extraembryonic mesoderm

Cytotrophoblast

Syncytiotrophoblast

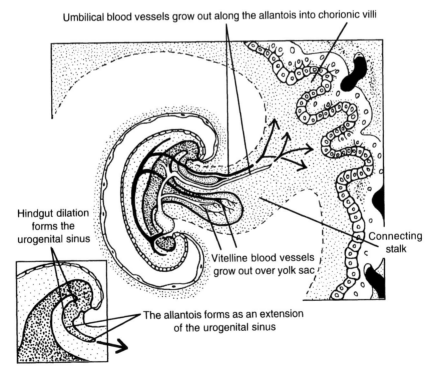

Umbilical blood vessels grow out along the allantois into chorionic villi

Hindgut dilation forms the urogenital sinus

Vitelline blood vessels grow out over yolk sac

Connecting stalk

The allantois forms as an extension of the urogenital sinus

Figure 18-3
Formation of placental vessels.

Development of the decidual (maternal) part of the placenta

The mature decidua entirely surrounds the uterine lumen (see Fig. 18-4). Initially, embryonic chorionic villi cover the entire decidual surface. Beginning in month 3, villi begin to degenerate everywhere except overlying the embryo. This starts the differentiation of the decidua into three separate regions. The *decidua basalis* is the portion of the decidua formed directly between the fetus and uterine wall. It is the only portion that becomes part of the placenta, and chorionic villi continue to proliferate only here. Portions of the decidua basalis coalesce to form septa that divide the fetal part of the placenta into 15 to 30 lobules, or *cotyledons*. Each cotyledon contains a main stem villus.

The portion of the decidua that overlies the developing fetus, and separates the fetus from the uterine lumen, forms a capsule around the fetus called the *decidua capsularis*. Finally, the *decidua parietalis* covers the remaining surface of the uterine wall. All decidua are shed at birth.

The growth of the placenta and fetal membranes changes the relationships of these portions of the decidua and fetal membranes. The decidua capsularis expands to meet the decidua parietalis. Both fuse together, forming a continuous layer of decidua surrounding the fetus. Within the chorionic part of the placenta, the amnion expands to meet the chorion and umbilical cord. As the amnion becomes plastered against their surfaces, it fuses with both. This obliterates the chorionic cavity.

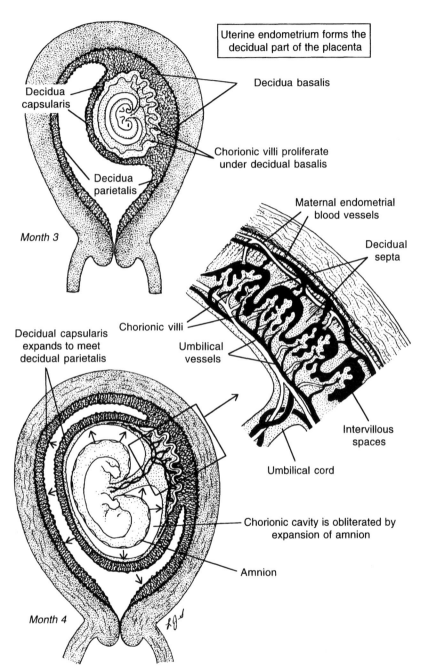

Figure 18-4
Development of the decidual part of the placenta.

MATURATION OF THE AMNION, YOLK SAC, AND UMBILICAL CORD

• **The amnion is formed in continuity with the ectoderm layer (see Fig. 18-5).**   The amniotic cavity forms between the embryonic ectoderm (epiblast) and the cytotrophoblast overlying it during week 2. An amniotic membrane then forms to line the trophoblast surface of this cavity, probably from outgrowth of the epiblast. As the embryo folds, the amniotic cavity expands, and its membrane expands along with it. This membrane is an avascular membrane. The amniotic cavity becomes filled with amniotic fluid, which is generated initially by trophoblast cells of the placenta.

• **The yolk sac is formed in continuity with the endoderm layer.**   The yolk sac is formed by cells from the early version of the endoderm layer, the hypoblast, migrating out over the surface of the blastula cavity, and transforming it into the yolk sac cavity. The yolk sac connection with the endoderm becomes narrowed in week 3 as the embryo folds, and the endoderm layer is folded into a long tube. The yolk sac is then continuous with the endoderm only in the future midgut region. The yolk sac and its connecting stalk, or vitelline duct, both become surrounded by extraembryonic mesoderm derived from the trophoblast layers. The major importance of the yolk sac lies in the formation of blood vessels called *vitelline vessels* in the mesoderm surrounding its walls, as well as the formation of the first embryonic blood cells within those forming vessels. These cells are essential for transport of oxygen in red blood cells from the first point at which a circulatory system is established in the embryo during week 3. The vitelline vessels themselves play a minor role in transporting materials into the embryo prior to establishment of the umbilical vessels late in week 3. Their major importance lies in their formation of most of the blood vessels supplying the intestinal tract and its mesenteries (see Chap. 12).

• **The connecting stalk surrounding the yolk sac forms the core of the umbilical cord.**   The extraembryonic mesoderm surrounding the yolk sac becomes confined to a stalk of mesoderm as a chorionic cavity forms within most of the wide extraembryonic mesoderm layer. This mesoderm stalk forms the core of the umbilical cord, which contains the yolk stalk from the outset. Late in week 3, the allantois grows out into the stalk, where it forms the epithelial structure around which the extraembryonic mesoderm forms the umbilical vessels. The connecting stalk matures into the umbilical cord as the umbilical vessels form. As the amniotic membrane expands, it becomes plastered against the surface of the connecting stalk mesoderm, forming its covering. During the fetal period, the loops of the small intestines temporarily herniate out of the body into the core of the umbilical cord.

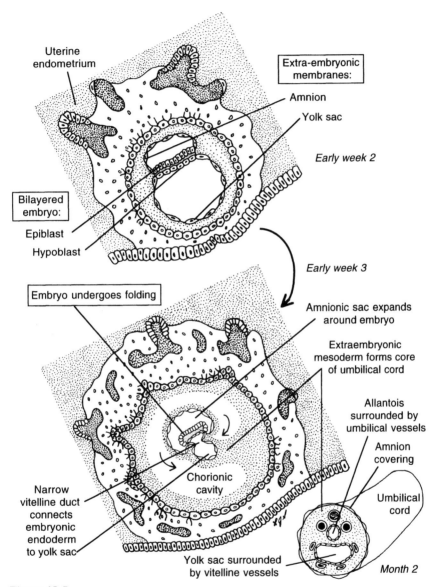

Figure 18-5
Maturation of the yolk sac, amnion, and umbilical cord.

PLACENTAL FUNCTIONS

• **The placenta transfers a number of substances between maternal and fetal circulations.**   Substances transferred to the embryo include gases (O_2 and CO), nutrients, electrolytes, vitamins, steroid hormones, and immunoglobulin (Ig) antibodies (primarily IgG, which confer passive immunity on the embryo). Most protein hormones do not cross in significant amounts, nor do immunoglobulin forms IgE, IgA, and IgM. In addition, many viruses, some bacteria and protozoa, and most drugs cross the placenta, demonstrating that the placenta is only a partial barrier to infectious or potentially teratogenic agents. Some cell types can cross the placenta, including some maternal white blood cells and fetal red blood cells. These fetal cells are the source of the maternal Rh reaction leading to *Rh incompatibility.*

If the fetus is Rh-positive but the mother is Rh-negative, fetal erythrocytes will generate a maternal immune response. These antibodies then enter the fetal circulation and initiate breakdown of fetal erythrocytes. Rh immunoglobin is now given to the mother to prevent this.

Substances transferred from the embryo to the maternal circulation for elimination include gaseous wastes (CO_2) and solid wastes (urea and uric acid derived from amino acid metabolism, and bilirubin from the breakdown of red blood cells). In addition, fetal blood volume is maintained at a proper level by elimination of water. This is particularly important in maintaining proper amniotic fluid volume (as covered also in Chaps. 12 and 14). The fetal components of the placenta are responsible for generating much of the amniotic fluid. This fluid is partially recycled by the fetal kidneys as they develop, since they become capable of processing a watery urine from the fetal blood that filters through the kidneys. Since amniotic fluid is constantly being generated, it must be constantly resorbed. The only way to eliminate the fluid is through the placenta into the maternal circulation. The fetus swallows amniotic fluid, the fetal intestinal epithelium resorbs much of it, and it is picked up by the fetal circulation and carried through the umbilical arteries to the placenta.

• **The placenta also plays a major role in manufacturing hormones and modifying others generated by the fetus.**   The placenta manufactures several glycoprotein hormones. These include human chorionic gonadotropin (HCG), which maintains the corpus luteum in the ovary. The corpus luteum in turn continues to manufacture hormones essential for the maintenance of pregnancy. In addition, the placenta directly manufactures the steroid hormones estrogen and progesterone. It becomes the primary source of these hormones supporting placental and fetal development through the last parts of the pregnancy. Its estrogen is also required for proper development of the reproductive system structures of both sexes. The placenta also manufactures human chorionic somatomammotropin (HCS) or placental lactogen (HPL), which has growth-hormone-like properties that are essential for development of the fetus before its endocrine organs become functional and begin to secrete hormones. Endocrine organs vary widely in the time of onset of secretion of functional hormones. Prior to that time, the placenta manufactures a range of other hormones that have yet to be completely identified, as well as activating others generated by fetal organs.

• I N D E X •

Locators for tables and figures are enclosed in brackets [ ].

Abdominal oblique muscles, formation, 134, [135]
Abortion, spontaneous
  chromosomal abnormalities, 11
  ectopic pregnancy, 34
Absent inferior vena cava, 280, [280]
Achondroplasia, 112, [113]
  single gene mutation, 13
Acquired immune deficiency disease (AIDS). *See* AIDS
Acrosomal vesicle, 24, [25]
  role in fertilization, 28
Adductor magnus, role as pelvic girdle muscle, 138, [139]
Adenohypophysis, 176. *See* Pituitary, anterior
Adrenal gland
  germ layer origins, 386, [387]
  structure, 386, [387]
Adrenal hyperplasia, 387
Adrenocorticotropin hormone, 378
Aganglionic megacolon. *See* Hirschsprung's disease
AIDS virus, placental transfer, 15
Alar plate, 156, [157]
  forebrain, 174
Alcohol, teratogenic effects, 14–15, 16
Allantois, 418, [419], 422, [423]
  role in urinary system defects, 344, [345]
Alphafetoprotein, neural tube defects, 17
Alveoli, 312, [313]
  development, 320, [321]
Amniocentesis, 17
Amnion, 2, 4, 44, 45, 422, [423]
Amnionic sac. *See* Amnion
Amniotic fluid
  fetal-placental circulation, 424
Amputations, intrauterine, 113
Anal canal, 294, [295], 296, [296]
Androgen binding proteins, role in reproduction, 394, [395]
Androgens
  effects, 14
  secretion by adrenal glands, 386
Anencephaly, 108, 122, [123], 184, [185], 242
Aneuploidy, 12
Angiogenesis, 268, [269]
Annular pancreas, 306, [307]
Anomalous pulmonary venous return, 280, [280]
Anorectal agenesis, 296
Anterior digastric muscle, 208, [209]

Antiacne medications, effects, 14, 15
Antibiotics, effects, 14
Anticoagulants, effects, 14
Anticonvulsants, effects, 14
Antitumor agents, effects, 14
Anus, 286, [287]
Aortic arch arteries, formation and derivatives, 204, [205], 268, [269], 270–271, [271], 297, [297]
  defects, [271]
  double, 272, [273]
  interrupted, 272, [273]
  right, 272, [273]
Apical ectodermal ridge (AER), role in limb development, 88, [89], 90, [91], 110
Appendicular girdle, skeletal development, 110, [111]
  muscle development, 136, 138, [139]
Aqueduct of Sylvius, 164, [165]
Arachnoid, 182, [183]
Arterial system, 246, [247], 270–271, [271]
  defects, 272, [273]
Association fibers, function, 178
Assortment, independent, homologous chromosomes, 22–23, [23]
Astrocytes, role in central nervous system, 152, [153]
Atresia
  bile duct, 306
  cervix, 364
  esophagus, 300, [300], 324, [325]
  gastrointestinal tube, 298
  mitral valve, 261
  pulmonary outflow, 266
  semilunar valves, 266
  tricuspid valve, 261
  vagina, 364, [365]
Atrial septation, 254, [255]
  defects, 254, [255]
Atrioventricular canal tube, partitioning, 250, [251], 258, [259]
Atrium, primitive, 250, [251], *see also* Heart
Auditory tube, 224, 236, [237], 238, [239]
Autosomal trisomies, effects, 12
AV canal, 250, [251]
AV node, function, 246
Axial muscles, formation, 134, [135]
Azygos veins, 276, [277]

B lymphocytes, role in humoral immune response, 398

Cerebral cortex, 180, [181]
Cerebral hemisphere
  lateral ventricle formation, 178, [179]
Cerebrum, [164], 164–165, [165]
Cervical vesicles, role in thymus formation,
  410, [411]
Chemoattractant growth factor molecules, role
  in nerve development, 150
Chicken pox, effects, 15
Chondroblasts, role in cartilage formation,
  100, [101]
Chondrocranium, 114, [115], 116, [117], 200,
  [201]
Chondrocytes, role in cartilage formation,
  100, [101]
Chondrogenesis, 101
Chordae tendineae, 246, 258, [259]
Chorion, 46, 416–417, [417]
Chorionic cavity, 46
Chorionic gonadotropins, production in pla-
  centa, 392, [393]
Chorionic plate, 416–417, [417]
Chorionic villi, 416–417, [417], 418, [419]
Chorionic villus sampling (CVS), 17
Choroid, eye, 234, [235]
Choroid plexus, brain, 178, [179]
Chromatid, 22
Chromosomal abnormalities, 11–13
Chromosome assortment, errors, 22
Chromosome duplication, errors, 22
Ciliary body, 232–233, 234, [235]
Circadian rhythm, pineal body role, 176, 380
Circulation patterns, fetal and neonatal, 282,
  [283]
Cleavage divisions, 32, [33]
Cleft lip, 216, [217]
  trisomies, 12
Cleft palate, 218–219, [219]
  etiology, 15
  trisomies, 12
Clitoris, 348, [349], 367, [367]
Cloaca
  endoderm origins, 69, [69]
  role in rectum and anal canal formation,
    296, [296]
  role in reproductive system formation, 366,
    [367]
  role in umbilical blood vessel formation,
    418
  role in urogenital system formation, 342
Club foot, etiology, 16, 113, [113]
Coarctation of the aorta, 272, [273]
Coccyx, 106
Cochlear duct, 236, 240, [241]
Colon, 294, [295]
  ascending, 294, [295]
  transverse, 294, [295]

Commissural fibers, 178
Commissures, 158, [159], 178, [179]
Compact bone, 102
Computed tomography, noninvasive fetal
  visualization, 17
Congenital defects, 3, 10
  cardiovascular, 12, 245, 250, 252–253, 260,
    [261], 262, [263], 264, 280, [280]
  central nervous system, 184, [185]
  chromosome assortment effects, 23
  face prominences, 216
  genetic causes, 11–12
  head and neck, 240, 242
  incidence in newborns/infants, 11
  kidneys, 338, [339]
  limbs, 112, [113]
  reproductive system, 364, [365], 366,
    [367], 368, [369]
  respiratory system, 324, [325]
  ribs, 108, [109]
  skeletal muscles, 144
  skull, 122, [123]
  trisomies and cardiac, 12
  urinary system, 344, [345]
  uterus and vagina, 364, [365]
  vertebrae, 108, [109]
Congenital hernia, 368, [369]
Conjunctiva, 232, [233], 234, [235]
Connective tissue
  mesoderm derivatives, 50, [51], 55, 76–77,
    [77], [78], 98, [99]
  pharyngeal arch derivative, 202, [203], 204
  role in skeletal muscle organ formation,
    126, [127]
  specialized, components, 56, [57]
Contraception, oral, 15
Convoluted tubules, kidney, 330, [331]
Copula, 222, [223]
Cornea, 232, 234, [235]
Corona radiata, role in oocyte maturation, 26,
  [29]
Coronary ligament, formation in ventral
  mesenteries, 309, [309]
Coronary sinus, 256, [257]
Corpora quadrigemina, alar region, 172
Corpus callosum, 178, [179]
Corpus striatum, 178, [179]
Cortex
  adrenal, 386, [387]
  cerebellar, 165, 170, [171]
  cerebral, 165, 180, [181]
Cortical cords, role in ovarian differentiation,
  358, [359]
Corticosteroids, secretion by adrenal glands,
  386
Corticotropin-releasing factors, production in
  placenta, 392, [393]

ISBN 0-07-063308-8

90000

9 780070 633087

SWEENEY: BASIC CONCEPTS/EMB.